First Aid
for
DOGS

An Owner's Veterinary Guide

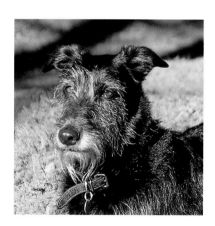

First Aid *for* DOGS

An Owner's Veterinary Guide

ANDREW GARDINER

BVM&S, CERT SAS, MRCVS

J.A. ALLEN · LONDON

British Library Cataloguing in Publication Data
A catalogue record for this book is available from the British Library

ISBN 0.85131.829.0

Published in Great Britain in 2002 by
J. A. Allen an imprint of Robert Hale Ltd.,
Clerkenwell House, 45–47 Clerkenwell Green,
London EC1R 0HT

Edited by John Beaton
Design and Typesetting by Paul Saunders
Line illustrations by Maggie Raynor

Colour processing by Tenon & Polert Colour Processing Ltd., Hong Kong
Printed in Singapore by Kyodo Printing Co (S'pore) Pte Ltd

CONTENTS

Preface

Most people who own a dog would say their life is enriched by it. For some, such as the elderly or lonely, their dog may be the most significant 'other' they come into contact with; more than just a pet, but a true companion and animal friend. Veterinary surgeons are privileged to witness this emotional bond and attachment on a daily basis, and to help preserve it in the face of accident or illness.

Just as with close human family or friends, so we may worry about our dog's health, especially since our canine companions cannot say exactly what is wrong or where it hurts. In writing this book, I have tried to imagine the concerned, enquiring owner and to keep this fictitious person in mind when explaining the sometimes complex nature of dog diseases. I have tried to answer the sorts of questions worried owners ask on a daily basis in veterinary consulting rooms, and to anticipate those further questions which only come to mind once they have returned home. Often, in the heat of the moment, complex information cannot be taken in properly or questions adequately formed, and it is here that turning to a reliable book can be useful and, very frequently, reassuring.

If this book can alert owners when to seek professional advice, give guidance on effective first aid to prevent any deterioration in their pet's condition (and even, on occasion, to save a life), and allow dog owners to understand and follow their pet's treatment in a knowledgeable way, then it will have fulfilled its main purpose.

It takes at least five years to train a veterinary surgeon and neither this book, nor any other, can be a substitute for professional veterinary care. Diseases are too complex, and our pet dogs too important, to take risks with their welfare. I have not written a guide to home diagnosis but instead, I hope, a general source of information on common dog diseases and disorders and their first aid, together with a little more technical background and explanation than is to be found in similar books, expressed in a jargon-free way.

Current increasing interest in alternative and complementary medicine is reflected in this book, with a useful section on basic homoeopathic first aid and a brief discussion of other complementary therapies given in the Introduction. While the acceptance and use of complementary medicine currently varies considerably between veterinary surgeons, this is a subject which is often of great interest to owners. It is important that the benefits and limitations of such therapies are understood and the background information provided here should help in that respect.

Writing this book has been both a challenge and a pleasure. I am indebted to the assistance and patience of my publisher, Caroline Burt at J. A. Allen, and to the generosity of veterinary colleagues, many of them busy specialists in their own disciplines, for kindly providing photographs which I did not have myself. They are all mentioned in the Acknowledgements.

Thanks are also due to John Beaton, Paul Saunders and Maggie Raynor for their expertise and advice in editorial matters, design and illustration respectively. I am also grateful for the support and encouragement provided by my family, especially my brother John whose photographic skills I drew on frequently to illustrate many sections of the book. Neither can I omit to mention my own uncomplaining dog, Tess. Her daily walks got progressively shorter as the deadline for the delivery of the manuscript approached. She also has a starring role as a patient and cooperative model for several of the photographs in the book, all done for the very reasonable fee of two Bonios.

ANDREW GARDINER
EDINBURGH

Acknowledgements

The Author and Publishers would like to thank the following for their kind permission to use copyright photographs in this book.

Mr Pip Boydell, The Animal Medical Centre, Manchester: page 185.

Celia Cox, ENT Referrals, Winchester, Hants: page 61.

Dr Sheila Crispin, Department of Ophthalmology, University of Bristol Veterinary School: pages 41, 44 [top], 48, 54, 280.

Cathy Curtis, Dermatology Referral Service, Ware, Herts: pages 77, 80 [bottom right], 92.

Mr J Ferguson, East Neuk Veterinary Clinic, St Monans, Fife: pages 160, 170, 186, 190.

Mr J E Gardiner, Portobello, Edinburgh: pages 9 [bottom], 12, 24, 25, 30, 31, 33 [top right], 44 [bottom], 53 [top], 62, 63, 70, 83 [right], 118, 125, 127, 129, 143, 164, 221, 222, 226, 268, 273, 276, 277.

Dr Cecilia Gorrel, Veterinary Dentistry and Oral Surgery Referrals, Pilley, Hants: pages 29, 33 [bottom right], 34.

Ann Gray, Kindu Basenjis, Pudsey: page 237.

Julie Henfrey, Dermatology Referrals, Rowlands Gill, Tyne & Wear: pages 68 [bottom], 82 [top], 90 [right], 225.

Dr John Mould, Department of Ophthalmology, University of Glasgow Veterinary School: pages 40, 43, 45, 51, 52 [left], 53 [bottom], 55.

Sue Paterson, Veterinary Dermatology Service, Altrincham, Cheshire: pages 82 [bottom], 83 [top], 90 [left], 197 [right].

James Smith, Leo Animal Health, Princes Risborough, Bucks: pages 66 [bottom], 75, 76 [bottom].

Barbara Sykes, Mainline Border Collie Centre, Eldwick, West Yorks: page 250.

Dr F J van Sluys, University of Utrecht, The Netherlands/Royal Veterinary College, University of London: pages 121, 230.

All other photographs are copyright of the Author. All illustrations are by Maggie Raynor and are copyright of the Publishers.

Using This Book

This book is arranged to discuss the health problems affecting all the different areas of the dog's body. This is a convenient way of discussing the many and varied illnesses, minor or major, that can affect dogs. Sometimes it is easier to consider the conditions affecting one specific part of the body, such as the eye (Chapter 3) or the ear (Chapter 4); at other times, looking at a body 'system' is more useful, such as the digestive, respiratory, and reproductive systems (Chapters 6, 7, 11 and 12).

Each chapter starts with some background information on the area under consideration, since it is often helpful to understand the basics before moving on to what can sometimes go wrong. This type of approach makes the diseases and their symptoms easier to understand fully. When the individual diseases are tackled, they are looked at under the headings of *Cause*, *Symptoms*, *Diagnosis*, *Treatment* and *Outlook*, so that all of the important points are covered logically. This sequence also closely follows the thought process that is gone through by the vet when you take your dog along for treatment.

The book should make interesting and educational reading at any time, and a thorough reading will give the reader a deep insight into their pet dog in health and disease. If a specific condition is diagnosed in your dog by the vet, then the book can be used to obtain further background information to aid understanding of the problem. When an owner fully understands an illness or injury, it is likely that he or she will be able to care for their dog better and work along with the veterinary staff to get a speedy return to normal health.

When searching for a disease, use the main contents list to locate the chapter corresponding to the appropriate area of the body that you want. Then turn to that chapter. The detailed contents list at the start of the chapter then outlines the main topics and conditions covered. More often than not, you will find the subject mentioned in this list. Alternatively, you can turn to the index when looking for explanation of a specific term or condition, or to discover where else in the book the subject of interest to you might be mentioned, perhaps in a slightly different context.

Throughout the book, attention is drawn to basic first aid and practical home nursing measures that owners can use to help their dog. Despite advances in modern medicine and techniques, some of them very 'high-tech' indeed, good nursing and patient care remain vital to the success of many treatments and can do wonders to improve a sick dog's demeanour and convalescence. Just like us, sick dogs can become depressed, and even give up the will to live, if good basic nursing and comfort are not attended to. These guidelines given in the first aid and nursing boxes should, of course, always be followed in conjunction with any specific advice from the veterinary surgeon who is looking after your pet.

In addition, Chapter 18 lists first aid and homoeopathic treatments for the common accident and emergency situations encountered in dogs. Try to become thoroughly familiar with this information – it could save your dog's life.

Introduction

Acquiring and Owning a Dog

Owning a pet dog is both a great pleasure and a responsibility. Dogs can offer many qualities which are considered important to our emotional and physical well-being, and surveys have consistently shown that dog owners are generally healthier and happier people. In some way, dogs help protect us against many of the minor physical and psychological disorders that seem common in modern societies. Perhaps this has something to do with recapturing our lost connections with nature and other animal species, and allowing us to pause and take a simpler perspective on life at least now and again. At any rate, dogs have had, and seem set to continue to have, an enduring relationship with people.

All this is important because human beings, like dogs, are social animals. Whilst not pretending that a dog offers the same quality of relationship as to be found in another person, there is no doubt that most dog owners value their relationship with their dog for what it is – a friendship that extends across the species barrier and that brings mutual pleasure and security.

In return for this, we have the responsibility to try to ensure that our dogs lead reasonably happy and healthy lives. We have to make sure that their basic physical and behavioural needs are met, and that their healthcare is attended to. Dogs cannot choose their owners; they are dependent on us for virtually everything, from protection against preventable diseases to dealing with life-threatening emergencies.

Benefits of dog ownership

- Companionship
- Provides exercise, routine and contact with other people
- Handling pets lowers blood pressure and stress levels
- Dogs are non-judgemental, loyal and dependable in their behaviour
- Dogs allow us to recapture lost connections with nature and the animal kingdom and provide us with a more straightforward perspective on life
- Caring for dogs teaches responsibility in children and usually allows them to come to terms with animal death before they experience human death

Some basic questions

Before acquiring a pet dog, the following points should be carefully considered:

- Is a dog the best type of pet for your circumstances and lifestyle?
- Think carefully about the size, breed and coat type of the dog you choose. Different breeds also have

different temperamental characteristics. Speak to knowledgeable owners or professionals and try to get to know individual dogs if you do have a specific breed in mind. Remember that cross-breeds can make excellent (and unique) pets and that rehoming kennels are usually staffed by very experienced dog handlers who can often match up suitable dogs with prospective owners with great skill.

- Have you the time, energy and patience to devote to a puppy or boisterous young dog, or would an adult dog be more appropriate? Dogs learn quickly but basic training does not happen overnight and some breeds are more trainable than others!

- Do other members of your family or household share your enthusiasm? Will they assist with the care and exercise of the dog?

- Are you prepared for food and vet bills, for wet evening walks in bad weather and for kenneling or other arrangements during holidays?

- Remember that most dogs cast hair, usually all the year round, and muddy pawprints can appear on carpets and furniture!

- Above all, try to make sure that the dog you choose has an even and predictable temperament. This is the single most important factor in any pet dog and is connected with good early socialisation and basic handling. These topics are covered in Chapter 16, which also gives advice on what to do when difficulties arise in this vital area.

Most people have automatically thought through several of the above points before coming to their decision, but it is surprising how many dogs are acquired on the spur of the moment. A forlorn face is spotted in a rescue kennels, you fall in love with it and take it home that day – many happy dog-owner bonds have started that way, but it does help if you have considered at least some of the main implications *before* visiting the rescue kennels or breeding establishment!

Remember that if a mistake is made at the time of acquiring a dog, it can cause much heartache later on because very strong emotional bonds can be formed, even to 'problem dogs' which cause disruption, mess

or sometimes even danger to their owners. There are no hard and fast rules however; some of the strongest bonds I have witnessed between dogs and owners have arisen in unusual circumstances: the homeless person whose dog eats better than they do; the elderly couple who take on a nervous dog to give it a second chance, getting nipped in the process, before gradually winning the dog over and turning it into a relaxed and sociable pet. If you are sure you want a particular dog and believe you can give it a good and loving home, then you should go ahead, but take all the advice you can get from books, other owners and veterinary professionals. Use their experience to help avoid common pitfalls in acquiring and caring for your new dog.

Health Risks from Dogs

At the stage of acquiring a pet dog, particularly if they have never had one before, some owners worry about potential risks to human health. In fact, a healthy dog poses very few health risks to people, whether adults or children: the benefits of pet ownership greatly outweigh any small risks. However there are a number of conditions that can be passed from dog to human and which should be recognised and treated promptly. People suffering from immune system diseases such as HIV/AIDS and other conditions can still enjoy the benefits of pet ownership but medical advice should be sought after diagnosis or before acquiring a dog.

It should also be borne in mind that certain of these conditions can be passed from human to dog – the dog may not always have been the culprit! The diseases below represent the main areas of concern for diseases transferable from dogs to people.

Virus infections

Rabies
Rabies affects a wide variety of species and is discussed on page 23. Many countries are rabies-free and movement of animals between them is subject to strict regulations. Dogs can be vaccinated against rabies but this is not usually carried out unless

international travel is planned. When abroad, care should always be taken when approached by stray dogs especially if they behave in an unpredictable way.

Other viruses

Other virus infections are theoretically possible. Some of these are asymptomatic, i.e. an infection takes place but no illness is produced. Several viral infections may result in diarrhoea. Whenever your dog and any family member has diarrhoea at the same time, medical and veterinary advice should be sought.

Bacterial infections

E. coli, Salmonella and Campylobacter

Although *E. coli* is an important cause of disease in people, and dogs suffer from their own form of *E. coli* infection, spread between the species has not been shown to occur. However, sensible hygiene precautions should always be taken should your dog be diagnosed with *E. coli* diarrhoea; this however is a rare cause of diarrhoea in dogs.

Dogs are affected by *Salmonella* and a very low percentage of healthy adult dogs can carry and excrete this bacterium. The percentage of excretion in young dogs is thought to be higher. Exactly how significant this is in terms of human disease is hard to tell but if *Salmonella* is diagnosed in your dog, medical advice should be sought. It is a rare occurrence in general veterinary practice to diagnose this disease in dogs.

Campylobacter affects both dogs and people. Once again, if diarrhoea is occurring simultaneously in dogs and humans in the same household, this condition needs to be ruled out by your doctor and veterinary surgeon. The dog may have infected the people, or vice versa.

Leptospirosis

This disease is discussed on page 22, however very few human cases come from dogs. Most people are infected when they participate in water sports where rat urine may have contaminated the water, e.g. canals.

Other bacteria: dog bite wounds in people

An important bacterial infection is that resulting from dog bites. Dogs may carry a variety of bacteria in their mouths and a bite from a dog can act like an injection of poison, meaning that dog bites should *always* been treated promptly by your doctor. A course of antibiotics is often prescribed. Dog bites occurring in people who are immunosuppressed due to HIV/AIDS or other conditions should be treated urgently.

Protozoa

Protozoa are minute parasites that can cause disease in dogs and people and may be transferred. *Giardia* is one such parasite that may cause diarrhoea in both species; medical and veterinary advice should be sought whenever this is suspected.

Cryptosporidiosis is an important disease in people with defective immune systems and those on chemotherapy. Dogs may occasionally harbour this disease. It is not known if they would pose a risk to human health but the possibility should be considered. Milder diarrhoea can be caused in healthy children and adults.

Intestinal parasites

Toxocariasis

Puppies and young dogs shed many eggs of the dog roundworm *Toxocara canis* in their faeces. When these faeces are allowed to lie on ground that may be used by children (e.g. play parks) there is a risk children could pick up the infection. The faeces are not immediately infective but become so if left on the ground and remain infective for some years.

Despite this apparent risk, disease caused by toxocariasis is very rare, but when it occurs it can cause eye injury in children. For this reason, dog faeces should always be picked up from communal areas (remember the faeces are not infective at the time they are passed by the dog). *Toxocara* infection and prevention is discussed in detail on page 116.

Fleas and mites

Fleas tend to prefer their own species but will also bite other animals they accidentally come into contact with. Thus the dog or cat flea will occasionally bite pet owners. Likewise, the human flea will bite the pet dog if infestation is present.

Owners may also exhibit skin lesions if their dog has sarcoptic mange (scabies). Medical treatment should be sought to clear up the skin infestation, which results in intensely itchy skin patches.

If you have skin problems at the same time as your dog, parasites should always be suspected as the cause. Mention your skin problems to the veterinary surgeon; it will often help in the diagnosis of both your problem and your dog's!

Parasitic skin problems are discussed fully in Chapter 5.

Your Veterinary Surgeon

Routine healthcare and preventative medicine

Most pet dogs lead long and relatively healthy lives. However even the healthiest dog is likely to require a visit to the veterinary surgeon at some stage for a minor or major health complaint. As well as this, yearly general health examinations and booster vaccination is carried out in most pet dogs and is to be recommended. Infectious diseases to which dogs are prone, and their prevention by vaccination, are discussed thoroughly in Chapter 1.

The other main emphasis in canine preventative medicine is routine worming against round and tapeworms, which is usually carried out two to four times yearly. Worms are discussed in Chapter 6 and the use of worming preparations obtained from the veterinary surgeon is the surest way to prevent this minor problem. Prevention of flea and tick infestation in the warmer months has been made possible due to the development of new drug therapies for these parasites. The important role of fleas in skin disease in dogs is covered in Chapter 5. In many cases, however, flea treatment is only resorted to when evidence of infestation is found or suspected in an itchy dog.

Routine neutering

Routine neutering – referred to as castration in male dogs and ovariohysterectomy (spay) in females – is performed in many dogs not intended for breeding. These operations prevent pet dogs from mating and from the sexual/reproductive behaviours associated with this. In western societies a high percentage of pet female dogs have been spayed; the percentage of pet male dogs that have been castrated is lower, although this is a less major operation than spaying and is to be

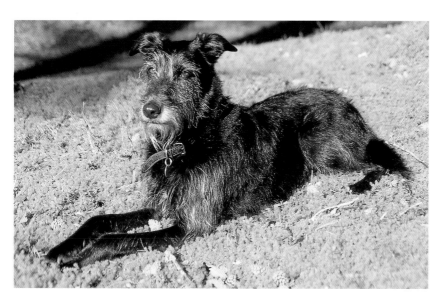

A healthy adult dog – the author's 8-year-old cross lurcher bitch 'Tess'.

encouraged. Castration and spaying are also required for certain medical conditions that usually arise in older, unneutered dogs.

On balance, most veterinary surgeons would agree that routine neutering of pets is a good thing. While to some it may seem 'unnatural', it is also in some ways unnatural to keep dogs and prevent them from exhibiting sexual behaviour and from breeding. In entire (unneutered) pet dogs, instincts and urges are denied which, especially in male dogs, may lead to undesirable or dangerous behaviours such as roaming and territorial aggression. The alternative – allowing dogs to mate indiscriminately – is irresponsible as it increases the stray dog population and can lead to great suffering in puppies and adult dogs. Many unwanted dogs end up in rehoming centres or dog pounds each year, and some of these have been seriously neglected or injured while straying.

If you decide to have an unneutered dog, and there is nothing inherently wrong in this, you have a responsibility to ensure that, if it is a male, it is not breeding with female dogs and creating unwanted litters, nor causing a nuisance to other pets or people by roaming. Similarly, owners of unneutered female dogs must be constantly alert to the possibility of straying and breeding during the twice yearly oestrus or heat cycles. If the bitch does become pregnant, then you must ensure that responsible homes are found for all of the puppies and that they will be properly cared for, vaccinated, etc. at the appropriate times.

When to spay female dogs

Despite many rumours to the contrary, there is no merit in letting a bitch have one litter of puppies. This neither alters the dog's temperament nor contributes to future health. The opposite could be said to be the case as all pregnancies carry the small risk of complications, necessity for caeserian section, etc. and it is well known that early neutering reduces the risk of mammary (breast) cancer in bitches. It is however thought that allowing a bitch to have one oestrus (heat) cycle may be advantageous in preventing the low incidence of urinary incontinence (page 148) and infantile vulva (a condition in which the external genital organs of the female are underdeveloped) in susceptible female dogs. This needs to be balanced against the effect of prevention of mammary (breast) cancer that early neutering affords: spaying *before* the first oestrus period reduces the risk of mammary cancer in later life to almost zero. The protective effect is still quite high if spaying occurs after the second oestrus, but is lost thereafter.

Thus the timing of spaying has pros and cons on both sides. A good compromise is to spay after the first oestrus has occurred but before the second; at this time, good protection against mammary cancer is still possible and the small risk of adverse effects of too early spaying is also avoided.

Dog breeding is discussed in Chapter 15 and problems particular to male and female dogs in Chapters 11 and 12.

Special problems of young and old dogs

Certain diseases are commoner in specific age groups. Cancer, for example, is diagnosed far oftener in older than in younger animals; the same applies to chronic diseases of the kidney and liver and to acquired heart valve disease. Abnormal bone development, however, is a problem of young dogs, although older dogs may have to live with the consequences of this. Infectious diseases are also generally far commoner in young dogs.

When acquiring a puppy be sure that you are aware of all the points mentioned in the checklist on page 246 to ensure that you get off to a good start with your new dog.

Particular health problems encountered more frequently in young dogs include:

• Infectious diseases (see Chapter 1)

• Bone or joint disease associated with certain breeds or with overfeeding or over-supplementing puppies and young dogs (Chapter 9)

• Behaviour problems (Chapter 16)

Older dogs are more likely to suffer from chronic or degenerative diseases, including:

• Mobility problems and arthritis (Chapter 9)

• Liver or kidney disease (Chapters 6 and 8)

• Heart disease (Chapter 7)

- Various diseases of the male and female reproductive systems (Chapters 11 and 12).

Veterinary Diagnosis and Treatment

The diagnosis of disease is a highly skilled process which is a mixture of science, art and experience, made more difficult in animals by their inability to describe symptoms subjectively. The famous vet James Herriot called one of his books *If Only They Could Talk*, referring to the problem of unravelling symptoms and diagnoses in veterinary medicine when the patient cannot speak to the doctor to explain what the problem is or exactly where it hurts.

When a veterinary surgeon examines your dog, he or she brings years of advanced training and experience to the task, such that in most cases it is possible to arrive at a diagnosis reasonably quickly. This may be evident on initial examination or may need to be supported by further tests such as blood tests, X-rays, scans, and so on. It can be physically impossible to diagnose some illnesses without recourse to extensive (and therefore expensive) tests, but only when a diagnosis is made can relevant treatment be prescribed, whether this takes the form of medicines to be given or a surgical operation.

Another problem is that dogs, like all animals, are individuals. Although many diseases and conditions have typical symptoms, not all of these may be present in every case so that in most instances a diagnosis ends up being a 'balance of probabilities'. More difficult diagnoses have a higher chance of being incorrect, and therefore the diagnosis may need to be changed as time passes or if treatment is not working as expected.

The prognosis is the expected outlook after a diagnosis or course of treatment. Most veterinary surgeons use words like: *excellent*, *good*, *fair*, *uncertain*, *guarded*, *poor* and *hopeless* to describe prognosis. This can help in weighing up treatment options and is important in giving owners a realistic expectation of the outcome after treatment. Remember that it is not always possible to be absolutely certain about the prognosis; words like 'fair', 'uncertain' and 'guarded' can often mean that there is room for manoeuvre in the prognosis. It simply isn't possible to be definite because so many variables can be involved.

The flow chart on page 8 illustrates the approach to diagnosis used by most veterinary surgeons and may help clarify what can be a confusing and at times frustrating process for the worried dog owner. It is important to realise that living bodies are not like mechanical objects such as cars! It is not always easy or straightforward to 'lift the bonnet', locate the problem, make a few adjustments and then guarantee absolute success, especially in complex or advanced disorders. Medicine – both animal and human – constantly throws up surprises: the very ill patient that is not expected to survive, but does, as well as the unexplained death after routine treatment (thankfully rare).

Diagnostic tests

The commonest diagnostic tests used in veterinary medicine are:

- X-rays
- Blood tests
- Ultrasound examinations
- Endoscopy

Increasingly, advanced computer-controlled scanning techniques (CT and MRI scans) are being used in pets as the cost of this technology falls and machines used in human medicine become available. Most scanners of this type are to be found in veterinary schools or in specialised practices to which veterinary surgeons may refer suitable patients.

X-rays

X-rays provide a picture of the inside of an animal's body shown as a collection of shades of grey. X-rays are a vital part of many diagnostic procedures but they, like other tests, are not always 100% conclusive. Some disorders do not show up well on X-ray; others require specialised X-rays using contrast materials such as barium to highlight them. Usually several X-rays taken at different angles need to be used to avoid confusing results.

In order to get high quality X-rays, complete

Veterinary examination and diagnosis flowchart

Vet takes clinical history
- Owner explains problem/symptoms to vet
- Vet listens and asks questions

Vet performs clinical examination
- Vet examines dog, concentrating on problems

Diagnosis
- May require diagnostic tests

Diagnostic tests
e.g.
- Blood tests
- X-rays
- Ultrasound
- Endoscopy

Treatment
- Drugs • Surgery • Hospitalisation

Follow-up
- Vet and owner assess response to treatment

Incomplete cure
- Reassess patient
- Perform more tests if required
- Revise diagnosis if required
- Continue or alter treatment
- Refer to specialist vet if required

Complete cure
- Stop all treatment

Incurable disease

No treatment available

Permanent treatment needed
- Treatment controls but cannot cure disease
- Regular reassessment to fine-tune treatment and pick up any complicating problems
- Revise diagnosis if required
- Owner education to fully understand the disease

Palliative therapy
- To control pain and distress
- To maintain quality of life

Euthanasia
- When quality of life is poor
- When dog is in permanent pain or distress that cannot be alleviated or controlled

immobility is required hence dogs are quite often sedated or anaesthetised to obtain the pictures.

Blood tests

By measuring the concentrations of chemicals in the blood, important information concerning likely diagnoses can often be obtained. For example, if the kidneys are not working well, substances which are normally filtered out of the blood by the kidneys are not removed from the body, hence an increased concentration of these substances could point towards kidney disease when the diagnosis is being made.

Sometimes, however, there can be more than one explanation for abnormal blood test results; additional tests or other investigations may be needed to narrow this down. Chronic diseases can be monitored effectively by repeated blood tests to assess how the patient is responding to treatment.

Ultrasound

Ultrasound is another means of 'looking inside' the body, but using sound waves instead of radiation (X-rays). Ultrasound is very safe and is useful for various diseases and conditions. It does not usually require sedation or an anaesthetic and is quite painless.

Endoscopy

This technique involves inserting a long flexible camera into the dog's body so that organs can be viewed directly. It is used in the respiratory (breathing) and

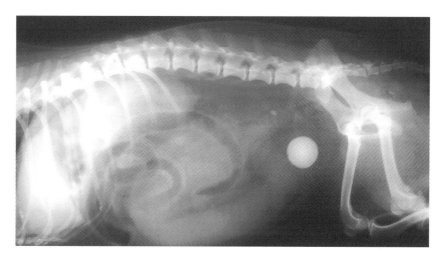

X-ray of a dog's abdomen. The X-ray resulted in the diagnosis of two unrelated problems: bladder stones and a uterine infection (pyometra). Both of these conditions are discussed later.

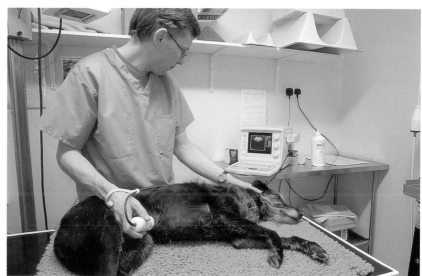

Ultrasound scans are painless and require no sedatives or anaesthetics.

gastrointestinal (digestive) tracts. It usually requires a general anaesthetic since the equipment is extremely fragile and expensive and could easily be damaged if the patient moved or bit it!

Endoscopy can be a very useful technique as it allows biopsy samples to be taken without recourse to surgery. Also, many dogs have had 'foreign bodies' (objects) removed from their throats, oesophagus, stomach and respiratory tract using endoscopy. Without this, major surgery would have been required.

Veterinary Costs and Insurance

The cost of treatment naturally varies according to the condition. Some conditions have a high initial cost but then no further costs if a cure is produced. Surgical treatment of pyometra (womb infection, see page 211) in an older unneutered female dog, or the successful repair of a bone fracture (page 156) are good examples of these. Other conditions have ongoing costs as the diseases are not curable, only controllable; chronic skin disease (page 69) or diabetes mellitus (page 219) would be good examples of these problems.

The cost of any course of treatment is usually made up of some or all of the following categories:

• Initial and review consultation fees

• Fees for diagnostic tests performed at the veterinary practice or sent away to specialist laboratories

• Fees for hospitalisation and surgery if needed

• Costs of medicines, dressings, etc. needed during treatment

• Specialist or referral fees if appropriate

• Costs of any special diet needed during recuperation or after diagnosis.

Variation in fees and choosing a practice

Fees vary between practices. To some extent this depends on which part of the country one lives in. Fees in major cities tend to be higher than in rural locations. An important consideration, however, is the type of practice attended. A specialist practice with high levels of equipment and intensive patient monitoring is bound to be more expensive than a smaller practice with only a few staff and less overheads. This does not mean that such a practice is necessarily always 'better', but facilities for more advanced investigation and diagnosis may be conveniently at hand, and you would have the advantage of already knowing and – hopefully – liking the staff.

On the other hand, a smaller practice may be able to provide a much more personal service simply because there are few staff and they will tend to get to know patients and clients very well. If you attend a small practice and your dog develops a serious problem requiring intensive treatment, then it is likely you could be referred to a centre with appropriate staff and facilities, in the same way as a general medical practitioner would refer a patient to hospital for tests or treatment. You would then return to your own practice once the specialist treatment had been completed.

The most important factor in determining which practice you attend is the impression you get of the staff and their approach.

• Are they welcoming and interested in you and your dog?

• Have they a caring and concerned approach?

• Are the staff approachable and willing to discuss possible diagnoses, treatments and costs in an open, unbiased way without exerting any pressure?

• Are the premises clean and well cared for?

The above are important qualities, possibly as important as the level of equipment and facilities that are at hand within the practice. Obviously, any practice must have a certain basic level of equipment to perform routine tasks, but skills in patient and client care can be as important as high tech facilities, especially when specialist referral practices are becoming much more available for the (infrequent) occasions when they are needed by any individual dog and its owner.

Many practices arrange open days or evenings, allowing clients to view the premises and meet staff in an informal way. These give a great opportunity to see 'behind the scenes' at the veterinary practice and most people who attend find them very interesting.

Pet insurance policies

Many companies now offer health insurance policies for pets, designed to cover unexpected costs due to accident, emergency or disease. Insurance companies will not pay for routine preventative treatment such as vaccination, worming or elective neutering operations. However most other diseases are covered, provided the animal is not suffering from any of these at the time the insurance policy is first taken out. In mosts cases, cover is started in puppies or young dogs. Insurers may refuse to start a policy on an older dog or may charge a higher premium.

If your dog is diagnosed with a chronic disease requiring on-going or life-long treatment, it is likely that this will become excluded from the policy and, after a variable period, you will need to meet these costs yourself. However, you should benefit from the policy cover in the initial phases of diagnosis and treatment, and in many diseases this is the most expensive period.

With the ever-growing complexity of modern veterinary treatment, more and more can be done for sick or injured dogs and pet insurance provides a guarantee that expensive treatment could be undertaken should the need arise. Even the basic policies are fairly wide-ranging and usually cover referral fees, complementary medicine and possibly physiotherapy should this be needed. However, as with all insurance policies, the small print should be carefully examined. There are so many policies on offer that it can be difficult to choose one, however chatting to other dog owners and, especially, the staff at your veterinary practice is a good idea. Veterinary staff deal with insurance companies on a daily basis and if a company is proving awkward at settling claims, then they could warn you against taking out a policy with that insurer. Various levels of cover are usually available, from basic (suitable for most pet dog owners) to more comprehensive policies. Certain breeds known to be susceptible to particular problems may need to be insured at a higher premium than others.

In most instances, the veterinary fees are intially paid to the practice by the dog owner. A claim form is then handed to the veterinary surgeon, who fills this in, and the fees are then reimbursed to the owner (minus any excess) by the insurance company. Most claims take several weeks to settle. Pet insurance comes into its own when a large unexpected bill is received (e.g. after treatment for a road accident, requiring major surgery) or when many diagnostic tests need to be carried out to identify a disease.

Complementary Medicine

Complementary medicine comprises a variety of approaches to injury and disease which can be used alongside conventional medical treatment. The term 'alternative medicine' is used when these other therapies are used *instead* of conventional medical treatment.

Complementary and alternative medicine can arouse strong feelings. Some people claim the therapies are of no use, even dangerous, and that they should never be used. Others maintain that conventional treatment is unnecessary and that it approaches illness and disease from the wrong perspective, whereas alternative approaches consider the 'whole animal' and are therefore better and safer.

As with most debates of this type, it is likely that the answer lies somewhere between the two extremes and that other forms of medicine do have a place in animal and human treatment, sometimes by themselves and sometimes working alongside conventional methods. Unfortunately, the nature of the debate sometimes presents the issue as an 'either/or' situation: either you agree with the conventional system of medicine and reject alternatives, or vice versa.

Regardless of your own viewpoints, it is always safest to have your dog examined by a qualified veterinary surgeon. If you are interested in complementary or alternative approaches, you may be able to be referred to a vet specialising in these techniques. The danger in using non-veterinary qualified therapists is that they may miss important symptoms which must be treated urgently in order to preserve life. Although there are undoubtedly skilled animal therapists who are not qualified vets, one can never be sure of their

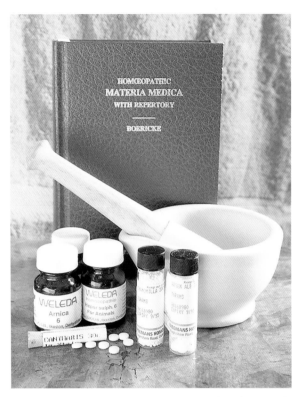

Homoeopathy can complement conventional medicine and surgery.

Of these, acupuncture is the most widely accepted mode of therapy. This ancient system of medicine uses very fine needles inserted into specific target points of the body to control or eliminate symptoms. It is a complex therapy and can be very successful in skilled hands. A growing number of veterinary surgeons are interested in and are using acupuncture. It is not applicable for home use.

Homoeopathy is another ancient form of medicine which has gained wider acceptance recently. It is more controversial than acupuncture but is generally a very safe form of medicine that can be used to good effect by owners in first aid situations. Homoeopathy and homoeopathic first aid for dogs is discussed more fully in Chapter 18. Homoeopathy can also be used for more complex diseases and conditions, but this application of homoeopathy requires years of specialist training. Not all homoeopaths are qualified veterinary surgeons or doctors as there are qualifications in homoeopathy which can be obtained by non-medically registered practitioners. However the initial assessment of an animal is always best performed by a veterinary surgeon.

Herbal medicine utilises the natural properties of plants and other products to cure disease. Many conventional medicines are, of course, derived from plants but the approach in herbal medicine is slightly different, in that the medicines are presented in a less purified and refined form and in lower concentrations. As with the others, this is a complex therapy which should only be undertaken by an experienced practitioner under veterinary supervision. Unlike homoeopathy, it is possible for owners to cause harm to their dog if they administer large doses of herbal products inappropriately and without adequate guidance.

Other complementary approaches are used less commonly at present but it is possible these may become more available in the future as the number of practitioners increases. In all cases, it is important to try to take an objective approach and not to risk your dog's health by trying alternative therapies without at least some input from a veterinary surgeon.

training or background or whether they have a firm grounding in the nature of all dog diseases. In this situation, it is possible that inappropriate therapy could not work or, even worse, endanger life.

Types of complementary therapy

The main types of complementary therapy for pets are:

- Acupuncture

- Homoeopathy

- Herbal/botanical medicine

Less frequently used therapies are:

- Aromatherapy

- Bach flower therapy

- Bioenergetic therapy (using magnetic fields)

- Physical therapy (massage, chiropractic, etc.)

CHAPTER 1

Major Infectious Diseases and Vaccination

Common symptoms of infectious disease
• Poor appetite • Vomiting/diarrhoea
• Lack of energy • High temperature • Coughing
• Contact with infectious dogs

Introduction

Infectious diseases are those that are passed between dogs, either directly (when a healthy dog comes into contact with an infected one) or indirectly (when a healthy dog encounters infection by means of contamination, e.g. contamination of the ground by faeces from an infected dog). Indirect infection obviously poses problems for control of the disease – simply making sure that a susceptible dog does not meet another one 'face to face' is not enough to guarantee that infection will not occur. The virus which causes parvovirus, for example, can easily survive in the ground for months and is resistant to most disinfectants. It can be inadvertently 'walked in' to the dog's environment on the feet of visitors, exposing the unvaccinated dog to risk of infection.

The major infectious diseases still exert a significant toll of disease and death amongst domestic dogs, and animal welfare charities treat many such cases every year, especially of parvovirus. When a disease is caused by a virus (such as parvovirus or distemper), it is not possible to give drugs that will quickly eliminate the virus and cure the disease; antibiotics are only effective against bacteria, not viruses. With viral infections, only supportive treatment can be given whilst, hopefully, waiting for the dog's own immune system to deal with the infection. Unfortunately, this does not always happen, especially in young dogs, and death from complications of the original infection can occur. In places where a significant number of dogs congregate (e.g. urban environments, kennels, etc.) control can be particularly difficult.

The diseases currently preventable by vaccination of dogs are:

- Parvovirus

- Distemper ('hard pad')

- Leptospirosis

- Infectious canine hepatitis

- Rabies

- Infectious tracheo-bronchitis ('kennel cough')

The last two are not part of the routine vaccination protocol of most pet dogs. Rabies is only given in countries where the disease is endemic, or in dogs travelling between countries, and kennel cough vaccination tends to be administered shortly before a dog enters a boarding kennel or attends a dog show.

Pros and Cons of Vaccination

An on-going debate

There is no doubt that routine vaccination has had an enormous impact in the control of a number of potentially fatal dog diseases, thus improving the health and welfare of millions of pet dogs – so much so that the once common 'killer diseases' are quite rarely seen amongst well managed dogs today. These diseases are, however, still present, and will cause serious illness or death in susceptible animals. Two days before writing this, the author treated parvovirus in three unvaccinated young dogs; one of these died from the disease. No one who witnesses a case of parvovirus would wish to expose their pet to this unpleasant condition.

Modern vaccines are very safe products but, like all medicines, absolute guarantees of freedom from side-effects cannot be given, only relative percentages and 'risk-benefit' assessments. Taken as a whole, current vaccines are very safe and their benefits far outweigh

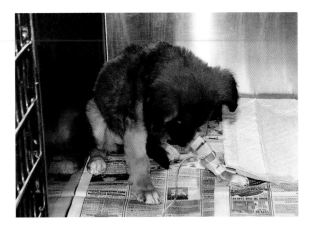

A very ill puppy under treatment for parvovirus. This puppy recovered after five days of intensive care but could easily have died.

Is a booster needed *every* year?

There is a fairly strong suggestion that yearly boosters are not needed for certain of the infectious diseases of dogs. The efficiency of modern vaccines is such that distemper, parvovirus and infectious canine hepatitis may be protected against after a primary course of two injections while a puppy, followed by a complete booster given at one year of age. Leptospirosis, however, is not included in this category: the immunity from this vaccination is known to be of shorter duration and boosters are important.

In fact, many veterinary surgeons do not vaccinate for distemper every year (usually giving it every two years), but parvovirus and leptospirosis are routinely given annually. An argument could be put forward to vaccinate only for leptospirosis once a dog is over one year of age.

There are, however, several problems with this viewpoint:

- Although there is scientific suggestion that boosters may not be necessary, carefully controlled long term studies have not been carried out. Most veterinary surgeons suggest yearly boosters 'to be on the safe side' and follow the guidelines issued by vaccine manufacturers in doing this.

- Boarding kennels require evidence of up-to-date booster vaccinations, as do dog shows. Without regular full boosters, dogs may not be admitted.

- Pet insurance policies may require annual boosters and health examinations otherwise they could be invalidated should a claim be required.

- Dogs do vary and it is not possible to guarantee that each and every dog will have an adequate immunity without annual boosters – or even, for that matter, with them. Rightly or wrongly, the yearly booster has simply grown to become the accepted practice across most veterinary clinics.

The final decision rests with the owner of the dog, who must decide whether to vaccinate, and how often to attend for boosters. The lack of available data is frustrating for all concerned. Most responsible dog owners do currently take their pets for annual boosters and incidences of adverse effects are very rare.

the risks of non-vaccination in pet dogs. Nevertheless, concerns have been raised about the need for repeated booster vaccinations in dogs and claims made about possible adverse effects of this.

Principles and side-effects of vaccination

Vaccination works by exposing the body's immune system to disease in a 'safe' form, allowing the body to mount an effective immune response so that, should the real disease be encountered in the future, symptoms will not appear. The discovery of vaccination was one of the major landmarks in human and veterinary medicine. Since that time, vaccines have been developed and refined to a high degree of safety and efficiency.

For a vaccine to work effectively, it must 'show' the body enough about the disease to allow the body's immune system to recognise the virus or bacterium that causes it in the future. However, at the same time, the vaccine must not actually *cause* the disease itself – otherwise there would be no point in vaccinating in the first place. The overall aim is to create a solid immunity to the disease, which acts like the immunity an animal obtains after suffering from the disease (assuming it survives), but *without* causing major symptoms.

This is, in fact, a tall order and there is no doubt that initial attempts at human and animal vaccines often created unwanted symptoms – not usually as bad as the disease itself, but unpleasant nevertheless. With improving technologies, it has been possible to manufacture vaccines that produce virtually no side-effects after vaccination but which still effectively protect against diseases.

What side-effects can occur?

Tissue reaction

A minor side-effect is irritation at the site of the vaccination injection – in dogs, vaccines are often given underneath the loose skin of the scruff or along the top of the back. The animal may show some pain here

How vaccination works

Unvaccinated dogs

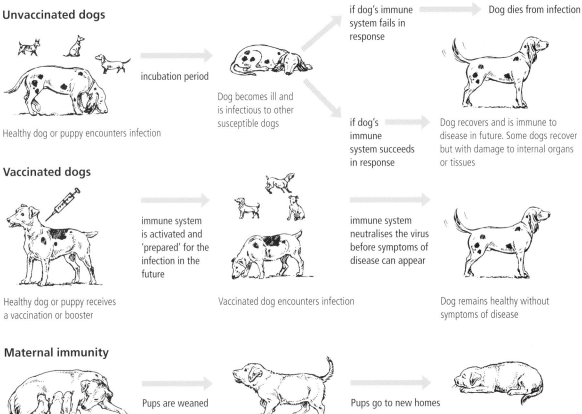

Healthy dog or puppy encounters infection

incubation period

Dog becomes ill and is infectious to other susceptible dogs

if dog's immune system fails in response

Dog dies from infection

if dog's immune system succeeds in response

Dog recovers and is immune to disease in future. Some dogs recover but with damage to internal organs or tissues

Vaccinated dogs

Healthy dog or puppy receives a vaccination or booster

immune system is activated and 'prepared' for the infection in the future

Vaccinated dog encounters infection

immune system neutralises the virus before symptoms of disease can appear

Dog remains healthy without symptoms of disease

Maternal immunity

Immune or vaccinated bitch passes on protection to her puppies in milk as they suckle

Pups are weaned

Puppies lose this maternal protection by 12 weeks of age

Pups go to new homes

If pups have not been vaccinated (usually at 8 and 12 weeks) and they encounter infection, they may become ill and die (or, if lucky, recover and be immune)

and the area may swell up. Usually, this reaction subsides after a few days and no treatment is required. The vaccine is just as effective as if no reaction had occurred. Very few vaccinated dogs develop a reaction like this.

Very occasionally, an abscess can occur at the site of a vaccination. This results from skin contamination and would require specific treatment such as antibiotics or surgical drainage. Any injection given to a dog carries a slight risk of abscess formation if infection is inadvertently introduced when the needle is inserted.

Dullness and raised temperature

Some owners notice subtle changes in behaviour, especially after first vaccinations. Puppies may sleep a

little more and perhaps miss one meal. These mild symptoms, which may be associated with a slightly high temperature, pass over in a few hours. Such responses are not of concern provided they are temporary in nature.

Encephalitis

A very rare reaction is the development of encephalitis (brain inflammation) after vaccination. This has been reported after rabies and distemper vaccinations. Some days after vaccination, neurological signs develop, including weakness, incoordination and behavioural changes. This is a highly unusual reaction and is not considered by most veterinary surgeons as a reason to withold vaccination. Cases which arose in response to a certain strain of vaccine led to that vaccine being immediately withdrawn and replaced by safe vaccines.

Problems in pregnancy

Veterinary advice should be sought if vaccination is required during pregnancy, as this may influence the type of vaccine used. Problems are however unlikely.

Anaphylaxis

This is a severe allergic reaction that may occur to any medical or non-medical product. Symptoms include breathlessness, vomiting, diarrhoea and collapse and may start within several hours of a vaccine being given. Anaphylaxis has been associated with certain leptospirosis vaccines in some dogs, but fortunately is a rare reaction. Prompt treatment usually stops symptoms quickly. Suspected anaphylaxis should be treated as an emergency and the dog returned to the veterinary surgery immediately.

Anemia and platelet deficiency

Platelets are small blood cells which assist in the formation of blood clots, and hence stop bleeding. Very rare reactions to vaccination may involve the destruction of the dog's own red blood cells and platelets by the activated immune system. A few cases of such disorders have been reported in the medical literature, but are considered extremely rare. Nevertheless, extra caution is exercised in dogs already suffering from diseases which involve destruction of blood cells by the immune system; in these patients, different types of vaccine may be employed.

Failure of vaccination

This side-effect occurs when a vaccinated dog contracts the disease it is supposed to be protected against. This is a distressing situation that can arise from a number of causes. Note that vaccination against kennel cough (infectious tracheo-bronchitis) is not always 100% effective due to the complexity of this disease; however kennel cough is far less harmful than other infectious diseases such as parvovirus or distemper.

Occasionally, symptoms of one disease can mimic another. For example, a vaccinated dog may develop bloody diarrhoea and an assumption will be made that this is parvovirus and that vaccination has failed; however, there are other causes of bloody diarrhoea to consider. Definite proof of failure of the vaccination requires specific laboratory tests.

Genuine failure of vaccination may mean:

1. The dog was already infected with the disease when vaccination was given.

2. The dog has an abnormal immune system and does not respond as expected to the vaccine.

3. The vaccine itself is defective or was not administered as directed. (Vaccines should only be given by veterinary surgeons or under their supervision and control.)

4. First vaccination was carried out before 12 weeks, as recommended, but the second component of the vaccine (given at 12 weeks or older) was missed. 12 weeks is a crucial age: a vaccination must be given on or after this date to produce lasting immunity (see maternal immunity below).

5. The dog was continually exposed to a very high degree of infection – an unusual situation, but one which may cause vaccine protection to eventually break down.

Maternal Immunity

Maternal immunity is the natural immunity that is passed from mother to offspring in the milk, and especially in the initial milk produced by the mother shortly after birth (colostrum). Colostrum is a very important substance as it is rich in antibodies and provides newborn puppies with protection against serious diseases. If a puppy does not receive colostrum for any reason (e.g. the bitch dies during whelping) the risks of infection are higher.

Maternal immunity is not permanent, it simply provides a 'stop gap' between birth and, in pet dogs, initial vaccinations against major infectious diseases. Maternal immunity also depends on the diseases the bitch has encountered or been vaccinated against. If a bitch has not suffered and recovered from a certain disease, nor been vaccinated against it, no protection can be passed onto her puppies; indeed, the bitch herself is susceptible to the disease.

As maternal immunity disappears, but before vaccination takes place, puppies can be left exposed to risk from diseases. The problem is that the strength and duration of maternal immunity varies somewhat. It is not possible to say that by, for example, 8 weeks all maternal immunity will have gone. This has two important implications:

1. When maternal immunity disappears, puppies are susceptible to diseases unless vaccination has been carried out.

2. If vaccination is carried out too early (before maternal immunity disappears) the vaccine does not work so efficiently – it may, in fact, be cancelled out by the maternal antibodies still in the puppy's body.

Thus maternal immunity, whilst important for puppy health, poses problems for the timing of vaccination: a vaccine given too early may not last, but one given too late may leave the puppy open to a 'window of opportunity' for infection.

To tackle this problem, puppies are usually given two initial vaccinations (or more than two in situations of high risk of infection). Studies have shown that in the majority of puppies maternal immunity has disappeared by 12 weeks so, as long as a vaccination is given on or after this time, immunity should be long-lasting. Risk of infection for puppies younger than 12 weeks is provided by the first vaccination, which can be given at an early age – usually around 8 weeks.

Major Infectious Diseases of Dogs

PARVOVIRUS

CAUSE The cause is a small virus, invisible to the naked eye, which first caused disease in dogs in the 1970s and 80s. The virus is a very resistant one and is difficult to kill using disinfectants. It can survive in the environment for many months and millions of virus particles are present in the faeces of infected dogs.

Parvovirus is the commonest infectious disease of young dogs and is always potentially serious. Rottweilers and Dobermans seem even more susceptible than most other breeds.

SYMPTOMS Symptoms are commonest in young dogs up to 6 months of age. The incubation period (time from infection to development of symptoms) is approximately 7 days. The commonest pattern of symptoms is: depression and lethargy, with poor appetite, leading onto vomiting and then frequent diarrhoea, which may contain blood. In severe cases, the diarrhoea consists almost entirely of blood and affected dogs may die of shock.

Dehydration can be rapid and severe, leading quickly to death in puppies. Symptoms may be provoked or worsened by a period of stress (e.g. seen in puppies moving into a new home environment, experiencing a new diet, etc.).

Milder infections also occur, usually in older or adult dogs, and in these cases the only sign may be a period of being 'off colour' with mild diarrhoea. Most adult dogs have an immunity to the infection, either through vaccination or from encountering the disease (and surviving) while younger.

Is my dog vaccinated?

All dogs older than 12 weeks of age should be fully vaccinated, with an up-to-date vaccination record card clearly identifying the dog, the veterinary practice attended and the vaccines administered, together with the dates given and, usually, the vaccine manufacturer's batch numbers. The card should be signed by a veterinary surgeon.

If you acquire a dog, you should not take for granted that it has been vaccinated unless you are given a completed vaccination card. This is the only guarantee that protection is present. Blood tests can be performed to check on antibody levels, but these represent an additional expense. If there is any doubt about vaccination, you should discuss the situation with your veterinary surgeon. Additional vaccination may be preferable to living with any uncertainty about the vaccination schedule.

First aid and home nursing for infectious diseases, especially parvovirus

Basics
In all cases of serious infectious diseases, e.g. parvovirus, the dog nursed at home must be allowed to rest in a quiet area. Avoid overheating the surroundings. Room temperature is fine unless the dog is shivering. If you think the dog is cold, turn the room heating up and use additional blankets or 'bubble wrap' packaging, which has good insulating properties, as covering until the dog seems more comfortable. Plenty of clean bedding underneath the dog is important and in illnesses causing vomiting and diarrhoea, this may need to be changed many times during the day if it becomes soiled. A thick plastic sheet under the bedding or basket is a good idea to protect the floor and make cleaning easier.

Toileting
If possible, the dog should be encouraged to go out 4 times daily, supported in a blanket sling if necessary, to pass urine and faeces. This often helps to cheer dogs up during the convalescence phase as it provides some fresh air and interaction with the owner.

Eating and drinking
If fluids can be tolerated without vomiting, small frequent drinks of water or glucose solution, should be offered. If food can be tolerated 'light diets' (e.g. cooked chicken/rice, cooked fish/rice, scrambled egg/ rice) are best. Give 4–6 small meals throughout the day. Dogs unable to tolerate water or food by mouth usually need to be hospitalised and put on a drip to prevent dehydration.

Other nursing
Any discharges accumulating around the eyes and nose must be bathed away using lukewarm water. If the area around the anus or prepuce/vulva becomes soiled, this must be carefully cleaned and dried. In very ill dogs, it is inadvisable to give them a bath; instead, use large amounts of paper towel to clean and dry the area and wait until the dog is fitter before giving a full bath or shower. Administer medication as directed by the veterinary surgeon and report any changes in the dog's condition to the practice in case further examination, treatment or hospitalisation is needed. Remember to give plenty of TLC as dogs with these illnesses are frequently miserable and dejected.

Prevention of infection
Avoid contact with all other dogs and practice good basic hygiene. Plastic gloves and aprons are sensible precautions. Wash hands after dealing with the sick dog. Disinfectants effective against viruses are usually available from veterinary practices.

Very occasionally, heart problems (myocarditis) are caused by parvovirus in puppies. This can cause sudden death in apparently healthy young puppies, or, if they survive, heart problems may develop later in life. Myocarditis is much rarer than the other symptoms of parvovirus however and is hardly seen now.

DIAGNOSIS Parvovirus can be proved by isolation of the virus itself from faeces samples or by other laboratory tests. Blood samples, looking for antibodies to the disease, can be useful in addition to this to provide confirmation. In practice, the characteristic symptoms in a young dog which has not been vaccinated provide sufficient basis to start treatment. Time can be of the essence.

TREATMENT There is no straightforward cure for parvovirus. Treatment aims to support the dog's organs while its own immune system copes with the disease. The main aim is to prevent or treat dehydration while the enteritis caused by the virus resolves. Severe cases may require hospitalisation for intravenous drips, antibiotics (to prevent complicating bacterial infections) and drugs to control persistent vomiting. Blood transfusions are occasionally given.

Some dogs may be able to be treated as outpatients. They require careful nursing and are likely to have frequent diarrhoea at home. Meticulous attention to keeping the patient clean, dry and warm is required, together with administration of fluid replacement drinks and any other medication

Environmental contamination and risks

Faeces from dogs with parvovirus contains literally millions of virus particles and is therefore highly infectious to other dogs (not to people). Coupled with this, the virus itself is very durable and can easily survive for months in the environment. It is also resistant to many common disinfectants and cleaning agents. These properties can make the disease extremely difficult to eradicate from kennel situations where many dogs are housed together.

Cleaning procedure for the kennel or home
- Remove all trace of faeces and debris by carefully lifting it and then by repeated washing of contaminated areas using warm soapy water followed by rinsing. The aim is to create a perfectly clean surface, including all cracks, corners and crevices. Allow the area to dry thoroughly.

- Apply a disinfectant known to be effective against parvovirus to the area (available from veterinary practices). Bleach works well provided there is no debris collected in corners or surface cracks. Rinse well after bleach and allow to air dry. (Use 1 part household bleach to 32 parts water.)

- Ensure that any healthy dogs introduced to the area are immune to the disease, i.e. they have suffered from it and are now fully recovered or they have been vaccinated.

supplied by the veterinary surgeon. If fluids cannot, or will not, be taken and kept down by mouth, intravenous drips are required either as an outpatient or combined with hospitalisation.

OUTLOOK The outlook is reasonable in older dogs treated promptly, but puppies and younger dogs may succumb to this disease very quickly. Parvovirus is a highly unpleasant condition and in severely affected puppies unlikely to survive, euthanasia may be recommended to prevent further suffering.

PREVENTION In most cases, routine vaccination of puppies at 8 weeks and again at 12 weeks is carried out, with annual booster vaccinations thereafter. Occasionally, a further dose is given at 16 or 18 weeks of age to ensure complete protection.

Prior to the first vaccination at 8 weeks, immunity provided by the bitch in her milk affords protection against the disease to the puppies. However, when infection is known to be present or a particular threat, and earlier protection of puppies is required, vaccination may be started at a younger age. Repeat doses will still be needed up to 12 weeks in order to ensure that immunity from vaccination remains good.

Illness in newly acquired puppies

Puppies are vulnerable to parvovirus at the time of rehoming, usually around 8 weeks. The stress of being separated from mother and litter, coupled with changes in environment and diet, may contribute. Occasionally, puppies are infected with the virus and only show signs once they are in their new home – this must be suspected if they have not come into contact with other dogs since they left the litter, and if the timing fits in with the incubation period of the disease. The explanation is that the puppy's maternal immunity to the disease has lapsed before vaccination could be started.

DISTEMPER

CAUSE Distemper is another viral disease of dogs and is related to the virus which causes measles in humans. Unlike parvovirus, it is a fragile virus, easily killed using standard disinfectants or even sunlight. Despite its fragility, however, this virus can cause devastating disease in young dogs particularly.

Spread requires quite close contact between dogs as the virus is usually inhaled directly into the respiratory system. The incubation period is around 2 weeks.

SYMPTOMS Mild forms of the disease occur and probably go unnoticed in most cases. In more serious cases, typical symptoms include high temperature, nasal and eye discharges and a troublesome cough caused by respiratory infection or pneumonia. Diarrhoea is often seen and there may be occasional vomiting. These symptoms often 'wax and wane' as the dog's temperature rises and falls. Other general symptoms such as lack of energy and poor appetite are very common in the early stages.

Distemper can affect many organs of the body. It causes a painful thickening of the foot pad which led to the term 'hard pad' being used for the disease. Similar crusty thickenings may be seen on the nose area, which is often caked with discharges. The teeth of young dogs may be affected, resulting in cavities forming in the enamel layer of the teeth. This tooth damage persists for the rest of the dog's life.

An important aspect of distemper is its effect on the central nervous system. These symptoms are seen later on in the disease. They may appear when the dog appears to be starting to make a recovery from the other symptoms and may, unfortunately, prove permanent. Fits/convulsions can occur or else spasmodic twitches affecting certain areas of the body may be present: a condition known as chorea. Jaw clamping and a variety of other spasmodic nervous symptoms may occur. Some dogs suffer partial or complete paralysis of the hind limbs.

DIAGNOSIS Characteristic symptoms lead to the suspicion of distemper, especially a respiratory infection progressing to include other symptoms over a period of a few weeks. The wide spectrum of possible signs means that usually several associated symptoms will be seen in individual dogs.

Confirmation of the diagnosis is very difficult. Certain laboratory tests are available, but these are not 100% reliable and their specialised nature means that many diagnoses are made on the basis of typical symptoms alone.

TREATMENT As with parvovirus, there is no cure. Only supportive treatment and nursing is possible whilst waiting for the dog's own immune system to cope with the infection. Antibiotics may be given to prevent complications arising from bacterial infection. Some dogs require intravenous fluids and drugs to help with vomiting and diarrhoea. All discharges are carefully cleaned away and eyelids and nostrils kept moist and clean. Palatable, easily digested food is given.

If fits occur, these will be treated using anticonvulsant drugs. Such treatment may need to be permanent if the fits persist. Unfortunately, fits may prove difficult or impossible to control with drugs, in which case euthanasia may be recommended.

OUTLOOK Recovery can take weeks to months, and some of the effects of distemper may be permanent. Severely affected dogs may require humane euthanasia, usually for progressive pneumonia or uncontrollable nervous symptoms.

PREVENTION Very effective vaccines are available for distemper. These are normally given at 8 weeks and again at 12 weeks, with earlier vaccinations given if there is particular risk. A booster vaccination for distemper given after one year should ensure good immunity for the rest of the dog's life, however distemper is frequently included in booster vaccinations for other diseases when combined vaccines are used.

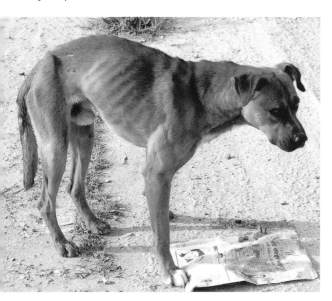

Stray dog in Greece with partial hindlimb paralysis, probably caused by distemper (see opposite).

INFECTIOUS CANINE HEPATITIS

CAUSE This is another viral illness of dogs, but is less common than parvovirus. The illness is spread via contaminated urine, faeces or saliva. Spread in the urine can continue for as long as six months after infection in recovered dogs. Young dogs are affected most and the incubation period is around 5 days.

The adenovirus which causes infectious canine hepatitis is a fairly tough virus and will survive in the environment for several weeks, so close contact between dogs is not necessary for transmission to occur (unlike distemper).

SYMPTOMS Infection causes a very high temperature, with dullness, poor appetite and enlarged lymphatic glands in the neck area. Vomiting and diarrhoea is often seen and there is abdominal pain due to liver inflammation (hepatitis). Respiratory and heart rates can be elevated and gums may be very pale. Severely affected dogs can suffer internal haemorrhages, seizures or coma and may die at this stage.

Symptoms usually last about one week. During recovery, a 'blue eye' may develop. This reaction in the clear window of the eye (the cornea) is a result of the dog's immune response to the infection, and usually indicates that the immune system is coping with the disease. In mild cases, development of a 'blue eye' may be the only indication that infection has occurred. The discolouration of the cornea normally disappears after several weeks.

DIAGNOSIS A variety of laboratory tests, taken in conjunction with the characteristic symptoms, can point towards infectious canine hepatitis. Measuring antibody levels in the blood and isolating the virus itself from inflamed tonsils confirms that the cause is the adenovirus of infectious canine hepatitis.

TREATMENT As with the other viral illnesses discussed here, there is no cure for this disease; rather, supportive treatment is given whilst hopefully waiting for the dog's immune system to cope with the virus. Typical hospitalisation treatments include intra-venous fluid drips, drugs given to control vomiting and general nursing care. Antibiotics are not usually given as they have no effect on the virus.

OUTLOOK This can be a rapidly fatal disease in severe cases. Milder cases normally recover well, though this may take up to two weeks.

PREVENTION Good protection is available from vaccination. The vaccine for infectious canine hepatitis is usually combined with other vaccines in a single injection.

LEPTOSPIROSIS

Possible risk of infection to human beings

CAUSE Unlike the diseases mentioned above, leptospirosis is caused by a bacterium (rather than a virus). Actually, two bacteria are capable of producing symptoms of this disease: one of these (*L. canicola*) is a true virus of dogs, the other (*L. icterohaemorrhagiae*) is a rat virus which can also infect dogs. Both are transmitted in urine. *L. canicola* is more likely in town dogs, where there is likely to be more proximity to dog urine, and *L. icterohaemorrhagiae* is more likely in country situations (e.g. on farms), where contact with rat urine may occur.

The rat species may be picked up if contaminated water is drunk or if food is contaminated with rat urine and the dog species may enter the body if contaminated dog urine is sniffed or licked. The organisms can also enter the body through small cuts or grazes which come into contact with infected urine. Such a situation could result from a dog swimming in a stagnant pool which was frequented by rats, for example, when infected water could be drunk or enter a small skin wound.

Both bacteria are fairly fragile and do not survive well in light or dry conditions. Most disinfectants are efficient at killing them.

Leptospirosis can also infect human beings and may cause serious disease. Fortunately, the disease is quite rare, but if it is suspected medical advice should also be sought from the family doctor.

SYMPTOMS Initial signs are vague, with dullness, a high temperature and poor appetite occurring. Symptoms then progress to vomiting, abdominal pain, diarrhoea and haemorrhages. Severe dehydration can occur as a result of kidney and liver failure. Jaundice can be present (a sign of severe liver disease).

The rat form of the disease causes mainly signs of liver failure whereas the dog form causes mainly kidney damage or failure.

DIAGNOSIS Blood tests can reveal the extent of liver or kidney damage and examination of urine samples may reveal the bacteria. If an unvaccinated dog shows typical signs, the veterinary surgeon may suspect leptospirosis.

TREATMENT If severe kidney or liver damage has occurred, hospitalisation for intensive treatment using intravenous drip fluids will be required. The bacteria can be killed using antibiotics.

OUTLOOK This depends on the severity of organ damage which has occurred prior to treatment being started. Both the liver and the kidneys have a good capacity to compensate for damage but if a critical amount of tissue is destroyed permanent symptoms or progressive deterioration can occur.

PREVENTION Vaccination is used to prevent this disease. Annual boosters are important with leptospirosis as the immunity achieved from vaccination is not permanent. The vaccine is often given as a single injection incorporating other infectious diseases.

Dogs should not be allowed access to stagnant pools.

RABIES

Possible risk of infection to human beings

CAUSE Rabies is a fatal viral illness which affects a wide range of mammals, including human beings. The virus itself is fragile and cannot survive outside a host, so transmission of the disease requires close contact between animals and is almost always passed on by a bite from an infected animal.

Certain areas of the world, such as the United Kingdom, Australia and Sweden are free from rabies. In other countries the disease is maintained in wild animals such as raccoons and bats, occasionally infecting man via domestic animals. In countries with large numbers of stray or feral dogs, these populations can also harbour the disease and may pose a threat to man when they are in close proximity to human habitations.

SYMPTOMS A bite acts as an injection of rabies into the bitten animal. The virus then affects the nervous system and brain. It becomes concentrated in the bitten animal's saliva so that it, too, becomes infectious.

Symptoms appear some time after being bitten – the exact time depends on how close the bite wound is to the nervous system and brain. Wounds nearer the brain result in major symptoms appearing sooner but delays of up to several months are possible.

Symptoms initially show as subtle changes in behaviour. Nervous dogs may become more confident and friendly. Alternatively, a friendly dog may become withdrawn and nervous. Dogs may chew at or traumatise their bite wound. The behaviour becomes more abnormal and unpredictable.

The 'furious' phase follows, although only about a quarter of infected dogs show this phase. This is the dangerous period when rabid dogs may attack other animals, including people. Their behaviour is totally unpredictable and they react to stimuli such as light or sound, even attacking inanimate objects. Extensive wandering is possible – rabid dogs have been known to travel over 20 miles.

Commoner than 'furious' rabies in dogs is so-called 'dumb' rabies. Here, symptoms are fairly vague, but muscle weakness, drooling and eye problems develop. Biting may occur if the dog is approached or surprised.

Finally, the unfortunate animal becomes progressively paralysed, unable to swallow, before collpasing and entering a coma, eventually dying of respiratory failure. It is a highly unpleasant illness and death.

DIAGNOSIS Unusual behaviour of a dog in a country where rabies is present should always be viewed with suspicion. Most countries have stringent regulations concerning the action to be taken, which usually involves confinement and observation of the dog and, in suspect cases, euthanasia.

TREATMENT There is no effective treatment for rabies. Affected animals are destroyed.

OUTLOOK The disease is fatal.

PREVENTION Vaccination is available against rabies but in rabies-free countries, vaccination of dogs is not normally carried out unless foreign travel is anticipated. Strict regulations exist concerning the transport of dogs between countries. It is possible, provided all regulatory procedures have been fol-

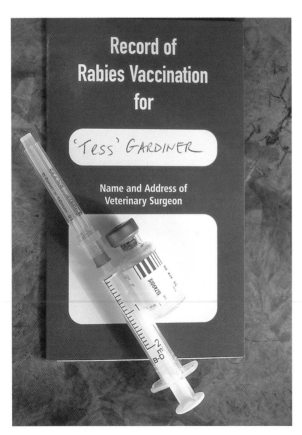

Vaccination means that international travel between certain rabies-free countries is now possible without lengthy quarantine.

lowed, to travel with pet dogs between rabies-free countries once vaccination, blood testing and microchip identification procedures have been undertaken. Otherwise, lengthy periods of quarantine are required.

KENNEL COUGH

CAUSE This is a very common infectious disease of dogs which is usually caused by several different organisms, both bacteria and viruses, acting together. In many dogs 'mixed infections' of this type are present which, together, are given the name infectious tracheo-bronchitis or 'kennel cough'.

Despite the name, the disease is not restricted to dogs kept in kennel environments. It can be picked up anywhere that dogs congregate: grooming parlours, dog shows, training classes and even veterinary surgeries. It is however commonest in boarding and rescue kennels. Sometimes, dogs which have not had direct contact with other dogs do pick up the disease, although this is fairly unusual and other conditions might be suspected in this situation.

The disease is transmitted in exhaled or coughed breath and via feeding utensils and equipment.

SYMPTOMS 3–4 days after exposure to infection a cough develops. This is usually a harsh and loud dry cough, worse after excitement or changes in environment. Coughing bouts can be protracted and sometimes the dog will retch up clear fluid or foam afterwards, leading the owner to believe that something is stuck in the throat. A mild nasal discharge may also be present.

Other than this, there are few symptoms. Most dogs remain bright, keen to eat and exercise and generally their 'usual selves'. Usually only old, sick or very young dogs are at risk of complications such as pneumonia, but dogs which suffer from tracheal collapse (see page 133) or other respiratory or heart diseases need careful observation and more comprehensive treatment.

DIAGNOSIS The symptoms are fairly typical of this condition and most dogs have been in contact with other coughing dogs within the previous 7–10 days. Gently touching the trachea during examination of the dog usually produces a bout of coughing. Provided no other symptoms are present, serious diseases like distemper and pneumonia can be ruled out (distemper is easily ruled out if the dog has been vaccinated).

TREATMENT Mild cases resolve well by themselves, although this can take several weeks. During this time, the best advice is to limit exercise and keep the dog away from dusty environments. Antibiotics are not usually needed. Changing from a collar to a harness or headcollar may help relieve coughing from lead pressure exerted on the neck, but walks should anyway be minimal while the cough is present.

When the coughing is frequent and irritating, drugs to suppress the cough may be given provided the dog is otherwise healthy.

OUTLOOK The outlook is good; this is not a fatal disease but repeated infections are possible. A few dogs develop a chronic tracheo-bronchial syndrome after kennel cough and may experience recurrent mild episodes of similar symptoms.

PREVENTION Some degree of prevention is possible by vaccinating dogs 1–2 weeks before they are due to enter kennels, and many boarding kennels insist on

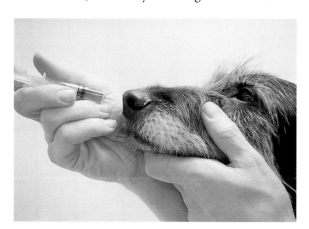

Intra-nasal vaccination against 'kennel cough', a troublesome but rarely serious infectious disease of dogs.

this before dogs are admitted. The vaccine for kennel cough takes the form of drops of vaccine instilled into the nose (the more usual kind of vaccine is an injection given under the skin). While most dogs tolerate this very well, there is no doubt that a few animals become distressed by the procedure which can, unfortunately, lead them to develop a phobia about the veterinary surgery. In these cases, the relative advantages and disadvantages of the vaccination should be discussed with the veterinary surgeon in advance. Nearly always, however, the vaccine can be given without problems. If it is vital that a very uncooperative dog receive the vaccine, mild sedation may be considered before the appointment.

Vaccination is not 100% reliable for this disease but if symptoms do appear, they are usually milder than in unvaccinated dogs.

Other Infectious Diseases

HEARTWORM

This is a parasitic condition found in some parts of the world (not the United Kingdom). Parasitic worms are present within the heart and associated large blood vessels. Serious infections can lead to respiratory and heart problems, even heart failure. The condition is diagnosed from X-rays and from results of blood tests. Treatment is given to kill the parasites and future infestations are prevented by monthly drug treatment. Heartworm is found in parts of Europe, the USA, Australia and Japan.

TOXOPLASMOSIS AND NEOSPOROSIS

These diseases are caused by minute parasites (protozoa) which forms cysts within muscles. Muscle weakness, incoordination and paralysis can be caused. Diagnosis usually involves muscle biopsies and blood tests. Treatment is likely to be successful if started early and consists of antibiotics and, sometimes, an anti-malarial drug used in humans.

LYME DISEASE

This is a parasitic disease which can be transmitted to dogs infested with ticks. The main symptoms are of joint pain and high temperature. Diagnosis can be difficult and often relies on excluding other possibilities, together with evidence of recent tick infestation. Fortunately, the disease is effectively treated using antibiotics and tick infestation can be prevented using veterinary-approved products prior to possible exposure to ticks.

TETANUS

Tetanus is not found commonly in dogs. When it does occur, it follows deep puncture wounds which are contaminated by the bacterium which causes tetanus. Nervous symptoms follow with muscle rigidity and 'lockjaw', caused by spasm of the jaw muscles. The gait of the dog is often jerky and mechanical and the ears and tail are held in an erect position. Death can occur from respiratory paralysis in severe cases.

Most infected, deep puncture wounds in dogs are treated using antibiotics, which would kill the tetanus organism if it was present. Other cases, provided not too severe, can still be treated – but the disease is rarely encountered in veterinary practice.

HERPES VIRUS INFECTION

This disease can be important in breeding dogs and in puppies. The virus is widely present within the dog population and puppies are normally infected from their mothers. If infection happens when the bitch is pregnant, abortion or stillbirth can occur. If infection is acquired by the puppies after birth, illness and death usually result. Affected puppies stop feeding, cry continually and may have a nasal discharge and difficulty breathing. They are unable to maintain their body temperature and may become hypothermic if there is insufficient warmth. The illness worsens over 1–2 days and puppies eventually lose consciousness and die despite treatment.

Bitches which have previously encountered the infection and recovered from it pass on immunity to their puppies within the first week of suckling, so once a bitch has had one episode of infection with death of puppies, future litters should be protected. The symptoms in adult dogs are fairly minor – usually a respiratory or genital infection.

There is no vaccine available for this disease.

CHAPTER 2

The Mouth and Nose

Common symptoms of mouth and nose disease
• Eating or swallowing problems
• Nasal discharge • Abnormal swellings
• Coughing, choking or snorting
• Bad breath

Structure and Function

There is great variation in the overall shape of the dog's mouth and nose area since different breeds have been altered during generations of selective breeding by man. Perhaps two extremes are the very shortened mouths and noses of breeds like the Boxer and Pekinese compared to the much longer mouths and noses of 'hound' breeds such as the Greyhound and Saluki. Many dogs (e.g. Labradors) lie somewhere between these two extremes.

Compressed faces are prone to certain problems such as teeth crowding and the production of folds and pockets of skin, especially around the lips, which can become inflamed and infected. Drainage of tears from the eye may also be inefficient, causing persistent tear overflow onto the face area. In Pekinese, especially, the hair on the nose area may rub against the eye surface, causing irritation and damage.

Breathing problems are also very common in squash-faced dogs, and this sometimes requires treatment involving surgery to the upper airways. Because

Several variations in dog face shape: the Boxer, Greyhound and Spaniel.

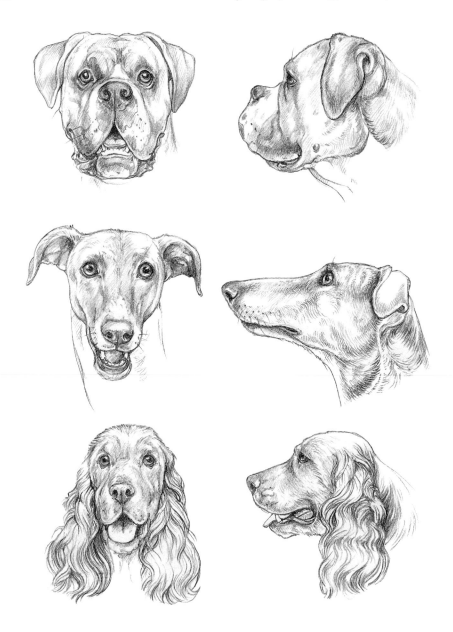

of the problems with their upper airways, these dogs are especially prone to heat stress. Panting is the main mechanism of heat loss in dogs, which do not sweat apart from on their feet. Care should be taken to ensure that brachycephalic (short-faced) dogs do not overheat during the summer months as this can cause collapse and death.

Longer-nosed breeds generally have fewer problems although studies on nasal cancer and fungal infections have found these problems to be commoner in longer-nosed breeds.

The teeth

Dogs should have their full set of permanent teeth by age 7 months. Retained primary (milk) teeth are common in smaller breeds; if these cause crowding problems in the mouth they should be removed. The 'dental formula' of the adult dog is:

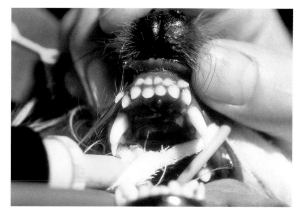

Retained primary (milk) teeth in a young dog. Removal is usually recommended.

	Upper jaw	Lower jaw
Incisors	3 each side	3 each side
Canines	1 each side	1 each side
Premolars	4 each side	4 each side
Molars	2 each side	3 each side

giving the dog 42 teeth in total.

The different teeth evolved to do different jobs: the incisor teeth have developed to allow nibbling and grooming; the canines allow tearing actions, while the premolars and molars are designed to shear food into fragments that can be swallowed. These functions have arisen through thousands of years of evolution but the modern pet dog, fed on tinned or dried food, eats a diet that is very different from its wild counterparts, e.g. wolves.

Dental disease is extremely common in dogs and while part of this is undoubtedly due to the fact that pet dogs live far longer than wild ones, diet also plays

Skull and teeth of a dog

1. incisors
2. canines
3. premolars
4. molars

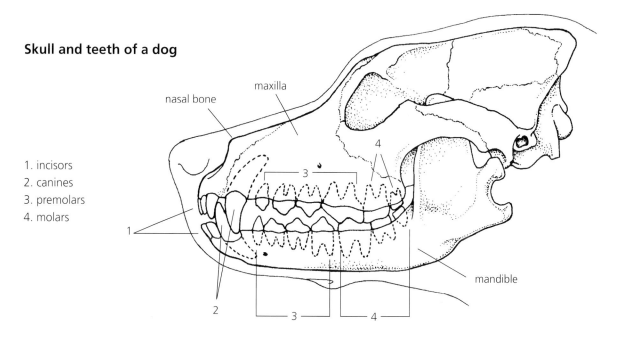

a role and in some respects modern pet food leads on to certain dental and gum diseases.

In the natural state, tough gristle and fibrous tissue exercise the gums and teeth and keep them healthy. Raw or semi-digested vegetable matter also has a cleansing action. Soft and sticky tinned pet foods, while completely balanced nutritionally, do not provide these essential actions to keep teeth healthy and thus may contribute to dental disease, especially if no biscuit is fed. However, for most dog owners it is impractical to feed a diet of raw meat and vegetables which would approximate to the diet of a wild carnivore such as the wolf, and so a compromise needs to be reached. Whilst bones do allow good teeth exercise, they also carry certain risks especially if they are small or brittle. Many dogs are admitted for emergency surgery to remove chop bones which have been swallowed and caused major damage to the oesophagus or bowel. Obstructions to the stomach and small intestine may also be caused by these.

The nose

Many people think you can tell how healthy a dog is by looking at its nose. A healthy dog, they say, has a cool wet nose. There may be a little truth in this, but in fact ill dogs can often have cool moist noses, so this isn't a very accurate guide! A healthy nose, however, should be free from blemishes and there should be no cloudy or blood-tinged discharge from either nostril, nor signs of accumulated matter. The skin of the nose should be smooth and even with no red or ulcerated areas.

The tongue and gums

The tongue, gums and lining of the mouth should be moist and salmon-pink in colour. This colour is important because it indicates the health of the respiratory and heart systems. Vets check the colour of mucous membranes during routine clinical examination and also press the gum and measure how long it takes for the pink colour to return after blanching of the gums – this test assesses the circulation and is known as the 'capillary refill time', an important measurement in sick dogs. It should be less than 3 seconds.

Signs of respiratory or cardiovascular failure are

 Bones can be dangerous

In most cases, bones are probably best avoided in pet dogs as they carry several risks. Chop bones, in particular, are notorious for becoming stuck and perforating internal organs. Large knuckle bones are relatively safe but some dogs manage to remove splinters of bone which, if swallowed, could cause damage.

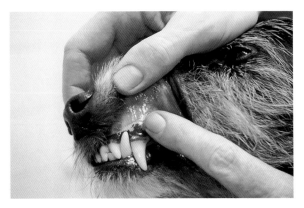

Testing the capillary refill time. The blanched gum re-colours in several seconds in a healthy dog.

bluish-tinged gums, and in dogs suffering from severe haemorrhage (bleeding) or anaemia, whether internal or external, the gums may be pale or even white.

The tongue is important not only for lapping fluids but also as a means of heat loss during panting.

 Muzzles

Whenever a dog is muzzled great care should be taken to ensure that it does not overheat because of inability to pant effectively. See first aid treatment for hyperthermia/heatstroke in Chapter 18.

Caring for Your Dog's Teeth

Dental disease is widespread in dogs and many pets suffer in silence for months or years. Toothache is highly unpleasant for any animal so it is not surprising that dogs with the most severe symptoms become lethargic, irritable and suffer from a poor appetite,

A large variety of hard biscuits and chews are available to encourage chewing and healthy teeth/gums.

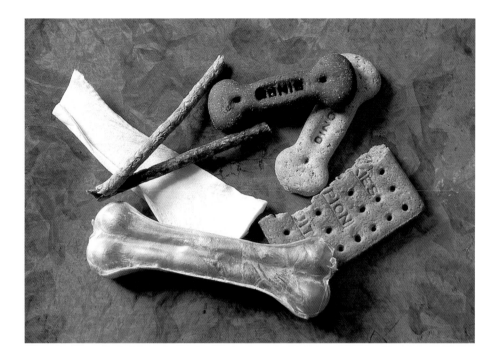

resulting in weight loss. Severe mouth infections including abscesses are frequently seen in dogs and the only indication of how unpleasant these problems can be is the improvement that is noticed in many dogs' demeanour when the mouth is treated. Owners often say that their dog seems years younger after dental treatment for severe disease.

Reducing tooth and gum disease

To some extent, tooth and gum disease is inevitable. It is a natural consequence of ageing and is due to wear and tear as well as the gradual build up of mineral deposits from food. Gradual accumulation of dental plaque and tartar leads to gum inflammation (*gingivitis*), decay and eventual weakening of the supporting structures of the tooth and tooth root disease. Accidents such as cracks in the teeth (e.g. from chewing stones) cause further problems and if infection is severe, dental abscesses may form in the jaw bones. These may show up as firm painful swellings on the side of the face and are highly unpleasant for the dog.

Feeding a balanced diet and including elements within this which are especially good for teeth will help reduce tooth and gum problems (as described in the box), but there is no doubt that the best method of

 Feeding and playing for healthy teeth

All dogs require a balanced diet but consideration should also be given to feeding foods that keep teeth and gums healthy. Dogs receiving only tinned food are likely to develop severe dental disease early in life. This is a particular problem with small breeds, who tend to be fussy eaters and can soon become accustomed to eating nothing but pâté-type foods from tins. All dogs should receive some of the following items:

- Mixer biscuits with tinned foods

- Hard biscuits

- Dog chews

- Fresh fruit or vegetables if they like these, e.g. carrots, turnips, apples, etc.

Pull-type toys are excellent for keeping dogs' teeth clean, especially if they move through the mouth during the tugging game. This acts just like brushing the teeth (see page 32) and is probably more fun for the dog!

Six steps to successful tooth brushing in dogs

1. Start **gradually**. At first, simply get your dog to sit quietly and still while you gently lift up the lip and inspect the teeth. Good basic training pays dividends here. Allow your dog to get thoroughly used to this. Do not brush or use toothpastes at this stage, simply inspect and gently touch the teeth and gums. The session should last no more than 5 minutes and should be repeated for 3 or 4 days before progressing.

2. **Reward** your dog after every session. This is to emphasise quiet and calm behaviour. It is useful to carry out the exercise at roughly the same time and in the same place every day. Most dogs respond well to routines like this.

3. **Use dog toothpaste**. Dogs do not appreciate fluoride toothpaste, which foams and is not designed to be swallowed. Special dog toothpastes in attractive flavours (e.g. chicken) are available. Once your dog has performed well at stage 1, introduce the toothpaste by smearing a little on the gums with your finger. Do not use the brush at this stage. Repeat this process for several days, spending a little more time smearing toothpaste along the lines of the teeth and rubbing gently.

4. Next, introduce the **toothbrush**. Different designs are avilable. Use the one which suits you best. Some owners prefer the small brush that fits over one finger, whereas others use a brush with a handle. Use the brush gently and concentrate on the gum margin areas.Gradually build up to 5 minute sessions each day.

5. Be **regular**. Not everyone manages to brush their dog's teeth every day, but aim for a minimum of three times per week. In the initial stages, when you are getting your dog used to the technique, daily sessions are best.

6. At all times treat the process quietly and calmly. It is not a game but an exercise in obedience and should be approached in this way. Very young children are best not involved. Most dogs quickly become used to toothbrushing and it becomes a normal part of their grooming routine.

---

slowing the process is the method we use on ourselves – tooth brushing. Brushing serves to dislodge tiny particles of food which adhere to the gum margins and act as triggers for inflammation and decay, stopping the process before it becomes established and progressive.

Veterinary Diagnosis and Treatment

Dental conditions

Some assessment of a dog's teeth can be made in the awake animal but quite often detailed examination has to wait until a general anaesthetic can be given. In most cases, treatment will be carried out at the same time. Dental X-rays may be necessary to fully assess tooth root problems and decide on the best line of treatment.

Most dental treatments in dogs take the form of 'descaling and polishing' and extractions. Whilst cosmetic effects are important in human dentistry, in dogs the emphasis is on relieving pain and discomfort and in preventing future problems. Descaling is the removal of accumulated tartar (the mineral deposits from food which cause gum disease and, eventually, tooth damage). This is carried out by hand instrument or, more often, with the aid of an ultrasonic descaler. Polishing smooths the tooth surface after descaling and helps prevent adherence of minute food particles to the tooth face.

Extractions are carried out when the tooth cannot be saved or when the presence of the tooth is causing problems for other reasons, e.g. retained primary teeth, or following jaw fractures. More complex procedures are also carried out when they would benefit the dog concerned and help improve its oral health.

Nose conditions

In examination of nasal passage problems X-rays are frequently used. Biopsies may be taken and in some

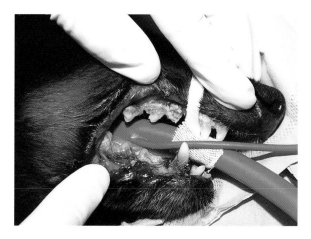

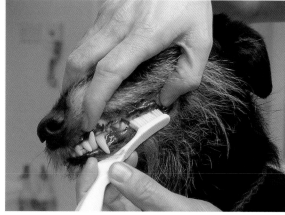

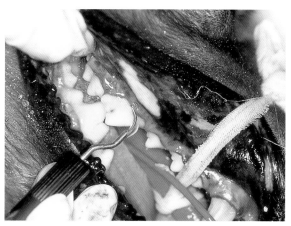

ABOVE *Excessive tartar build up in an 11-year-old dog.*

ABOVE RIGHT *Brushing the teeth and gum margins. Specially designed toothbrushes help.*

BELOW RIGHT *Ultrasonic removal of accumulated tartar is followed by polishing of the tooth enamel to leave a smooth surface.*

conditions, such as suspected fungal infections, blood tests are indicated. Conditions affecting the skin of the nose may also be biopsied, and may be related to skin problems elsewhere.

The throat area

Proper examination of the throat almost always requires a general anaesthetic as only a very limited amount can be seen in the awake animal. X-rays and endoscopy may be used in addition.

Costs and prognosis in mouth and nose diseases

Dentistry

The final cost of any course of dental treatment depends on the severity of the problem. There is no doubt that many dogs require extensive treatment to make their mouths healthy again. The most expensive course of treatment could involve:

1. Multiple tooth extractions

2. Antibiotics and painkillers before and after surgery

3. Dental X-rays

4. In old dogs, blood tests before the anaesthetic and intravenous fluids (a 'drip') during and after surgery

5. Hospitalisation overnight

Such comprehensive treatment would be relatively expensive, but would be neccesary for thorough treatment of a severely affected mouth.

Routine scaling and polishing for mild tartar accumulation would be far less costly and several extractions would be somewhere between the two costs. Throughout any dog's life, it is likely that routine

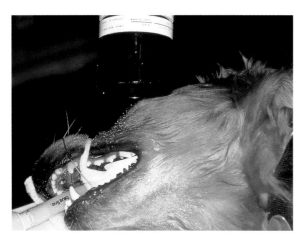

Dental X-ray being taken in an anaesthetised dog.

scaling and polishing may need to be repeated several times – unless the owners are extremely efficient at brushing their dog's teeth. Good home brushing can therefore save money that would otherwise need to be spent on dental treatment.

Precautionary blood tests are usually advised for all older animals since hidden kidney problems, especially, can complicate anaesthesia and surgery in these patients. Knowing about them in advance allows the vet to take action to limit the effects of anaesthesia and surgery. These do also add to the overall cost.

Nasal diseases

Nasal diseases are quite varied in nature. Anaesthetic and X-ray costs are likely to be involved at some stage in many cases, and if surgery is required then this would increase fees substantially. Nasal tumours are encountered in dogs and these have a poor outlook, although the symptoms can be alleviated for some time while quality of life remains good.

Throat diseases

These are fairly rare. Simple infections or inflammations may occur and are usually treated easily and quickly. Sometimes, objects get stuck and may need anaesthesia or surgery for removal, and several diseases exist which lead to abnormal swallowing.

Cysts can arise in the throat area, and certain tumours may also show here. The condition of laryngeal paralysis, seen typically in older medium to large breed dogs, is discussed on page 137.

Commonest Mouth and Nose Problems in Dogs

DENTAL AND GUM PROBLEMS

CAUSE A certain amount of dental disease arises inevitably as animals grow older. It is caused by accumulation of food particles, inflammation and infection. Poor diet plays a part, especially lack of hard or fibrous foods in smaller breed dogs that are fussy eaters.

Certain breeds are prone to teeth crowding and dental disease is then more likely where the teeth lie against or overlap each other. Trauma (e.g. tooth damage from stone chewing, road traffic accidents) can also cause tooth injury.

Gingivitis (inflammation of the gums) and stomatitis (inflammation of the mouth) can be caused by conditions other than dental disease. The commonest one is kidney insufficiency and chronic renal failure (see Chapter 8).

Sometimes, gum tissue proliferates and thickens, resembling a tumour or epulis (see under Cancer of the jaw, mouth and throat area). This can become very extensive, almost burying the teeth, and may require surgery to reduce the overgrown gum, but it is not malignant and is more correctly termed gingival (gum) hyperplasia (thickening).

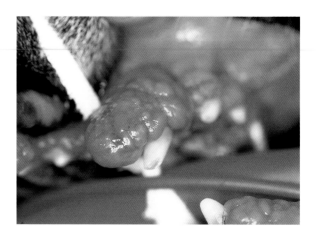

Epulis – a benign growth of the gum which is quite common in certain breeds. Bleeding may occur if the dog accidentally bites on it.

First aid and nursing for tooth loss and sore mouth

Complete loss of an intact tooth is fairly unusual in dogs, but if this were to occur the tooth should be placed in milk and the dog taken to the vet as soon as possible. It may sometimes be possible to replace the tooth. In most cases, however, the loss of the tooth will be accepted and will cause the dog no problems at all.

For dogs with sore mouths before or after dental treatment, softer food should be given. Tinned dog food can be completely liquidised if extra water is added. Specially prepared and highly palatable liquid or soft diets are also available from the veterinary surgery. These diets may encourage dogs with tender mouths to eat and avoids the need to use a human food blender for dog food, which is not advisable.

Homoeopathic treatment with Arnica is often very helpful before and after dental treatment. Dosages and further information are given in Chapter 18.

If other medication is to be given (such as antibiotics and painkillers), tablets can often be ground up and mixed into liquidised or soft food. This avoids handling a sore mouth or struggling with the dog to try to get it to take the whole tablet. When using this technique, give the tablets in a small amount of food, while the dog is still hungry, and then give the rest of the food afterwards. If you mix the tablet into the whole quantity of food, some of it may be left!

SYMPTOMS These can range from no obvious symptoms to severe facial swelling from a dental abscess. Dogs may be careful about eating or may yelp occasionally when chewing on food. There may be bad breath (halitosis) or excess salivation. The dog may simply be subdued and miserable if there is severe pain, e.g. from major infection or a recently fractured tooth.

Dental problems are often picked up during routine examination before the annual booster vaccinations. It is likely that many dogs 'suffer in silence' from grumbling dental disease. Relief in these cases is often apparent after suitable treatment.

DIAGNOSIS This is based on visual examination, examination under anaesthetic and dental X-rays, when needed.

TREATMENT The common treatment involves descaling and polishing healthy teeth and extracting diseased ones. More sophisticated treatment may be suggested for specific problems. Antibiotics and painkillers may be given for gingivitis and pain before and after surgery.

PREVENTION Regular brushing as described on page 32 is the key to preventing dental disease, together with attention to the diet. Various toothpastes,

brushes and mouthwashes are available for dogs. Tugging games also help to naturally clean the teeth.

OUTLOOK Good. Dogs can cope well with few or even no teeth. Obviously, it is best that as many teeth as possible are kept healthy and functional however. Sometimes teeth that have been completely and cleanly dislodged from the tooth socket can be saved and replaced with appropriate emergency dental surgery.

NASAL DISCHARGE/SNEEZING

CAUSE Many different problems can cause a nasal discharge. The more common ones include fungal infections, allergic or infective conditions and nasal tumours. Foreign bodies such as grass awns can become trapped in the nasal passages, causing infection and discharge. If the symptoms start after your dog has been exercised amongst tall grass, be sure to tell your vet. Occasionally, severe dental infections cause a one-sided nasal discharge of cloudy material.

Dogs with longer noses are more prone to nasal diseases than short-nosed dogs.

'Rhinitis' is the term used to describe inflammation in the nose area, from any of the above causes.

SYMPTOMS The discharge can vary from clear, cloudy to bloody depending on the cause. Other symptoms may include sneezing/snorting, gagging and excessive mouth breathing. One or both nostrils may be affected. Note that as many dogs tend to lick away discharges, careful observation can be required to notice them.

DIAGNOSIS X-rays are usually employed and examination using an illuminated scope/endoscope may be carried out. Blood tests and biopsies are also helpful in many cases to arrive at a final diagnosis.

TREATMENT Some nasal conditions can be difficult or impossible to treat. Fungal infections and nasal foreign bodies can usually be cured but nasal tumours and chronic inflammatory disorders carry a poorer outlook. As access to radiotherapy improves for pet owners, nasal tumours may be able to be slowed down in their growth rate.

OUTLOOK Poor for nasal tumours.

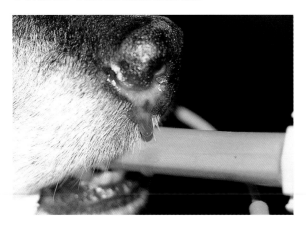

Nasal discharge in an 8-year-old dog. A grass awn was removed from the nostril but tumours often produce similar symptoms.

JAW FRACTURE/DISLOCATION

CAUSE Severe trauma, usually from a road traffic accident.

SYMPTOMS Pain, swelling, inability to close the jaw. The external appearance of the jaw (upper or lower) may be abnormal. Injuries to the hard palate may also be present and tooth loss may have occurred.

DIAGNOSIS X-rays are likely, requiring an anaesthetic.

TREATMENT Treatment is usually surgical and may make use of acrylic splints or external fixation devices. During this time, liquidised or very soft food may need to be fed.

OUTLOOK Generally good with correct treatment; jaw fractures tend to heal well as infection is limited by the cleansing and antibacterial properties of saliva.

OVER- OR UNDERSHOT JAW

CAUSE These are congenital problems which may be detected in puppies or young dogs.

SYMPTOMS Overshot jaw is where the upper jaw is longer than the lower; undershot jaw is when the lower jaw is the longer. Most dogs have no symptoms.

DIAGNOSIS This is easy as the condition is immediately obvious. Checking jaw alignment is one of the checks which should be carried out in puppies.

TREATMENT None is necessary unless the incisor teeth cause problems by rubbing on the tissues next to them (the hard palate or the area behind the lower incisor teeth). It is a cosmetic problem and most dogs live a perfectly normal life. It is considered a fault in show dogs however.

OUTLOOK Good.

CANCER OF THE JAW, MOUTH AND THROAT AREA

CAUSE The cause of most cancers remains obscure; they arise sporadically in all breeds and may affect the gums, lining of the mouth, jaw bones and tonsils, as well as the lymph glands of the throat area. Nasal tumours are also seen and are a fairly common cause of nasal discharge in the dog.

SYMPTOMS A visible growth may be seen (e.g. on the gums), or else symptoms of mouth pain or swallowing disorders may be seen, e.g. drooling blood-tinged saliva, weight loss, bad breath (halitosis).

A harmless gum growth called an epulis (see page 34) is encountered quite frequently, especially in Boxer dogs. There are often removed if large, because they may bleed and interfere with chewing, but they are not malignant cancers.

DIAGNOSIS These problems nearly always require a general anaesthetic, X-rays and biopsy of tissue to reach a firm diagnosis. X-rays of other parts of the body (e.g. lungs) may be required to check for tumour spread as, unfortunately, many tumours in this area are malignant and spread very quickly. Lymph gland tumours may be first picked up in the throat area but then, after tests, are found to involve other areas of the body.

TREATMENT Treatment, other than pain relief, may not be feasible for cancers which have spread. For those which have not spread and are confined to the jaw area, removal of portions of the jaw bone may be possible. Although major surgery, and not to be undertaken lightly, such operations can be very successful in dogs and patients normally adapt quickly to the loss of part of the jaw area and go on to lead a good quality of life.

Certain tumours are amenable to chemotherapy or radiation therapy, which can prolong life.

OUTLOOK Depends very much on the tumour type and whether spread has occurred. Some tumours are more sensitive to treatment than others. The best prognosis is with those that can be completely removed surgically.

OTHER SWELLINGS/FOREIGN BODIES

CAUSE Swellings around the mouth, nose and throat area are not always tumours. They may be caused by abscesses, cysts (containing saliva from a leaking salivary gland or duct) or foreign bodies. Rarer immune system problems can cause ulceration around the nose and lips.

SYMPTOMS Bones/sticks may get stuck across the roof of the mouth, where they become firmly wedged between the upper teeth. The discomfort can cause great agitation in affected dogs, who will paw frantically at the mouth area and drool saliva. In contrast to objects obstructing the airway, respiratory distress is not seen: the dogs can breathe adequately, but they have intense discomfort in and around the mouth. It is worth making an attempt to dislodge these yourself (taking care not to get bitten) but safe removal, together with checking for other damage, may require a general anaesthetic at the veterinary surgery.

DIAGNOSIS Tests to distinguish abscesses, cysts and other causes of swellings may be required. X-rays, ultrasound, biopsies and exploratory surgery are all used, depending on the precise condition.

TREATMENT Salivary cysts usually require surgery; abscesses may require surgery to establish drainage, followed by antibiotics. Foreign bodies are removed. Sometimes, small sharp objects can 'track' through tissues, causing excessive inflammation and fibrosis, and be extremely difficult to find and remove. More than one surgical procedure may be required as, until the offending object is found, continued swelling and infection is likely. This can persist for many months.

OUTLOOK Good for salivary cysts, removed foreign bodies and tumours that have been excised completely before spread. Partial or complete obstruction

 Obstruction of airway

Any foreign body obstructing the airway is a life-threatening emergency. See Chapter 18 for how to deal with this serious problem in a first aid situation. Common objects found stuck are bones, rubber balls/toys, sticks and occasionally stones.

This dog has a salivary cyst – a large pouch-like swelling full of leaked saliva. Treatment by surgery proved successful.

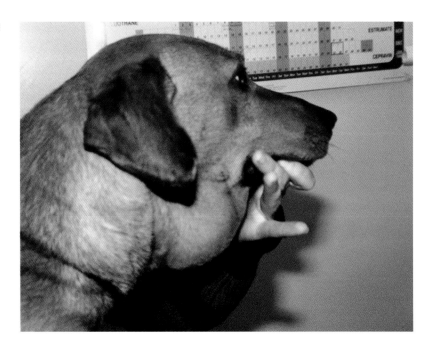

of the respiratory system caused by a foreign body requires very prompt removal of the object if the dog's life is to be saved.

STENOTIC NARES (NARROW NOSTRILS)

CAUSE This is a problem found in certain breeds where the nostril opening (nares) is too narrow (stenotic), producing interference with breathing. It is often found in conjunction with other breathing/respiratory problems such as laryngeal paralysis and narrowing of the trachea (see pages 137 and 133) and is commonest in short-nosed dogs such as Boxers, Bulldogs and certain other breeds such as Pekinese.

SYMPTOMS The narrowed nostril opening results in air turbulence and extra effort in breathing as well as noisy breathing.

DIAGNOSIS This is obvious from examination of the nostrils and watching the animal breathe; the nostrils may become easily blocked with mucus. Tests to discover whether any of the related conditions are also present may be required since these dogs often have several abnormalities.

TREATMENT Surgery to improve the anatomy of the nostril may be required, and treatment of other related problems at the soft palate, in the larynx and in the trachea may also be neccesary as it is often a combination of problems that leads to the overall condition.

OUTLOOK Good, if surgery is successful and the related conditions are also treated. There is usually considerable improvement in breathing after correction of these anatomical problems.

CHAPTER 3

The Eye

Common symptoms of eye disease
• Reddened eye • Discharge from eye
• Painful blinking • Eye held closed • Poor vision
• Swelling around eye

Structure and Function

The eye and its structure is one of the wonders of nature. Dogs see differently from human beings – their quality of colour vision, for example, is not the same and they are relatively short-sighted. In perceiving the world around them dogs also make use of their highly developed senses of smell and hearing, which are far superior to the same senses in people. Nevertheless, vision remains a vital function and a dog that is blind in both eyes leads a difficult and dangerous life. Loss of hearing can be coped with more easily than complete loss of vision.

The eye exists to capture and focus light waves and then project these onto a 'screen' – the retina – at the back of the eye, where the light energy is transferred into nerve impulses which are relayed to the brain, thus creating the perception of vision. Anything which disturbs any part of this process therefore threatens sight. Dogs adapt well to gradual deteriorations in the quality of vision, as occurs during the normal ageing process for example, and they can also cope well if one eye has to be removed due to disease or injury, but bilateral (both sides) blindness is a daunting prospect for both dog and owner.

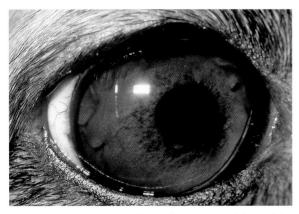

The normal dog eye. Note the perfect position of the eyelids, the bright, clear cornea and lack of any eye discharges. The third eyelid is on the right hand side.

Parts of the eye

Eyelids

The eyelids have a vital role to play. Blinking is the eye's main defence mechanism and serves to prevent or limit injury to the senstive structures of the eye. The blink reflex is therefore a very important response. It is easily tested (see box on page 42) and checking the blink reflex is an important part of any neurological (brain or nerve) examination. A poor or

The structure of the eye (left eye)

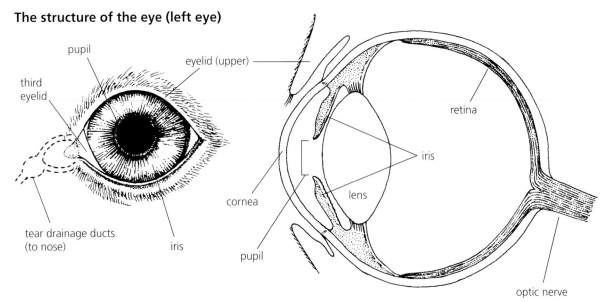

Different parts of the eye when viewed straight on and in cross-section.

Eye injuries

Due to the great sensitivity and importance of the eye, any condition affecting it must be taken seriously and veterinary advice sought promptly. Time can be of the essence, since the eye has only a limited ability to withstand inflammatory conditions or anything which causes a change of pressure within the eyeball itself. Most eye injuries are therefore classed as emergencies.

absent blink reflex can indicate damage to the nervous system, as well as being dangerous for the eye concerned. Certain breeds (e.g. Pekinese) do not blink well, making them prone to diseases of the eye associated with drying-out of the eye surfaces.

Blinking also serves to spread the tear film across the eye surface. Tears are crucial to the health of the eye. They provide lubrication and constant cleansing of the eye surface and they also contain natural substances which deter bacteria. Defects in tear production (especially too few tears) cause problems and eye disease in many dogs as will be described later.

In addition to the upper and lower eyelids, dogs have an additional eyelid known as the third eyelid, also called the nictitating membrane. Only the corner of this structure is visible in the normal eye. In order to examine it, the vet gently presses on the eyeball while everting (turning out) the lower eyelid. The third eyelid is important because it can become inflamed, torn or 'foreign bodies' (e.g. grass seed) may become trapped behind it. Its normal function is in protecting and lubricating the eye: it produces part of the tear film and helps disperse this across the surface of the eye with blinking.

Eyelashes

Eyelashes are very sensitive hairs located on the edges of the eyelids.They serve a protective function and when anything touches them, a blink response is stimulated. Eyelashes occasionally cause problems if they grow in the wrong place or direction. If this happens, they can irritate the eye surface, causing a profuse watery discharge or even an eye ulcer (see pages 49 and 53).

Conjunctiva

The conjunctiva is the thin, almost transparent protective covering of the eye. It lines the eyelids and the eye surface itself and contains minute blood vessels. During inflammation, these blood vessels enlarge in size and number, causing the characteristic reddness of conjunctivitis.

Cornea

The cornea is the clear 'window' of the eye against which the eyelids close. It is a sensitive structure and, because it is in contact with the environment, it occasionally suffers injury, such as ulcers or damage from objects entering the eye. Corneal problems are fairly common in dogs and are discussed later.

Iris

The iris is the structure which gives eyes their colour, although some dogs have a non-pigmented iris. There is no loss of vision in these 'wall' eyes, nor are there any problems when different eyes have different-coloured irises, as occasionally happens in some breeds.

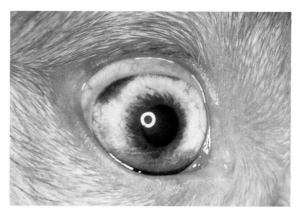

Eye of a Collie dog showing a blue iris. Vision is normal.

The iris is capable of opening and closing in a circular fashion to control the amount of light entering the eye via the pupil.

Pupil

The pupil is the space through which light enters the eye on its way to the 'screen' (retina) at the back of the eye. The size of the pupil can be adjusted to accommodate for bright or dim light, very much like the way the diaphragm of a camera operates to control the exposure under different lighting conditions. Assessment of pupil size is an important part of eye examination and is also studied closely during neurological tests on dogs.

The pupils react in a predictable way to changes in light intensity: pupils are small in bright light (e.g. outside on a sunny day) and large in dim light (e.g. darkness). When a dog moves from bright to dim light or vice versa the size of the pupil changes over the course of a few seconds. This is an important reflex called the pupillary light reflex and it can be affected both by disorders of the eye and disorders of the central nervous system (brain and spinal cord and associated nerves).

Abnormal pupils would be:

- Pupils that are large (dilated) in bright light

- Pupils that are small (constricted) in dim light

 ## Can my dog see properly?

Many owners become aware of failing sight in elderly dogs. The signs may be subtle at first but can include occasionally walking into objects, misjudging distances and failing to see their owner unless he or she moves or makes a signal. Although this deterioration cannot be reversed, most dogs compensate well providing their owners make allowances for the problem. For example, it is best not to make sudden, major changes to the arrangement of furniture in the house if you have an old dog with poor vision – it will most probably be quite disorientating for them.

An easy way to test vision is to set up a small obstacle course and check to see if your dog can negotiate it in normal and subdued lighting conditions. When vets carry out this test, they often blindfold one eye to check the vision on each side separately. Dropping balls of cotton wool near your dog and checking to see if he follows them with his head and eyes is also useful. Pay attention to his behaviour out of doors: if you look carefully, you can often detect poor vision by the way your dog reacts to the environment.

Blink reflex

This is also called the menace response and is an important neurological test, as well as a test of vision. The test is simply carried out by making a (careful) threatening gesture towards the eye with your hand. Try to avoid creating air currents. The normal response is a blink from the eye. The movement does not need to be particularly fast. Take care not to hit your dog's face!

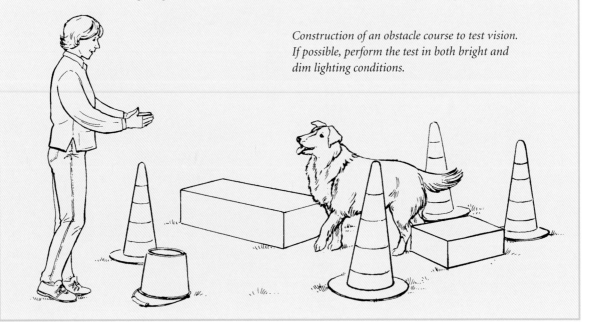

Construction of an obstacle course to test vision. If possible, perform the test in both bright and dim lighting conditions.

- Pupils that fail to change (accommodate) when the light intensity changes

- Right and left pupils that are of different sizes.

In order to conduct a full examination of the internal structures of the eye, it is sometimes necessary for the veterinary surgeon to insert drops into the eye which cause the pupil to dilate. This allows easy and clear examination of the back of the eye through a wide pupil. It takes some time for the effects of these drops to wear off and during this period, the pupils will be of unequal size (unless drops were put in both eyes at the same time).

Lens

The lens lies immediately behind the pupil. Its job is to focus light rays and allow the animal to adjust its eyesight in order to see near or far objects. The lens is a transparent structure and cannot normally be seen. Cataract (see page 55) is an eye condition in which the lens becomes opaque. Vision is affected by cataract because light does not pass through an opaque structure as well as through a transparent one.

Retina

The retina lines the inner surface of the back of the eye. It is the 'screen' on which images are made by light after it has entered the eye and been focussed by the lens. Nerve cells associated with the retina then convert these images into eletrical signals which are relayed to the brain in the optic nerve. The brain then 'decodes' these signals and this results in the animal being aware of visual images.

Part of the back of the eye is covered by a layer of very reflective cells called the tapetum. This structure helps to concentrate light within the eye and improves the efficiency of the eye. In animals the tapetum is often highly coloured. At night, if light enters the eye (e.g. headlights from a car, a torch) then this bright reflection can often be seen. The colour varies enormously. Often, the bright tapetal reflection of roadside nocturnal animals, such as foxes, can be seen while driving through the countryside at night.

Fluids – the 'humours' of the eye

The roughly spherical shape of the eye is maintained by fluids (called humours) located in the front (behind the cornea) and back (behind the lens) compartments of the eye. The production and distribution of these fluids is important. Too much, and the pressure in the eye raises, threatening all the sensitive structures (this happens in glaucoma); too little fluid pressure, and the eye ceases to function well as a processor of light.

 ## Does my dog have cataracts?

Many owners of older dogs think their pet has developed cataracts because they notice that the lens of the eye has taken on a greyish bluish colour at its centre. Any such changes in the eye should always be checked out by the vet but, in fact, in the vast majority of cases the condition is not cataract – it is a much less serious condition called nuclear sclerosis, which is considered part of the normal ageing process in dogs. A simple test in the veterinary surgery can confirm this. No treatment is needed for nuclear sclerosis and vision is not significantly impaired. Cataract is discussed later.

RIGHT *Old dogs often have a bluish or opaque lens. A simple test performed by the vet can rule out cataract.*

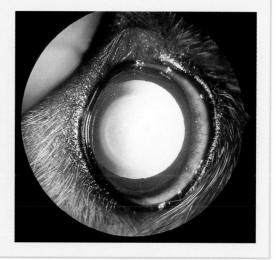

Caring for Your Dog's Eyes

The healthy eye requires no routine care from the dog owner apart from regular checking for signs of injury or disease. Nature has provided cleansing and protective mechanisms to keep the eye functioning normally: the eyelids, blinking and the production of tears are very efficient at keeping the eye healthy. Tears are much more than the fluids we associate with grief and hay fever. They are complex substances, designed to lubricate and protect the eye and to provide antibacterial actions. There is therefore no need to use eye wipes or drops in the healthy eye – it simply doesn't require them.

Accumulation of matter in eyes

Certain breeds (e.g. Yorkshire Terriers) are prone to accumulation of dried material at the corners of the eye. This tends to mat up the hair and, if allowed to accumulate, it can become very troublesome to remove, causing dermatitis on the surrounding skin, and maybe even requiring sedation or an anesthetic for adequate treatment. If you have a dog like this, first get your vet to check out the problem. If it is simply matter accumulation, then this should be wiped away once or twice daily. The best method is to use sterile saline, available from your veterinary surgery or chemist, soaked into a disposable swab or cotton wool. When removing the material, always wipe *away* from the eye rather than towards it.

Dogs with deep set eyes (e.g. Dobermans) often have a small blob of mucus present in the corner of the eye. Again, have your vet check this out. It is usually quite harmless and no action need be taken other than occasionally careful wiping *away* of excessive amounts.

Application of eye drops/ointments

If drops or ointment are prescribed, make sure you follow the instructions carefully. Many drops need to be kept in the fridge once opened. It is usually easier – especially at first – if you ask someone to steady your dog's head to allow you to have both hands free while applying drops or ointment.

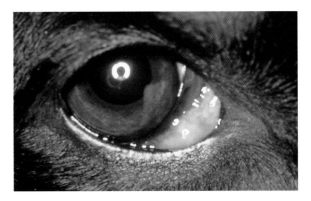

Dobermans often have blobs of mucus which collect in the corners of both eyes. No treatment is needed.

Your vet or nurse will probably have demonstrated the process to you in the clinic. Most products are easiest to apply by slightly everting the lower eyelid and then placing the medication here. It will rapidly spread over the eye with blinking. Take care not to let the nozzle of the tube contact your dog's eye. An easy way to apply ointment is to place some on your finger (it is best to wear gloves) and smear in onto the eyelid this way.

 Eye medication

Only ever apply eye drops or medications supplied or recommended by your vet. Even then, if you suspect the eye has reacted badly to them, contact the surgery or clinic for advice.

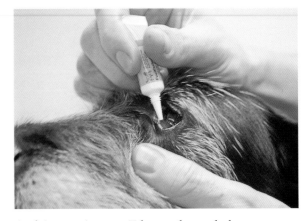

Applying eye ointment. Take care the nozzle does not contact the eye surface.

Thick ointments can be made easier to apply by placing them in a cup of warm water before using them (make sure the cap is on tightly and keep the nozzle of the tube out of the water). This makes them more liquid and they disperse over the eye more easily. Check with your vet to ensure you can do this with the product supplied. If your dog objects to cold eyedrops, warm the bottle between your hands for a few minutes before application.

Ensure that all medication is applied at the correct frequency. Some conditions require very frequent application, and this may have to be continued overnight, at least in the early stages.

Veterinary Diagnosis and Treatment

The most valuable tool in examining the dog eye is the trained *human* eye of your vet. Many eye conditions can be diagnosed readily by the naked human eye, perhaps aided by a small pen torch. Vets often also use an ophthalmoscope, an illuminated instrument which allows all structures in the eye to be examined closely. It may be necessary to darken the room while the ophthalmoscope is in use, and sometimes the pupils will be artificially dilated (using drops) to allow the observer to see clearly the back of the eye and the retina.

A number of other tests may also be carried out. As these are simple, painless and provide quick results, they may be done in the consulting room while the owner is present.

Fluorescent dye tests

Vets often use harmless coloured dyes to assess the clear 'front window' of the eye, the cornea. Dyes are required because scratches and even ulcers on the cornea can be very difficult to detect, but if there is any damage, the dye particles will adhere to the area and will show up as a bright patch (usually green) on the eye surface. The dye is usually applied from impregnated paper strips or from a small bottle of solution.

Another reason for applying dye to the eye is to check that the naso-lacrimal duct is not blocked. This duct is a fine tube which runs from the corner of the eye to the nose region. Its purpose is to drain away excess tears, which are eventually swallowed. Blockage of the duct can result in overflow of tears down the face or other problems. By placing coloured dye into the eye, and then waiting 5 to 10 minutes, the vet can then look carefully at the dog's nostril area. If the duct is working properly, the nostrils should be greenish because the dye has been washed down the duct with the tears in the normal fashion. If no dye appears then either the duct is blocked or the dog has been licking his nose and removing the dye! Careful observation is required.

If you see green dye at the nostrils after your dog's eye has been checked, it is therefore nothing to worry about. It shows that the naso-lacrimal duct is working normally.

Measuring tear production

Your dog's ability to produce tears may need to be checked because poor tear production is a common cause of recurrent eye problems. This test involves another type of paper strip. This one is left in the eye for a period of time. Tears move up the dry paper strip by capillary action and draw a dye marker with them as they go. At the end of the alloted time, the length of the dye on the strip (or the length of wetted strip) is measured against an indicator ruler to see if tear production is within the normal range.

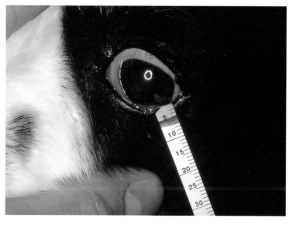

The Schirmer tear test is a painless way of measuring tear production. Tears wick up the paper strip and impregnated dye produces a reading.

Specialised tests

If your dog is referred for specialised diagnosis and treatment, veterinary ophthalmologists may use additional instruments to perform further tests on the eyes, e.g. measuring the fluid pressure within the eyeball or using special viewing devices to gain highly magnified images of certain parts of the eye.

Cost and prognosis in eye diseases

Any condition requiring specialised referral and treatment such as surgery will be relatively expensive. However this has to be weighed up against the benefits of preserving sight, and any alternative treatments that may be cheaper in the short term but not so effective in the longer term. Since eye diseases are so important to a dog's quality of life, such matters are discussed with the vet for each individual case.

Treatment for poor tear production (a common problem often referred to as 'dry eye' – see page 51) can be very effective but the cost of the best medication is currently quite high. However, once dogs show an improvement sometimes the frequency of application of the treatment can be reduced, saving money. Unfortunately the condition cannot be cured completely and treatment is likely to be on-going for the rest of the dog's life. Surgery is occasionally possible for this problem and avoids the need for on-going application of drops, but is not the favoured course of action for many vets.

Simple eye infections and irritations normally respond very quickly to appropriate treatment. These conditions are much less expensive to treat and are usually completely cured within 5–10 days.

Commonest Eye Problems in Dogs

Certain basic symptoms appear commonly in the eyes in response to injury or disease. These are:

• **Reddness**: the whole or parts of the eyes may be reddened. This is most noticeable on the white part of the eye (the sclera), on the cornea or in the lining of the eyelids, but reddness can also be present in other locations such as the iris and in the fluid-filled chamber in the front of the eye. Reddness indicates inflammation or haemorrhage (bleeding).

• **Eye discharge**: this may be watery, yellowish (often indicating infection) or red-tinged (indicating inflammation or bleeding).

• **Difficulty blinking or eyelid spasms**: severe eyelid spasms, usually caused by pain, can make the eye very difficult to examine.

• **Pain**: eye conditions often cause pain and some, such as iritis, are very painful indeed. Dogs suffering from painful eye disease are often subdued, reluctant to eat and may be irritable.

These symptoms alone are not specific for any one eye problem; in fact, many eye conditions have quite similar symptoms – this is why veterinary attention needs to be sought promptly. For example, a red eye can be caused by something relatively straightforward, such as conjunctivitis or mild bruising, but it can also be a symptom of much more serious, sight-threatening conditions such as glaucoma or iritis.

Eye conditions affecting the various parts of the eye are summarised below.

EYE INJURIES – GENERAL

CAUSE These include blunt trauma (e.g. road traffic accidents, accidental injuries with bats or balls) and sharp trauma (e.g. penetrating injuries). Of the two, blunt injuries are usually the more serious in that they more often cause damage that threatens sight. Although sharp penetrating injuries may sound more serious, they tend to cause localised damage which may be more amenable to healing or repair.

Prolapse (forwards displacement) of the eyeball can occur in squash-faced breeds (especially Pekinese). These dogs should not be picked up or held by the scruff as this can cause the eyeball to prolapse if the dog struggles. If these dogs are involved in a dog fight, eyeball prolapse may occur for the same reason.

SYMPTOMS Pain, eyelid closure, reddening of the eye, swelling.

Basic first aid for eye injuries

All eye problems should be seen by a veterinary surgeon. The eye is a sensitive organ and injury is always painful. An eye may not be able to sustain severe trauma or disease and the result could be blindness or necessity for removal of the eye.

First aid in the following situations can help limit damage. In addition, several homoeopathic remedies appropriate for general eye injuries are mentioned in Chapter 18. In all cases veterinary help should be sought as soon as possible.

Object in the eye

Have an assistant steady the dog's head firmly. Reassure the dog and use a muzzle or tie the nose if necessary, for safety. With one hand, part the eyelids and use the fingers of the other hand to remove the object, if this can be done easily. Objects in the corner of the eye may be easier to remove if wiped out using a moistened piece of cotton or gauze. If you cannot remove the object, ensure the dog doesn't rub its face or paw the eye while you seek veterinary help.

Severe injury to the eye, e.g. hit by stone or ball

If possible cover the eye with a sterile or clean pad moistened with saline. Hold this across the eye while transporting the dog to the clinic or hospital.

Prolapse of the eyeball

This alarming condition can occur in breeds such as the Pekinese, which have large, protruding eyes. As a result of injury or accident the eye displaces forwards out of the face and the eyelids partly close behind it. Usually this occurs after a fight with a larger dog but it can also occur if a Pekinese is lifted up by the scruff. Speed is of the essence. Very few owners would feel confident about parting the eyelids and gently pushing the eyeball back into its normal position using a moistened pad of gauze, but this is the ideal form of first aid treatment and should be attempted if you feel able to. Otherwise, the eye should be covered and kept moist during transportation.

Liquid, dust or fine material in the eye

Flush the eye repeatedly with large amounts of saline or water. Use of a syringe or eye dropper makes this easy.

Swollen eyelids, bites or stings around the eye

Bathe the eyelids in cool saline or water. Do not allow the dog to paw or rub the face.

DIAGNOSIS The severity of the damage must be assessed – this may require sedation. It is helpful to provide the vet with clear details of how the injury occurred.

TREATMENT A wide variety of injuries is possible, from superficial scrapes and bruises to dislocation of the lens and complete rupture of the eye. Treatment will be geared towards preserving vision whenever possible.

OUTLOOK This very much depends on the severity of the injury and the speed with which veterinary attention is sought. Prompt treatment or referral to a specialist may be able to save eyes that would otherwise be lost.

EYELID INJURIES, STINGS AND FOREIGN BODIES

CAUSE Injuries to the eyelids can be caused by sharp undergrowth, by running into fences or as a result of fights. The third eyelid may also be affected – this is also the place where grass seeds or other small foreign bodies get lodged.

SYMPTOMS Usually the injury is obvious, although if only the third eyelid is affected the problem may not be noticeable until the third eyelid itself is exposed. Large injuries affecting the eyelid margins are the most serious, but all eye damage in this area should be considered an emergency.

Foreign bodies may show as a profuse eye discharge, pain and reluctance to open the eyelids which may be very swollen and red. Obviously, there is the risk of damage to the eye itself here with any penetrating foreign body.

Stings on the eyelids are not very common but if they occur, the eyelids may swell up severely and the situation could resemble that described for foreign bodies above.

DIAGNOSIS Careful examination is carried out by the vet, often using local anaesthetic drops to relieve pain in the eye and permit proper assessment of the damaged areas.

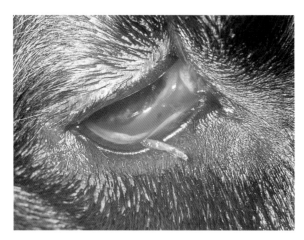

A grass seed lodged in the eye is a painful and distressing condition. Prompt removal is important and will often require an anaesthetic or sedative.

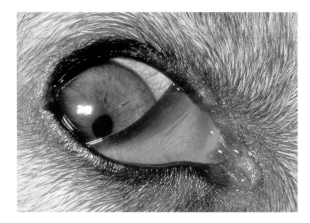

This dog showed intense eye pain after digging in the garden. Careful examination shows a tiny fragment of rose thorn embedded in the cornea.

TREATMENT Eyelid injuries are sutured; this is especially important when the eyelid margin has been disrupted because it must be repositioned extremely carefully to allow for normal blinking.

Foreign bodies are removed, often under sedation or anaesthesia, and stings are treated with anti-inflammatory drops and possibly injections/tablets.

Antibiotic treatment and painkillers are often provided for eye injuries. The dog may have to wear a protective lampshade-like shield (known as an Elizabethan collar) for a few days after treatment to prevent interference with the damaged areas.

OUTLOOK If treated promptly, most of these conditions have a good outlook but some scarring of the eyelid or the eye itself may remain after healing.

CONJUNCTIVITIS

CAUSE Conjunctivitis means inflammation of the delicate transparent membrane which lines the eyelids and covers the eye. Many things can cause the conjunctiva to become inflamed. Common causes of conjunctivitis are:

• Allergies

• Irritation, e.g. dust, smoke

• Foreign bodies, e.g. grass seeds

• Wrongly directed hairs on the eyelids or eyelashes

• Poor tear production

• Infections.

SYMPTOMS The commonest symptom is a reddened eye and there may also be an eye discharge and signs of pain/irritation.

DIAGNOSIS Examination of the eye should help to establish the cause of the conjunctivitis. Simple tests (see page 45) may be performed, and sometimes swabs are taken if infection is thought to be present.

TREATMENT This usually involves drops or ointments of some description. The precise ingredients

The reddened eye

Several other conditions, some of them more serious than conjunctivitis, can also cause a reddened eye, so whenever your dog has this symptom do not delay seeking advice.

depend on the cause (which is why you should never use drops that have been prescribed for a previous disease or for another dog).

OUTLOOK Most cases of conjunctivitis respond well to treatment however those caused by allergies may require lengthy or even, in a few cases, permanent treatment using drops or ointments.

ENTROPION AND ECTROPION

CAUSE These two problems represent abnormal eyelids. In entropion, the eyelids are inward-turning and in ectropion they are outward-turning. Entropion is the commoner of the two. They are hereditary conditions although sometimes similar problems can be caused when the eyelids are damaged and heal with a major scar, which distorts their shape.

SYMPTOMS Entropion causes irritation of the eye by the lashes and the usual sign is a chronic eye discharge and conjunctivitis in a young dog. This is the most troublesome of the two disorders. Occasionally in very young dogs the situation may improve such that surgical treatment (see below) is not needed.

Ectropion causes exposure of the lining of the eyelids and recurrent infections. It occurs most frequently in Spaniels.

DIAGNOSIS The conditions are easy to detect by careful observation of the eyelids. Entropion can be temporarily corrected by gently pushing on the skin above or below the eyelid: the inward-folded skin is straightened out and the lashes move away from the eye. Unfortunately, the problem resumes as soon as the tension on the skin is released.

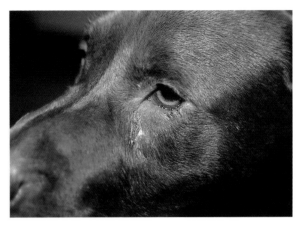

A dog suffering from in-turning eyelid (entropion). Eyelashes constantly irritate the cornea, producing pain and eye discharge.

TREATMENT Both problems are very effectively treated by plastic surgery to correct the eyelid shape. Entropion is treated by removing a crescent-shaped wedge of skin above the top eyelid and below the bottom one. When the new edges are sutured together after removal of the wedge, the in-turned eyelids and eyelashes are pulled up and away from the eye, giving instant relief from the chronic irritation and pain.

Medical treatment may be required until young puppies are old enough for anaesthesia and surgery, or (occasionally) until the condition resolves itself as the dog grows.

OUTLOOK The outlook is excellent after successful surgery.

HAIR IRRITATION

CAUSE Several problems are caused by hairs growing in the wrong place or rubbing against the eye surface. Particular problems can be caused by short stout hairs growing on the inner surface of the eyelid (ectopic cilia). Only one of these culprits is necessary to cause intense eye irritation and persistent discharge.

Hairs elsewhere may or may not be the cause of eye problems. Many dogs have a number of extra hairs along the eyelid margin which seem to lie gently against the eye. This is particularly common in the

American Cocker Spaniel breed and is also seen in several others. These hairs float on the tear film and do not cause problems in most cases.

Breeds with 'squash' faces, such as the Pekinese, may suffer from nasal hair rubbing the eye. This, combined with the poor blinking that is very often seen in these breeds, can lead to chronic eye irritation and pigmentation of the eye surface.

Symptoms Eye discharge, painful blinking and reddening or ulceration of the eye surface may be seen. Pekinese and similar breeds may develop dark pigmentation from chronic dryness and irritation.

Diagnosis This involves close examination of the eyelid margin and also the inner surface of the eyelid, usually with the help of a magnified light source. Nasal folds rubbing against the eye in short-faced breeds are best seen with the dog relaxed and not held around the face area (this can distort the position of the skin).

Treatment The culprit hairs can be plucked out; unfortunately, they tend to regrow, however permanent cures can be obtained using electrolysis treatment, cryosurgery (freezing) or surgery to remove individual hairs or clusters.

For irritation from nasal fold hairs, surgical removal of the extra skin making up the fold provides an effective cure.

Outlook They can occasionally be troublesome to treat but after surgery most of these conditions carry a good outlook.

'CHERRY EYE'

Cause This is a problem of the third eyelid occasionally encountered in puppies and young dogs. The eyelid has a swollen appearance and appears prominently in the corner of the eye, somewhat resembling a cherry. The exact cause is unknown but the condition is seen more frequently in certain breeds (e.g. American Cocker Spaniel, Lhasa Apso, Bulldog and Beagle).

Symptoms There may be no definite symptoms. Sometimes the protruding tissue can become damaged and there may be a slight eye discharge. The condition does not seem to result in any discomfort to most dogs although some appear to find it irritating and will rub or scratch. It can occur in one or both eyes.

Diagnosis Diagnosis is straightforward in young dogs. If an older animal developed a swelling like this, a tumour might be suspected.

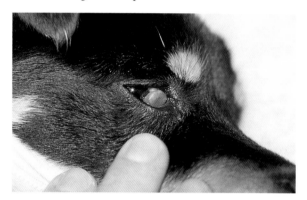

'Cherry eye' is caused by protrusion of a gland associated with the dog's third eyelid. Replacement of the protruded gland requires surgery.

Treatment Surgery is usually performed to tuck and secure the protuding tissue into a more normal location. Occasionally, part of the third eyelid may need to be removed, though most vets prefer to leave the structure intact if they can since it has an important protective and lubricating function in the eye.

Outlook Surgery is the only treatment for this problem. It can sometimes be tricky to ensure that the prolapsed gland is retained – they have a tendency to pop back out again. If removal is required, the dog may develop problems associated with low tear production in the affected eye (see 'Dry eye' opposite).

EYELID TUMOURS (GROWTHS)

Cause Tumours of the eyelid are common in dogs. A variety of tumours occur, but fortunately most (70 to

80%) are benign. Most eyelid tumours affect the edges of the upper or lower eyelids, but tumours of the third eyelid occasionally occur. However, even a benign tumour can grow to be large and cause considerable trouble in the eyelid region.

SYMPTOMS Sometimes there are no symptoms other than the presence of the tumour itself. Other tumours may cause eye irritation and discharge, occasionally leading to corneal ulcers (see below), and some tumours may bleed if accidentally knocked or scratched by the dog.

DIAGNOSIS This is usually straightforward but determining the exact type of tumour may not be possible until it is biopsied or (more usually) removed completely. Often, the vet will be able to provide an 'educated guess' as to the type and likely behaviour of the tumour from its overall appearance, taking into account the type and age of dog. This can help in deciding what treatment, if any, should be pursued.

TREATMENT This depends on the size, position and behaviour of the tumour. For example, small growths causing no problems, and which do not seem to be enlarging, may frequently be left alone in very old dogs. Growths causing eye irritation, ulceration or bleeding, or growths which are very unsightly and appear to be enlarging and interfering with blinking,

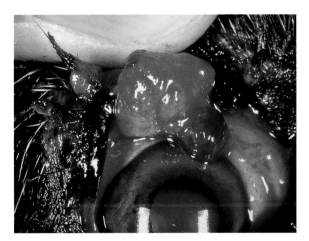

Most eyelid tumours turn out to be benign, neverthless they can grow to a large size. In old dogs, very small growths which are not changing in size may just be left alone.

are removed and often sent off for analysis to determine exactly what type of cells they consist of.

Very large growths may require more complex surgery to prevent problems developing after removal of large sections of the eyelid. Up to about one third of the width of the eyelid can be safely removed; beyond this, re-shaping the eyelid after excision of the tumour becomes a problem.

OUTLOOK The majority of eyelid tumours are successfully removed by surgery when they are at a small size. As most are benign, recurrence is unlikely. If a decision to leave the tumour alone is made, then regular observation is required so that further action can be taken as needed if the situation changes.

'DRY EYE'

CAUSE The cause is a disease or condition which damages the tear-producing glands, resulting in insufficient tear production to keep the eye lubricated and healthy. Various things can lead to this result. Distemper (in unvaccinated dogs), nerve damage, and a reaction to certain drugs have all been identified as causes of 'dry eye'. However the commonest cause seems to be an immune-mediated problem, whereby the dog's own immune system destroys the glands that normally produce tears.

Dogs frequently affected by the immune system cause include West Highland White Terriers, Cocker Spaniels and Lhasa Apsos.

SYMPTOMS This disease tends to start off quietly and gradually get worse. It can cause an eye discharge with conjunctivitis, ulceration of the eye and changes in the colour of the clear cornea – it may become a dark colour or small blood vessels may be noticeable. In many cases the cornea looks dull and there is frequently an accumulation of sticky mucus on the surface of the cornea.

Both eyes are usually affected, though perhaps to different degrees.

DIAGNOSIS Tear production is measured (see page 45). Affected eyes produce less tears than normal.

Some severely affected dogs can produce virtually no tears at all.

TREATMENT Immune suppressant eye ointments are used to good effect in most patients. These may be combined with other treatments, especially initially.

Severe cases which do not respond to the above treatment (most do) may require surgery. The surgery for this condition involves re-directing the course of a salivary gland duct so that it discharges into the eye. Thus saliva, instead of tears, moistens the eye. Although this can cause some complications, it is a desirable option when other treatments fail.

OUTLOOK In most cases, constant medication is necessary with periodic check-ups to ensure that the eye is not deteriorating.

PREVENTION All dogs should be vaccinated against distemper. The other causes are harder to prevent, and the commonest cause (the immune system cause) cannot be prevented or anticipated unfortunately.

 To help alleviate 'dry eye'

Regular cleaning of the eyelids and corners of the eye combined with frequent application of 'artificial tears' can greatly help this condition.

WATERY EYE/TEAR OVERFLOW

CAUSE In the absence of any signs of pain (e.g. redness, eyelids held partly closed) and when the discharge from the eye appears to be normal tears, the problem may be poor tear drainage. This usually means that the duct which carries tears away from the corner of the eye to the nose is too narrow or completely blocked.

Sometimes dogs lack one of the two tiny drainage holes that allow tears to enter the duct from the corner of the eye. This is a congenital problem seen in Cocker Spaniels and Golden Retrievers. Usually the lower of the two drainage holes is missing or improperly formed. Tear overflow is also quite common in small breed dogs.

Foreign bodies may become trapped in the naso-lacrimal duct, thus blocking it. This can occur in any breed or size of dog.

SYMPTOMS There are excess tears which may run down the side of the face and stain the hair coat. Note that excess tears can also be caused by irritation to the eye, so other problems must also be ruled out, e.g. abnormally positioned eyelashes or hairs, pain from deeper within the eye, etc.

DIAGNOSIS This is likely to involve a full eye examination and tests under sedation or anaesthesia to try to find an underlying cause. X-rays may be used.

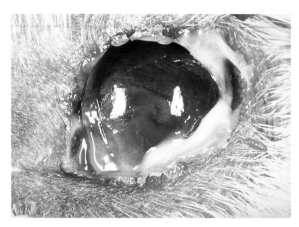

Severe 'dry eye' in a West Highland White terrier. Lack of normal tear production causes this unpleasant condition.

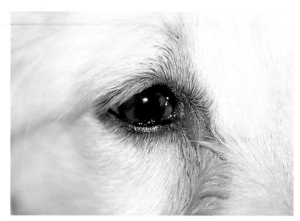

Watery eye (epiphora) in a cross-breed dog caused by chronic irritation from a wrongly directed eyelash.

TREATMENT Lack of a drainage hole can be corrected by surgery and blocked ducts can be flushed; sometimes a thin tube may be left in the duct for several weeks to encourage it to stay open.

OUTLOOK Many cases can be helped considerably and if a blocked tear duct can be relieved, the symptoms should disappear.

EYE (CORNEAL) ULCERS

CAUSE Anything which damages the cornea (the clear window at the front of the eye) could potentially cause an ulcer, which is an inflammatory condition leading to destruction of layers of the cornea. Corneal ulcers are encountered frequenty in veterinary practice. Common causes include:

• Poor tear production

• Injuries and foreign bodies, e.g. thorns, grass seeds

• Entropion, eyelid injury or eyelid tumours

• Infection and allergy

• Irritation from abnormal hair growth

• Irritant substances coming into contact with the eye

Dogs which have large protruberant eyes (e.g. Pekinese) are more prone to corneal ulceration as a larger proportion of the cornea is exposed to the drying action of air, and such dogs frequently do not blink well.

Corneal ulcers may be very superficial and mild or so deep that the eye is in danger of complete rupture.

SYMPTOMS Corneal injuries and ulcers are painful. Affected dogs will often show eyelid spasms, eye discharge and may rub or paw the face. The cornea may be cloudy or reddened; sometimes the crater of the ulcer can be seen, surrounded by whitish material and enlarged blood vessels. Vision in the eye may be affected.

DIAGNOSIS Close examination by the vet and the use of dye-impregnated strips to check for corneal damage and to check tear production are usually carried out. Deep ulcers are emergencies as the eye could rupture at any time.

TREATMENT Depending on the severity of the ulcer this may range from the application of drops or ointments, to complex surgical procedures to repair the ulcer and protect the injured area while the eye heals.

OUTLOOK Provided treatment is prompt and appropriate, most corneal ulcers can be dealt with successfully. Sometimes a small pale scar remains on the cornea after ulcer healing. Very severe cases, with penetration of the eyeball, can lead to loss of the eye.

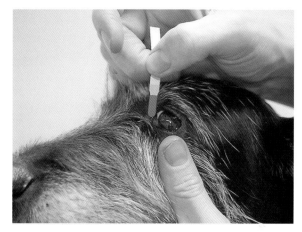

Applying fluorescein (fluorescent dye) to test for an ulcer on the cornea.

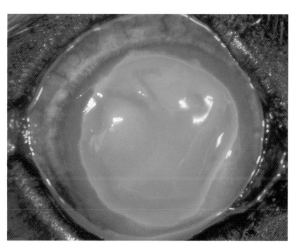

Large ulcer showing up green after fluorescein staining.

Lubrication for ulcers

Many minor ulcers benefit from the lubrication provided by frequent application of 'artificial tears'. Ask the veterinary surgeon for advice on their use and the best type to buy.

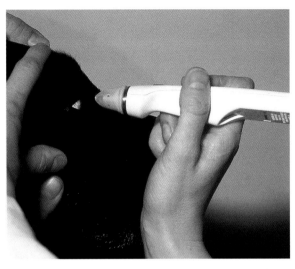

Measuring internal eye pressure to test for glaucoma after application of a local anaesthetic. The procedure causes no discomfort.

GLAUCOMA

CAUSE Glaucoma results from a build up of pressure within the eye. The normal circulation and drainage of eye fluids is disrupted, resulting in their accumulation within the eye. This leads to the dangerous increase in pressure. If this pressure build up is sustained, blindness results from damage to the optic nerve and the retina.

Glaucoma can be inherited or it can result from other forms of eye disease or injury which interfere with the drainage of eye fluids. Inherited glaucoma usually affects both eyes but not necessarily at the same time.

SYMPTOMS One of the problems is that the early stages may not be recognised, so glaucoma can be dangerously advanced by the time it is diagnosed. Common symptoms include sudden blindness, reddening of the eye and pain, cloudiness of the cornea (the clear window at the front of the eye) and a large pupil.

DIAGNOSIS The eye will be examined and its pressure checked. A high pressure indicates glaucoma. Suspected glaucoma cases may be referred to a veterinary ophthalmologist for investigation/treatment.

TREATMENT Numerous factors are taken into account including the type of glaucoma and its severity and whether the dog is blind and likely to remain so. Various medications may need to be applied to the eye or given by mouth; sometimes, surgery to improve eye fluid drainage may be required.

Glaucoma is a condition which may eventually lead to removal of the eye in order to alleviate chronic pain from an eye that can no longer see.

OUTLOOK Glaucoma is a very serious eye condition. Many cases receive treatment from specialist veterinary ophthalmologists in an attempt to limit the damage caused to the eye by severe pressure changes.

Breeds in which glaucoma is found more frequently

- Cocker Spaniels
- Poodles (Miniature and Toy)
- Basset Hounds
- Samoyed
- Husky
- Beagle
- Terrier breeds

 Seek help early

Glaucoma provides a good example of why it is important to seek veterinary help early on in any eye condition that involves reddening or pain.

CATARACT

CAUSE Cataracts result in the lens of the eye becoming whitish and opaque. The dog's vision is reduced as a result. Most cataracts are inherited but occasionally the condition arises as a result of other diseases, e.g. diabetes.

SYMPTOMS A whitish discolouration of the lens is seen and poor vision may be noticed if the condition is advanced. In inherited cataract, both eyes are affected. The problem is usually first seen in young dogs of 1–3 years old. Sometimes puppies are born with cataracts and occasionally the problem develops in more mature dogs.

When cataracts arise in response to other diseases of the body or eye, then a single eye may be affected and this can occur at any age.

DIAGNOSIS The diagnosis is straightforward but underlying or complicating factors often need to be investigated.

TREATMENT Surgery is performed by a specialist ophthalmologist. This involves removing the cataracts in both eyes; sometimes an artificial lens is placed into the eyes. Underlying diseases will also need to be treated (e.g. diabetes) and this will usually be undertaken before the cataract lenses are removed.

 Cataract diagnosis

Note that many older dogs have a harmless condition that resembles cataract called nuclear sclerosis (see page 43). A simple check at the veterinary surgery can provide the necessary reassurance. Similar symptoms in a young dog would be more likely to be cataract however.

OUTLOOK Although the lens is removed, dogs retain functional vision and the outlook for most cases is good.

Breeds suffering from inherited cataract

- American Cocker Spaniel
- Golden Retriever
- Labrador Retriever
- Standard and Miniature Poodle
- Miniature Schnauzer
- Welsh Springer Spaniel
- Boston Terrier
- and other breeds

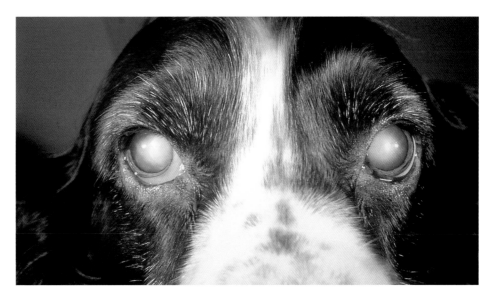

Bilateral (both sides) cataract in a spaniel.

IRITIS OR ANTERIOR UVEITIS

CAUSE This is a painful inflammatory condition of the eye that has a wide range of causes. Sometimes it arises as a result of another disease or injury to the eye, but it may also occur on its own. One or both eyes may be affected.

SYMPTOMS Pain is the main feature and the eye may be reddened. The pain may be intense enough to make the dog shy away from any approach to the head; the eyelids may be held partly closed or undergo spasms and the eye may water.

DIAGNOSIS Careful examination of the eye is carried out. Often, as with glaucoma, the pressure in the eye is estimated. (Iritis/uveitis results in a lower than normal pressure, allowing the vet to distinguish the condition from glaucoma.)

If both eyes are affected, a wide variety of further tests may be required to try to pin-point a cause.

TREATMENT If a definite cause is found, this will be treated. Most cases are assumed to be caused by an immune system problem and are treated with potent steroid drops and sometimes tablets to halt the damaging inflammation in the eye. Drugs which artificially dilate the pupil may also be used in order to try to prevent adhesions developing within the eye.

 A red, painful eye

Iritis/anterior uveitis is another serious condition that may simply appear as a red and painful eye. It is sometimes misdiagnosed as conjunctivitis by owners and prompt action is not taken. Neglecting this condition is extremely unpleasant for the dog, and may have poor consequences for vision. Once diagnosed, it is crucial that any drops are applied exactly as prescribed. It is normal for treatment to be continued for several weeks, gradually reducing the dosage if the eye responds well.

OUTLOOK Prompt treatment usually results in the inflammation being brought under control. The eye becomes 'quiet' and the dog is much more comfortable. However a vigilant watch needs to be kept for recurrences, as this problem does tend to come back again. At the earliest sign of eye reddening or pain, veterinary attention should be sought.

RETINAL DISEASES

CAUSE The retina is the 'screen' at the back of the eye on which the visual image is projected. Special nerve cells here transmit the image to the brain and allow the dog to see. Problems with the retina can therefore jeopardise vision. Many of these problems are inherited and are the subject of current research in order to improve understanding and, eventually, treatment. Some problems are associated with particular breeds of dog.

SYMPTOMS Unfortunately, because the retina is hidden from view, problems here are not usually detected until they are severe enough to seriously interfere with vision. Poor vision or blindness is therefore the most common symptom.

DIAGNOSIS Examination of the back (fundus) of the eye using an ophthalmoscope as well as other more specialised tests are carried out.

TREATMENT Many of these problems currently have no effective treatment. Where the condition is caused by some other underlying disease (e.g. inflammation), treatment may be able to slow or halt progression of the vision loss.

OUTLOOK Unfortunately, due to the advanced nature of these diseases at the time of diagnosis the outlook for good vision may be poor.

PREVENTION In inherited diseases, carrier animals should not be bred from in order to try to eliminate the problem in specific breeds. Testing schemes are available to try to detect carrier dogs for certain of these diseases. One such scheme screens Collie dogs for the condition known as Collie Eye Anomaly (CEA).

TUMOURS

CAUSE Like other organs in the body, the eye and its surrounding structures can be affected by tumours (see above for eyelid tumours, which are common in dogs). The internal and external parts of the eye may be affected and the tumours can be benign or malignant.

SYMPTOMS There are no specific symptoms for tumours. As with other eye problems, pain, reddening, altered appearance, loss of vision or abnormal discharges may all point to an underlying diagnosis of an eye tumour. Apart from eyelid tumours, cancer of the eye is diagnosed less frequently than some of the other problems mentioned above.

DIAGNOSIS Observation, X-rays/ultrasound and biopsy techniques may all play a part. To completely diagnose a tumour, a biopsy technique is normally required. This allows treatment to be planned.

TREATMENT Surgical removal may be feasible, or else treatment may be directed towards limiting the effects of the tumour.

OUTLOOK If a tumour is confined to the structures of the eye, and the eye is completely removed, a cure should be possible. Tumours which have spread to other areas may only be able to be controlled in an attempt to minimise unpleasant effects.

BLINDNESS

CAUSE Blindness can be caused by any injury or disease which damages the eye or interferes with the nervous system structures involved in seeing. Several of the conditions described above are common causes of blindness, e.g.:

- Glaucoma

- Retinal disease

- Persistent iritis/uveitis

- Severe (especially blunt) injury to the eye

- Ulceration which causes rupture of the eye

- Tumours

In addition, brain diseases or injury can also lead to blindness.

SYMPTOMS Blindness in one eye can be difficult to detect in dogs. Unlike human beings, they cannot voice their problems. If the underlying cause results in changes in the appearance of the eye (e.g. reddness, pain, swelling) observant owners can pick this up at an early stage and ensure treatment is started promptly. However, when there are no obvious external changes to notice (e.g. in retinal disease) the condition can progress silently until irreversible damage has been done.

DIAGNOSIS Diagnostic techniques used in each case depend on the information the vet receives from the owner (the dog's 'history'), on the appearance of the eye and on the likelihood of underlying disease problems which might be showing up in the eye first, but actually are present elsewhere in the body too as yet undetected.

TREATMENT The aim is always to treat the underlying cause whenever this can be found since this carries the best chance of a complete cure. In some instances, however, where a cure is not known or not possible,

 Test your dog's vision

If you suspect poor vision, perform the vision test described on page 42 (perform in bright and dim light and with right and left eyes separately blindfolded), note down your results and discuss them with your vet.

treatment has to concentrate on alleviating symptoms or on preventing a severe situation from getting even worse, i.e. the treatment may aim to *control* the disease rather than completely *cure* it.

If one eye has to be removed and the other eye remains functional, dogs usually cope extremely well. The altered appearance can, to some extent, be compensated for by the use of silicone prostheses which resemble the shape of the lost eye.

Totally blind dogs can be kept but demand constant care and attention. Success depends on the temperament of the dog, the commitment of the owner and on full discussion with the vet or ophthalmic specialist. It is a major undertaking and emphasis should always be placed on the dog's quality of life.

CHAPTER 4

The Ear

Common symptoms of ear disease
• Scratching/rubbing the ear • Head shaking
• Discharge from ear • Ear odour
• Swellings on the ear flap
• Head held to one side • Falling or circling to one side
• Pain when approach or touch head

Structure and Function

The ear is a sensitive organ of hearing and balance. The parts of the ear which we see are the ear flap (the pinna) and the outer opening of the ear (the external ear canal). The main function of the pinna is to collect and focus sound waves and to direct them into the external canal and towards the organs of hearing, which lie deep within the ear. The pinna also provides some protection for the outer opening of the ear canal.

The 'natural' pinna shape is seen in wolves, other wild relatives of the dog and in breeds like German Shepherds. In these animals, upright pinnae act as efficient collectors of sound waves. Centuries of selective breeding by human beings has, of course, led to a great many different dog ear shapes. Some of the problems which dogs suffer with their ears are linked to these alterations in shape and structure. For example, drooping ear flaps result in poorer ventilation; the external ear canal can become humid and warm, and may result in an increased incidence of bacterial and yeast ear infections.

The external ear canal leads to the ear drum (the tympanum) – a thin membrane which vibrates when sound waves pass down the ear canal to reach it. The ear drum is connected to a series of tiny, linked bones. These ingenious structures transmit the sound vibrations across the middle ear cavity. In the inner ear, the vibrations are finally converted into electrical signals which are passed on to the brain via the auditory nerve. The brain 'decodes' these electrical messages and thus the animal hears recognisable sounds.

The inner ear also contains the important organs of balance, which explains why dogs with serious ear disorders often appear incoordinated: they may constantly fall to one or other side, hold their head at an angle (head tilt) or walk in circles because the specialised organs of balance have been damaged by the disease.

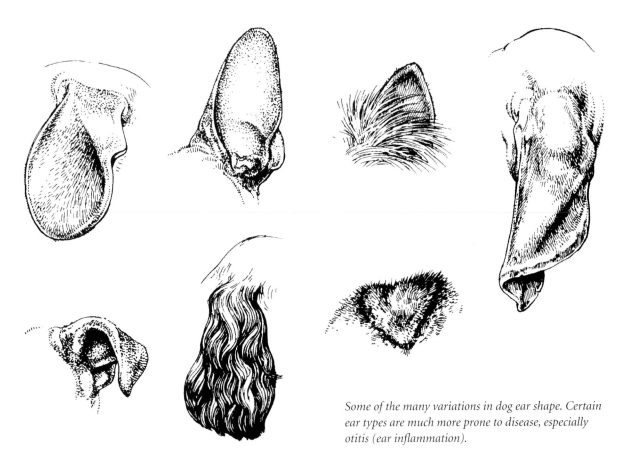

Some of the many variations in dog ear shape. Certain ear types are much more prone to disease, especially otitis (ear inflammation).

A small tube, the eustachian tube, links the middle ear with the throat. This tube opens up on swallowing and allows the pressure on both sides of the ear drum to become equal. This is the reason why sucking a sweet (and swallowing) helps alleviate the uncomfortable pressure changes people feel in their ears when aircraft are taking off or landing. Dogs rarely suffer problems with the eustachian tube.

Deafness in dogs

Dogs have extremely acute hearing and are sensitive to sound frequencies which the human ear cannot perceive at all.

It is quite difficult to tell whether a dog is deaf, especially if the deafness is only in one ear, because other senses, and the good ear, can compensate and hide the problem.

Certain breeds, such as Dalmatians, are prone to hereditary deafness. Research suggests that approximately 21% of Dalmatians are deaf in one ear and up to 7% are deaf in both ears. Screening for this problem is now being carried out to prevent breeding from affected dogs. Totally deaf dogs can be difficult to train and may often get themelves into dangerous situations, e.g. they would be unable to hear an approaching car. Such situations can be unsafe for dogs and humans alike.

Hereditary deafness has also been detected in many other breeds of dog, including the English Setter, Bulldog, Old English Sheedog and Boston Terrier. Performing the simple test described below allows you to determine only if there is *complete* absence of hearing; confirming partial deafness requires the use of specialised equipment to detect auditory evoked potentials (AEPs) – the electrical 'messages' being transmitted to the brain to register hearing. If dogs cannot transmit these messages (e.g. their auditory nerve is damaged in some way) then they will be unable to hear. This sophisticated technique provides a reliable way of detecting deafness when the patient cannot speak (a similar technique is also used in human babies).

 Is my dog deaf?

If you think your dog may be deaf, you can try a simple method to test his hearing. When he is not looking at you make a loud noise, e.g. clap your hands or blow a whistle. Take care not to create any air disturbances which may be detected by the highly sensitive muzzle whiskers and try to create the noise without excessive movement, which could be picked up by your dog's peripheral vision.

If your dog doesn't respond at all, he is likely to be profoundly deaf.

Partial deafness is much more difficult to detect.

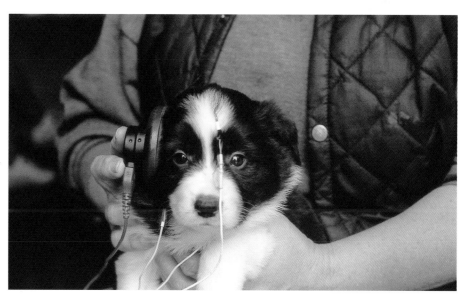

Hearing test being carried out in a puppy. The procedure is painless and is the only way to say for sure whether a dog is deaf.

Deafness and the older dog

Many owners notice a deterioration in their dog's hearing with advancing age. This is normal – and inevitable – but, as many ear diseases also interfere with hearing, other causes should be ruled out by the veterinary surgeon before you assume poor hearing is due to age alone. Most older dogs with failing hearing learn to respond to hand signals to encourage them to 'come' or 'stay'. As the hearing deteriorates, they may rely more and more on signals to communicate with their owner.

Caring for Your Dog's Ears

The healthy ear does not require any treatment or special care, other than regular checking to ensure that there is no discharge or irritation of the sensitive lining, or excessive accumulation of hair in breeds prone to this problem (e.g. Poodles).

Ear cleaners or medicated ear wipes should not be used on a routine basis unless your vet suggests this. The normal ear does not require them because the production, drying and gradual flaking out of wax is itself a cleansing process in the healthy ear and should not be interfered with. However, in dogs prone to wax accumulation ear cleaners may be useful to keep excess wax under control.

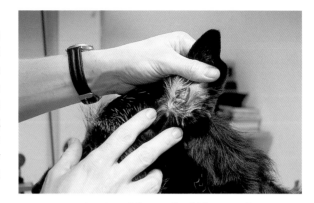

Routine examination of the ear should be carried out regularly in all dogs.

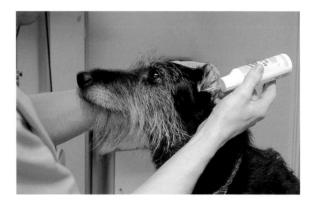

Applying ear cleaner or drops. The nozzle should not be inserted too far.

 Cleaning your dog's ears

Some dogs react badly to even very gentle and bland ear cleaners so, when using any new ear cleaner for the first time, only a very small quantity should be applied until you are sure your dog is not sensitive to it. Cotton buds, tweezers or other objects should never be used to clean a dog's ears. Damage to the sensitive ear canal lining can occur, and the buds tend simply to push any waxy material deeper into the ear canal, making the problem worse.

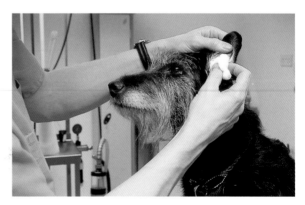

When using cotton wool, only swab from the top of the ear canal. Never push cotton wool or cotton buds into the ear canal. Debris or wax will rise to the surface naturally in most cases.

Veterinary Diagnosis and Treatment

Ear disease is common in dogs and, if untreated, it can become very serious. Chronic ear conditions can be extremely difficult to cure completely, so any ear problem should be treated quickly and thoroughly in order to try to avoid irreversible changes developing. As ear diseases are notoriously painful, this is another good reason to seek professional advice early.

Certain dogs are prone to ear disease and recurrences are inevitable. Recurrences, when they occur, should always be treated promptly, with veterinary advice, as the severity may alter during the course of time. Even if you have some medication left over from a previous treatment, you should contact your veterinary surgeon as it may not be appropriate to use the same product a second time.

Diagnostic techniques used by your vet

Common methods of diagnosis used by veterinary surgeons include:

- Visual inspection of the ear canals. The vet will often use a special illuminated torch for this purpose to allow inspection of the ear drum

- Swabs of any discharge coming from the ear may be taken and submitted to a laboratory for analysis

- Small biopsies may be taken if there is a growth present in the ear canals

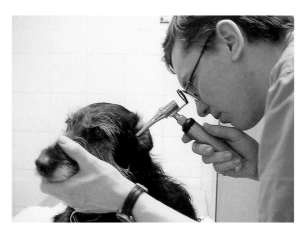

Using the auroscope may be too painful in severely inflamed ears and an anaesthetic or sedative could be required.

- X-rays may be used if the middle ear is thought to be affected by the disease

- Skin tests may also be carried out, since many ear problems are closely connected with skin disease.

Anaesthetics and sedatives are often required in severe and painful ear diseases, to allow a thorough examination without inflicting pain. This also enables pain-free and safe syringing and cleaning of the ears if required.

Ear surgery

Ear surgery can be divided into minor and major surgical procedures:

Minor surgery

- Simple suturing of ear flap wounds

- Treatment of haematomas (see below)

- Removal of small benign growths (e.g. warts)

- Removal of foreign bodies lodged in the ear (e.g. grass awns).

Major surgery

- Total removal of chronically diseased or inflamed ear tissue (known as total ablation of the ear canal). *Ablation* simply means 'surgical removal'.

- Modification of the shape of the ear to improve ventilation and make application of medication drops easier in chronic ear diseases (known as resection of the lateral wall of the ear canal). *Lateral* refers to the outer wall of the ear canal.

- Removal of ear canal tumours – the surgical technique used here depends on the severity of the tumour and its precise location.

Major surgery is reserved for what veterinary surgeons call 'end-stage ears' – in other words, ears in which all other treatments have failed. The surgery is undertaken to remove the inflamed tissue and

Basic first aid for ears

Constant shaking and scratching

Lift up the ear flap and examine the ear opening. If you can see something obvious near the very top of the ear canal, gently remove it with your fingers of a pair of blunt tipped tweezers if it is safe to do so. Never probe deeply into the ear. If in any doubt, do nothing until veterinary advice has been taken.

Constant scratching risks damage to the ear, ear flap or side of the face. Fit a protective Elizabethan collar until the problem can be dealt with properly.

Bleeding ear flap wounds

Even a small injury on the ear flap can cause persistent bleeding which is usually worsened by the dog repeatedly shaking its head and sending a fine spray of blood droplets everywhere. Major blood loss is unusual although the repeated shaking does create the impression of large volumes being lost. Many of these wounds benefit from being stitched closed but useful first aid measures include:

1. Apply gentle pressure across the bleeding area through cotton wool or gauze. Keep this up for 10 minutes and then see if bleeding has stopped. Unfortunately, it often tends to start up again as soon as the dog moves its head.

2. Fit a loose stocking or T-shirt over the dog's head to hold the ear flap close to the head and keep it still. Make sure this is loose enough to allow the dog to breathe, pant and see while you transport it to a clinic.

Stings and allergic reactions

These can be dealt with by bathing in cool water or applying an ice pack (e.g. bag of frozen peas or similar) to the ear flap. It is usually impossible to find and remove a sting. A homoeopathic treatment is mentioned in Chapter 18.

---

alleviate associated pain and distress. Very often, it is successful in these aims and dogs that have perhaps been suffering for months or even years take on a new lease of life when the source of chronic pain is finally removed.

The most severe form of surgery (total ablation of the ear canal) renders the dog unable to hear. However, most of the patients in which this procedure is performed are already deaf from chronic inflammatory disease and so this fact is of little relevance. The vast majority of dogs receiving this surgery from an experienced surgeon recover very well indeed and have a good quality of life afterwards.

Lateral wall resection does not cure chronic ear disease but, if used in the right cases, it makes the condition much easier for owner and veterinary surgeon to manage. Some dogs which have had a lateral wall resection may need to have total ablation carried out later if the first procedure does not work well.

Costs and prognosis in ear disease

Simple ear problems usually respond readily to treatment and a complete cure is expected, usually within 5–10 days. Treatment is unlikely to be on-going; it may involve 2–3 veterinary visits and sometimes a short anaesthetic for minor surgery in cases of wounds that require suturing.

More severe ear problems have a tendency to recur, even with the best treatment. Chronic ear disorders are often related to skin disease (which can also be very difficult to cure completely) but if the skin condition is ignored, the ears are unlikely to respond very well to local treatment alone.

There is no doubt that serious, chronic ear conditions can be expensive and frustrating to treat. Long courses of medication and repeated sedatives/anaesthetics for flushing the ears may be required. X-rays may be needed to assess the severity of the problem and some persistent conditions require major surgery (as described earlier).

In the most problematical cases, control of symptoms – rather than a complete cure – is all that can be realistically achieved and the emphasis is on making the dog comfortable and pain-free. These are the dogs which may benefit from surgery to literally remove all of the chronically diseased ear tissue. Afterwards they will be deaf in the affected ear – but comfortable.

Owners have a very important role to play in closely monitoring chronic ear conditions, and in making sure that simple reversible problems do not progress to more serious disorders.

Commonest Ear Problems in Dogs

HAIR BUILD-UP

CAUSE This is a common problem in Poodles, their crosses and many other breeds which contain excess hair in the ear canals.

SYMPTOMS Head shaking; ear scratching or rubbing; irritability.

DIAGNOSIS Gently lift the ear flap and look into the external ear canal. Often a mass of matted hair and trapped wax can be seen. This is intensely irritating for the dog.

TREATMENT The trapped hair/wax is removed. This is often easier said than done as plucking out the hair may be painful. Struggling risks damaging the ears, so if your dog won't tolerate plucking, a sedative or anaesthetic at the veterinary surgery will be required.

OUTLOOK Usually, immediate relief is obtained by the dog once the trapped material is removed.

EAR MITES

CAUSE The culprit is the dog ear mite, *Otodectes cynotis*, a tiny parasite only just visible to the naked eye. Much rarer is infestation with another species of mite, *Demodex canis*. Most cases are caused by the commoner *Otodectes*.

SYMPTOMS Ear pain and irritation due to otitis (inflammation within the ear canals); intense itch within the ears and on the surrounding skin areas; dark, dry waxy material within the ear is a common finding with ear mites.

The symptoms are caused by the dog reacting to the presence of the parasite within the ear. The irritation produced in the ear canal stimulates excess wax production and the walls of the ear canal can become inflamed and sore. An itchy cycle then develops. Scratching and rubbing by the dog makes the situation worse. Dogs with ear mites may come and ask for their ears to be rubbed. Lifting the ear flap will reveal the accumulated wax and source of the problem.

DIAGNOSIS The condition is diagnosed or suspected when the vet examines your dog's ears using an auroscope. Examination of samples of waxy material under the microscope will often reveal the tiny living parasites.

TREATMENT This usually inolves the application of ear drops for 1–2 weeks. Sometimes ear cleaners are prescribed first to disperse some of the excess wax

Prevention of hair build-up

Regular checking of the ears will help you detect this complaint at an early stage but unfortunately there is no means of preventing the hair growing in this awkward location in the first place. Once the condition is brought under control, try to limit future occurrences by regularly removing a small amount of hair. Wiping your fingertips with powder before you start will help you get a better grip on the fine hair that lines the ear canals. Don't persist for too long at a time and be sure to reward your dog well afterwards. It is best to avoid using tweezers even in the most placid dogs unless you are an experienced groomer (in which case blunt plastic tweezers are required) – it is very easy to damage the ear if the dog moves suddenly. Most of the hair occurs near the opening of the ear canal and can usually be reached using fingertips alone.

If your dog goes regularly for grooming or clipping, you could ask the groomer to do this job for you, but tell them not to persist if your dog struggles excessively as there is no doubt some dogs find this process extremely uncomfortable.

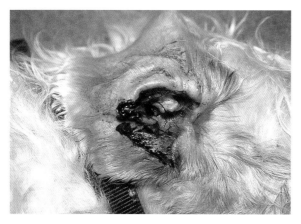

Otitis with production of excess wax. The dog constantly shook his head from irritation and pain.

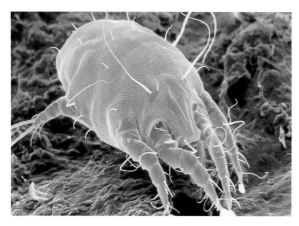

The ear mite Otodectes cynotis *is more commonly a problem in cats, but occasionally dogs will be found to be suffering from this parasite.*

before the medicated drops are used. Occasionally, this condition is treated by injection of anti-parasitic drugs if other methods do not seem effective or if dogs are unable to be treated in the usual way.

OUTLOOK The outlook for this problem is excellent.

AURAL HAEMATOMA

CAUSE An aural (ear) haematoma is a large blood blister occurring between the layers of skin that make up either side of the ear flap. The haematoma comprises a large swelling that may be very tense. It is fluid-filled, and the fluid consists of a type of watery blood. The cause is some damage to the blood vessels within the ear flap, causing bleeding into the space between the layers of skin and underlying cartilage. Common situations triggering haematomas are:

- Persistent head shaking (due to another ear condition, e.g. mites)

- Crushing injuries (e.g. ear trapped in a door, or a bite to the ear flap)

Most are caused by excessive shaking of the head and/or scratching at the ears.

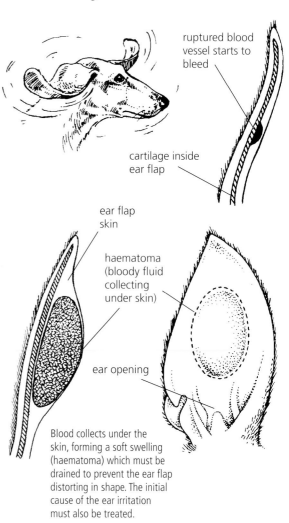

ruptured blood vessel starts to bleed

cartilage inside ear flap

ear flap skin

haematoma (bloody fluid collecting under skin)

ear opening

Blood collects under the skin, forming a soft swelling (haematoma) which must be drained to prevent the ear flap distorting in shape. The initial cause of the ear irritation must also be treated.

Constant shaking of the head carries the risk of haematoma formation. A large pocket filled with blood develops in the ear flap, following damage to a small blood vessel.

Symptoms The swellings are easy to notice when large, but smaller ones may be missed. Most dogs with haematomas have other signs of ear problems, usually head-shaking or ear pain, for some days before the haematoma appears.

Diagnosis This is very straightforward. Sometimes the vet may insert a fine needle into the haematoma to confirm that it is blood-based fluid present and not a fluid from infection (pus), but abscesses are encountered far less frequently than haematomas in this location.

Treatment The haemtoma, if small, may be drained using a needle and syringe. Sometimes sedation is required for this process. Steroid preparations may be injected into the ear. This process of drainage by fine needle aspiration may need to be repeated 1–2 times before the haematoma finally disappears completely.

Large haematomas are treated by minor surgery involving drainage through an incision made directly into the underside of the ear flap. Sutures or a soft plastic drain are then inserted into the ear for 5–7 days.

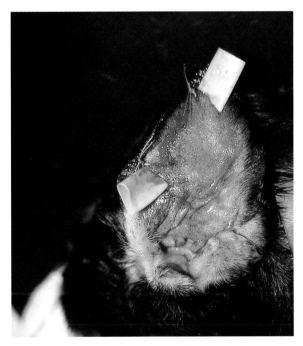

Large haematoma treated using a soft latex drain. The ear will drip reddish fluid for several days after surgery.

Ear drains and stitches for aural haematomas

If your dog has had sutures or a drain placed for an aural haematoma, keep him away from soft furnishings because the haematoma will leak fluid for several days and could cause stains. The purpose of the surgery is to establish drainage, hence it is intended that any fluid being formed will leak out of the ear rather than remain within it, forming another haematoma. This seepage, though a nuisance, usually stops after 2–3 days.

Prevention
Most haematomas could be prevented by catching ear disease at an early stage and starting correct treatment then. Those caused by bites or crushing injuries are however unavoidable.

The underlying problem must always be treated too, as a haematoma is only a symptom of some other condition causing ear discomfort.

Outlook Aural haematomas carry a good outlook. Most are cleared up within two weeks. Severe ones may cause some scarring and distortion of the ear flap however. This can also occur when treatment is delayed. The worst cases of delayed treatment result in a thickened, twisted ear flap which vets call 'cauliflower ear'.

FOREIGN BODY

Cause A 'foreign body' is an object from the outside world which has somehow found its way into an animal's body. In the ear, the commonest foreign body is a grass awn. Dogs running through long grass may pick up one of these and, because of the direction of the fibres of the awn, they tend to migrate down into the ear canal, causing pain and intense irritation. Sometimes several awns are found. Without treatment, large abscesses can form, the awn may migrate through surrounding tissues and many problems can then ensue.

SYMPTOMS Ear pain; constant irritation. Occasionally, dogs may become so agitated that they appear to be having a fit.

DIAGNOSIS Heavy sedation or general anaesthesia is required to allow careful examination of the ear canals.

TREATMENT Removal of the offending object is carried out under sedation or anaesthesia. The forward-directed spikes on grass awns makes retraction out of the ear difficult, however with the dog properly immobilised slender instruments can be inserted into the ear. Relief is instantaneous when the dog wakes up.

OUTLOOK The outlook after removal of the offending object is good provided no major damage has occurred to the sensitive ear structures.

OTITIS

CAUSE Otitis means inflammation of the ear, and has many causes including several of the conditions already mentioned. Foreign bodies, ear mites, bacterial and yeast infections and allergies all cause otitis. When the vet examines your dog, the main purpose is to try to establish what the precise cause of the otitis is.

Perhaps the commonest cause of chronic otitis in dogs is allergy – usually to grass pollens, but sometimes also to other agents or, occasionally, specific foods. Many dogs with allergic ear disease also have similar skin problems to a greater or lesser extent. Otitis can rapidly escalate and is an unpleasant condition since the lining of the ear has many sensitive nerve endings.

SYMPTOMS This depends how severe the otitis is and may range from mild ear discomfort with rubbing of the ears to intense pain that may be so severe as to make an otherwise placid dog agressive whenever the ears are touched or even approached.

DIAGNOSIS This will involve examination of the ears (perhaps under sedation or anaesthesia) and, often, collection of samples for further testing, espe-

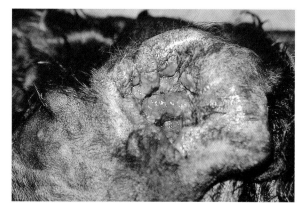

Otitis

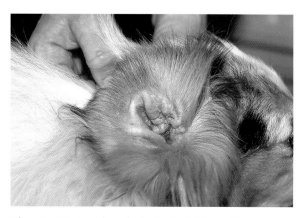

Chronic otitis in a dog which also had skin problems.

cially in the more complicated cases. Skin problems may also need to be investigated at the same time.

TREATMENT Specific treatment depends on the exact cause, but usually involves ear drops/washes, and sometimes courses of tablets. Severe cases may need to have the ears repeatedly syringed out under sedation or general anaesthetic. Surgery is recommended for those unfortunate dogs where the ear has been irreversibly damaged by chronic or unremitting inflammation.

OUTLOOK Otitis is always potentially serious since the enclosed space of the ear means that only a limited amount of inflammation can be tolerated before sensitive tissues begin to be damaged. Early treatment usually carries a good chance of success. Make sure a full treatment course is completed before assuming the problem has been cured.

CHAPTER 5

The Skin

Common symptoms of skin disease

• Itching • Hair loss • Crusty/scaly hair coat or skin • Greasy hair coat or skin
• Reddened/sore skin • Excessive licking of skin/hair • Parasites visible on coat
• Ear or feet problems • Growths on skin surface

Structure and Function

The skin is the largest organ in the body. It provides the body's outer covering, protecting all the underlying organs and tissues from damage, infection and changes in temperature and humidity. It is a complex structure and consists of many different parts. In dogs, of course, most of the skin is covered by hair, but the hair coat is thinner on the underside of the abdomen. In most dogs, the lining of the ear (which is modified skin) usually has no or very few hairs, although certain breeds such as Poodles suffer from excessive hair growth in the ear canals, which tends to trap wax and cause irritation (see page 65). The ear and the skin are very closely related; often, skin problems are closely associated with ear problems and are part of the same disease.

The type and colour of dogs' coats vary enormously. Both have been subject to the effects of many generations of selective breeding, sometimes for specific purposes, e.g. the dense coat layers of the Pyrenean Mountain Dog provide effective insulation against extremely low Alpine temperatures, while the Newfoundland's coat is highly waterproof and contributes to buoyancy in these dogs, which have been bred to be effective swimmers and rescuers.

The skin has many nerve endings within its upper layers. These nerves transmit pain and alert the animal to dangerous or damaging situations. This plentiful supply of nerves also means that skin diseases causing inflammation or itching can be intensely irritating for dogs, even making some dogs become uncharacteristically aggressive. Skin pain from burns is one of the most unpleasant forms of pain there is and can be difficult to control.

Glands are present in the skin which help to keep the hair coat and skin surface healthy and a layer of fat underneath the skin acts as insulation against both excessive heat and cold. Unlike human beings, dogs have very few sweat glands. The only places where dogs can really sweat is on their feet – this often shows up as damp footprints on the veterinary surgeon's consulting room table if the dog is nervous.

Nails

Dogs' nails are made of very tough specialised protein, designed to withstand constant wear and tear. The nails grow continuously and are worn down as the dog walks on harder abrasive surfaces.

Most dogs have five toes with nails on each forepaw and four on each hind paw. The small first toe or 'dew claw' on the inside of each forepaw is a rudimentary structure that serves no real purpose – it is occasionally removed in puppies, or in older dogs if it gets caught frequently. Because the nail on the dew claw is not in contact with the ground surface, it needs special checking to make sure it does not become overgrown and begin growing into the surrounding skin, causing inflammation and pain.

Most dogs don't have dew claws on the hind paws, but they are occasionally seen. When present, hind

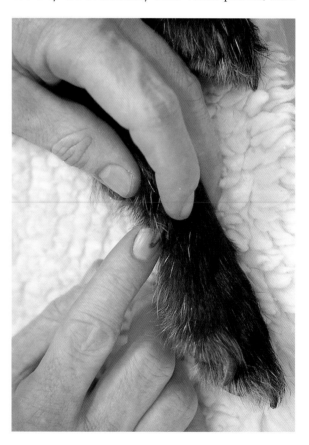

RIGHT *The dew claw, or short first toe, is present on the front foot (unless removed). Occasionally, hind foot dew claws are also present.*

dew claws often tend to hang rather loosely. These can be a nuisance in that they can get caught and torn in active or young dogs (much more often than front dew claws). Removal of hind dew claws may be best if they seem likely to cause problems.

Dogs' nails may be either black or white. When it comes to trimming, white ones are easier because the blood and nerve supply to the nail can be easily seen through the nail surface. This is impossible with black nails and occasionally leads to minor bleeding (and a loud yelp!) if a nail is trimmed too closely.

Foot pads

At the end of each toe the skin is modified to form the thick and tough digital pad, which acts as a protective cushion. Behind the digital pads is the large main (or metacarpal) pad and above this, not in contact with the ground, is the 'stopper' (or accessory carpal) pad.

These pads often become injured in dogs (e.g. by walking on glass) or else small sharp objects may become embedded in them or caustic substances, such as salt spread on roads in winter months, may damage them or the skin between them. Wounds to the pads may need to be sutured. If something is suspected to be stuck inside, X-rays or a minor operation may be needed.

Anal sacs

These skin-associated structures are well known to many dog owners as a source of occasional irritation to their pets. The anal sacs or anal glands are two scent glands, located under the skin on either side of the anus, with openings just inside. As the dog passes faeces, the foul-smelling secretion from the gland is smeared onto the faeces; this acts as a means of marking out territory.

 Tips on trimming the nails

- White ones are easier because the blood and nerve supply (the 'quick') can be seen. Always make the cut several millimetres below this (see diagram).

- With black nails, an 'educated guess' has to be made. Err on the side of caution.

- Use strong dog nail clippers, large enough for the size of your dog's nails. Larger dogs can have very tough nails and clippers that are too small or blunt just bend the nail, causing discomfort and resentment.

- Only trim a little: if the end of the nail rests just above the ground surface when the dog is standing flat, it does not need to be trimmed.

- Check the dew claws particularly since the nails here can curl inwards.

- Reward your dog well for staying still!

- Many dogs never need their nails trimmed if they get regular exercise on harder surfaces.

- Some dogs hate the process, especially if they have been hurt by it before – in these animals, it is best to let your veterinary surgeon or nurse do the trimming, or else take the dog for long walks on pavements or rocky surfaces.

If you cut too much and the nail bleeds, keep your dog quiet and apply some cotton wool and then a loose bandage or sock to the affected foot. The bleeding stops in 5–10 minutes, but could start up again if the dog was walked soon after that and the small blood clot at the end of the nail got disturbed.

Nails should be trimmed to avoid the 'quick' otherwise pain and bleeding will be caused.

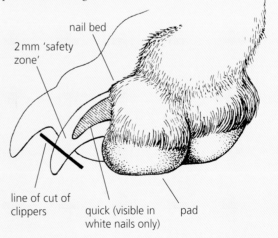

Minor problems with the anal sacs are very common (see later).

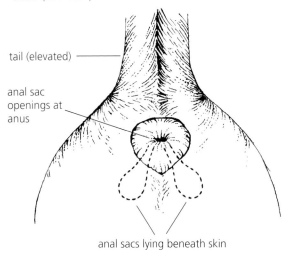

tail (elevated)

anal sac
openings at
anus

anal sacs lying beneath skin

Position of the anal sacs, which lie underneath the skin on both sides of the anal opening.

Caring for Your Dog's Skin and Coat

Should I bath my dog?

Since dogs sweat very little, they do not need bathed as often as people. The skin and hair of a normal dog remains clean and healthy with dry grooming by the dog (and owner). In fact, excessive bathing can be detrimental as it can strip the hair coat of natural oils and possibly dehydrate the skin, especially if strong substances are used.

Of course, there are situations where a bath is definitely necessary – some dogs have a tendency to roll in offensive things while out walking (a behavioural action designed to mask their own scent) and in these situations a bath is required for social reasons! Other dogs with skin conditions may need regularly bathing with prescribed shampoos. But for most dogs, a bath every two to three months is more than adequate.

Unless instructed otherwise by your vet, a mild hypoallergenic shampoo is best.

Perfumed shampoos designed for human use are likely to be very unpleasant for dogs with their much more acute sense of smell; also, these shampoos are designed for human skin, which has certain differences from canine skin. Therefore it is best to keep a bottle of mild hypoallergenic dog shampoo to hand for occasional baths if needed; these shampoos are available from most veterinary practices.

When bathing a dog, remember:

- Lukewarm water should be used. The bath temperature that a person might enjoy would be highly uncomfortable for most dogs.

- Avoid the head, eyes and ears area.

- A shower head is very useful, especially in rinsing, which must be thorough.

- Towel-dry thoroughly afterwards. Some dogs will tolerate a hairdryer, but again this should not be too hot.

- Take care when lifting dogs into and out of baths: some dogs tend to struggle and may panic on a slippery surface, so use a towel or rubber mat in the bath itself to provide a firm footing.

Grooming routine

Grooming is a useful exercise, not just for keeping the coat healthy, but also as a means of reinforcing basic

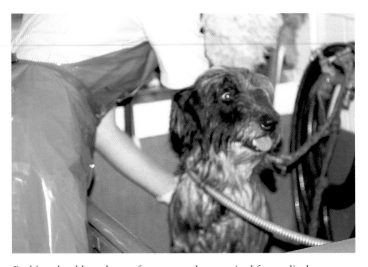

Bathing should not be too frequent, unless required for medical reasons.

training in sitting still and being handled. Grooming shouldn't be a 'game', it should be performed quietly and calmly and the dog should not object to being moved around for different body parts to be dealt with. Dogs that are regularly groomed in this way tend always to be calmer in the veterinary surgery as they are used to being handled.

Breeds vary enormously in the amount of grooming they require. Short-coated dogs require far less, although it should still be performed in these dogs since it allows the owner to check the dog thoroughly for potential problems such as small skin wounds or growths.

Various grooming tools are available for different coat types. In general, long or dense-haired dogs should be groomed 'little and often' rather than subjected to prolonged sessions every now and again. Many of these breeds may occasionally be clipped to conform to breed standards or to keep dense coats under control.

 Summer clip

Old dogs with long, dense hair often benefit from a short clip in the summer months as it prevents overheating.

If you encounter mats, these are better teased out with a comb or removed using grooming clippers. Scissors carry the risk of accidentally wounding the skin, as it can be extremely difficult to identify the skin clearly if heavy mats are present. Severely matted dogs are best clipped out professionally by a dog groomer.

Eyes and ears

Eye wipes or ear cleaning drops are not needed in most dogs, and if any condition of the eyes or ears is suspected a veterinary surgeon should be consulted. Some dogs with deep-set eyes (e.g. Dobermans) accumulate mucus in the corners of the eyes. This is quite harmless and can be removed with a cotton swab dampened in saline or water. It is best for a veterinary surgeon to check over the eyes first to confirm that this is the problem as infections can appear in a rather similar way in some dogs.

Yorkshire Terriers and other small breeds may also accumulate matter at the eye corners. This can be removed in the same way and is best done daily. If the material is allowed to dry and harden, removal becomes much more difficult.

Dogs which accumulate hair within the ear canals (especially Poodles) should be checked carefully at each grooming session. It is often possible to keep this under control by gently pulling out any hair seen with dry fingers but if a great deal is present, the task is better performed by a professional groomer or at the veterinary surgery (sometimes sedation is needed for this uncomfortable procedure).

Anal sacs (see page 95)

In dogs that are prone to developing full anal sacs, and if infection is not a problem, the veterinary surgeon may show the owner how to express these glands safely. It is a fairly simple – if unpleasant – procedure and many owners prefer to let their veterinary surgeon do it.

Teeth

A useful part of the grooming routine is to check the teeth, gums, tongue and lining of the lips for signs of disease or injury. Tooth brushing should be carried out (as described on page 32) and any abnormalities in the teeth or mouth reported to the veterinary surgeon.

Reward the dog!

Don't forget to reward your dog well when it has sat quietly to be groomed, inspected or have teeth brushed.

Veterinary Diagnosis and Treatment

Close examination of the skin can usually suggest a diagnosis to the veterinary surgeon, though often some tests may be carried out to confirm this. Common tests on the skin include:

- Examination of coat brushings or hairs plucked from the skin

- Skin scrapings

Helping the vet diagnose your dog's skin problem

So many different things can cause skin disease that it is helpful to give some thought to possible causes before your appointment at the surgery. If the veterinary surgeon asks any of these questions, you will then have the answers ready.

• Is this the first time the condition has occurred or has your dog suffered skin disease before?

• Are the ears or feet affected?

• Have you any other animals in the house, or have there been any new additions recently? Do any of these animals have symptoms of skin disease?

• Do any people in the house have symptoms of skin disease?

• Have carpets been changed recently or treated with chemicals/shampoos?

• Has different bedding material been used for your dog or have you changed brand of washing powder?

• Has your dog's diet been changed?

• Has your dog been treated for fleas?

• Is your dog bathed frequently? If so, what product is used?

• Have you recently moved to a new area?

• Are there any other symptoms present, apart from the skin ones?

The answers to several of these questions may point the way towards a diagnosis for more complicated causes of skin disease.

Don't ignore skin problems in the mistaken belief that they are not serious. If neglected, very lengthy courses of treatment may be required to put them right and in the meantime the dog will suffer considerable discomfort. Anyone who has suffered from an itchy, painful rash will confirm how unpleasant this can be.

• Skin biopsies

• Blood tests to check hormone levels

• Allergy sensitivity tests

Skin scrapes and biopsies (and allergy tests) usually require sedation to allow good samples or a proper test to be carried out. Sometimes these need to be repeated if an inconclusive result is obtained, or to monitor response to treatments.

Costs and prognosis in skin diseases

In some senses, diagnosing skin disease is easier than disease of other body systems because the evidence is easy to find. The whole organ can be examined easily with the naked eye, not requiring X-rays, ultrasound or other techniques.

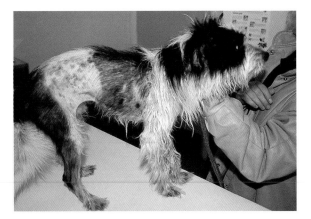

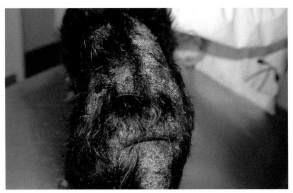

RIGHT, ABOVE *Neglected skin, in this case caused by untreated flea allergy.*

RIGHT, BELOW *The chronically inflamed skin has a thick, hairless appearance and is constantly sore and itchy.*

The problem of scratching

Dogs which scratch their skin excessively can inflict a lot of damage (called self-trauma) which can worsen the skin condition considerably and make diagnosis harder. The problem is the 'itch-scratch-itch' cycle which is set up in many cases of skin irritation. Scratching becomes irresistible to the dog, but this only worsens the problem.

Severe scratching can lead to hair loss, crusting, bleeding and intense inflammation – as well as considerable discomfort to the dog.

Many skin diseases cause pruritis (itchiness) in dogs – there is no single cause. The veterinary surgeon usually needs to do some detective work to find out what has been causing the itch in the first place. Then treatment can be given to deal with the cause and make the dog more comfortable.

itch   **scratch**

Itching leads to scratching, which in turn leads to more itching – a vicious circle.

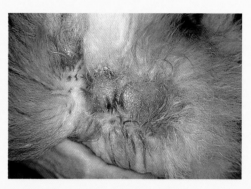

Skin damage caused by constant scratching. Sometimes, the initial damage to the skin remains unknown, but could be a sting, bite or allergy.

Treating skin disease, however, is not always so easy. A few conditions cause chronic problems. Often, these are caused by allergies which cannot be completely eliminated, only controlled. Flare-ups may occur from time to time.

A complete cure is possible for many of the simpler skin diseases, however, and treatment costs are relatively inexpensive compared to other disorders. Short courses of medication are often are all that is required once a definite diagnosis has been made.

Commonest Skin Diseases in Dogs

DERMATITIS

CAUSE Dermatitis means inflammation of the skin. Anything which irritates the skin can cause dermatitis, the commonest causes being:

- Skin allergies
- Skin infections
- Skin parasites (fleas, skin mites, lice)
- Skin fold problems

Most of the conditions in this chapter cause dermatitis of one form or another. Examples of the above problems are considered in more detail below.

SYMPTOMS Affected skin is usually reddened and inflamed and itchy or sore. The dermatitis can be confined to a very small area or else the whole skin surface may be affected. Symptoms are seen most easily where hair is thin, e.g. on the underside of the abdomen. Hair which appears moist and lifted up from the surface of the skin is likely to be lying over an area of severe dermatitis or a burn.

DIAGNOSIS In every case the veterinary surgeon aims to find out what has caused the dermatitis and to treat that. Common causes include flea irritation (probably the commonest) and acute moist dermatitis ('hot spot') seen in the summer months and following a bite, sting or allergic reaction. Less common causes include food allergy and contact allergy from lying on something which provokes an immune hypersensitivity reaction.

Another very common cause of dermatitis in dogs is atopic disease (see page 86).

TREATMENT Whenever the underlying cause is discovered this is treated and usually leads to prompt disappearance of the symptoms. Sometimes anti-inflammatory treatment in the form of creams, tablets or injections is also given to ease the intense discomfort in severe cases whilst waiting for the other treatment to take effect.

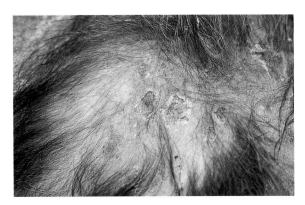

Dermatitis caused by an allergy to pollens.

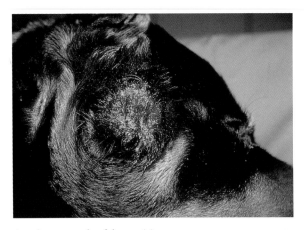

Another example of dermatitis.

Dogs suffering from the painful and irritating condition of acute moist dermatitis (or 'hot spot') often benefit from having a wide area around the sore and inflamed skin clipped free of hair. This allows easy application of any shampoo treatments. This condition should never be neglected as it is unpleasant and can spread quite rapidly.

Correct use of medication

Always ensure you complete the full course of medication in skin diseases. It is common practice to treat severe skin infections for a long time, often well after the symptoms have disappeared. This is to try and achieve an effective cure since if bacteria are not totally eliminated the problem could recur, even although the initial symptoms are no longer present.

OUTLOOK The outlook is good for most cases of dermatitis. That caused by allergy, however, may need on-going treatment to keep it under control and that caused by abnormal skin folds requires surgery for a permanent cure.

Parasitic Diseases

FLEAS

CAUSE Fleas are by far the commonest cause of dermatitis and skin problems in dogs, and are not restricted to stray or neglected dogs: any dog can pick up fleas. A great deal of skin disease is caused by fleas each year, despite increased efforts to control these parasites. The flea, however, is an adaptable animal and seems to be able to stay 'one jump ahead' of many products designed to control it.

Fleas in general are not particularly fussy about which animal they choose for their host and, in fact, it seems that the flea most often found on dogs is the cat flea, *Ctenocephalides felis*, rather than its dog cousin, *Ctenocephalides canis*. The dog flea is slightly more selective in that it rarely causes problems in cats and,

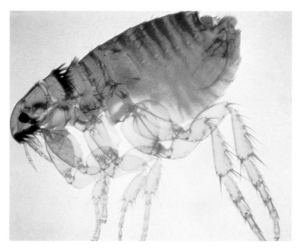

The cat flea – a very common cause of skin problems in dogs.

SYMPTOMS The main symptom is itchiness, and fleas can cause an intense reaction in sensitive dogs. The problem is that not only does the bite of the flea cause discomfort, but dogs which are repeatedly bitten may develop a hypersensitivity (allergic) reaction to flea saliva. They then become ultra-sensitive to future bites, a few bites sparking off a marked skin reaction and persistent itch. Thus there may be very few fleas around but the dog's reaction to them is exaggerated. A dog certainly need not be 'crawling' with fleas to show severe symptoms because of them, and great vigilance with flea control is needed in dogs which are prone to flea bite hypersensitivity reactions.

DIAGNOSIS Dogs with severe flea reactions often have a characteristic distribution of skin problems, which tend to be worse along the flanks and on the top of the body around the tail base. The skin here may be red, flaky and with scabs due to constant scratching. Hair loss will be seen. Touching the area may provoke skin twitches or a bout of scratching. Secondary skin infections are common. Less severely affected dogs may just be scratching more than usual, without any of the more pronounced signs that develop without treatment.

If a live flea is seen crawling over the skin, then the diagnosis is simple. It can be assumed that many more fleas and their larvae are present in the dog's environment. More often, live fleas are not seen but flea dirt is detected. Flea dirt consists of small granules of black material lying close to the skin surface. When some of this is placed on a white background and moistened, it blots out a reddish colour – indicating digested blood, which the flea has acquired from its host. The 'flea dirt' test provides conclusive evidence for an infestation.

TREATMENT The fleas both on the dog and in the home must be eliminated. Just treating the dog is unlikely to be successful in severe cases. To understand why, the complete life-cycle of the flea must be understood (see the diagram on page 78).

Careful combing with a flea comb will remove fleas, but it is a time-consuming and unpleasant task. A better solution is to obtain an effective flea-control product from a veterinary practice. Examination of

in dogs, it is commoner in those housed in kennels than in domestic pets. Occasionally other species of flea may be found on dogs, including the hedgehog one and even the human flea, but these are much rarer.

Flea infestation used to be a seasonal problem, worst in summer and autumn, but changes in human living conditions (especially fitted carpets and central heating) mean that fleas are able to survive year-round in our houses, and cause year-round problems for our dogs. It is however still worse in the warmer months.

 Can pet fleas infest people?

As mentioned, many fleas (unlike lice) are happy to land on and bite any animal and quite often dog owners whose pets have fleas may suffer an occasional bite themselves. A heavy infestation in the house could mean repeated bites, which are uncomfortable and itchy. Note that sarcoptic mange (scabies) in dogs can also affect owners – see page 80.

Fleas don't live permanently on their host (again, unlike lice). They spend much of their time in dark corners of our houses, breeding. This is why it is not always possible to demonstrate live fleas on a dog suffering from flea infestation, but usually other evidence is available (see Diagnosis).

Flea life cycle

Adult flea

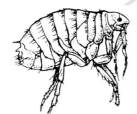

Adult flea seeks a host
to suck blood

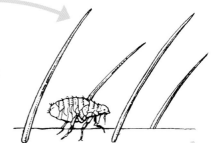

Flea bites dog, sucks blood, and causes
skin irritation (*note:* the flea only stays
on the dog for a few minutes at a time)

Larvae pupate
into adults

Larvae feed on debris
and adult flea faeces,
and moult twice

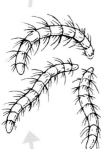

Flea moves on to another
host (dog, cat or human)
and feeds from it

Moulting and pupation
depend on temperature. In
warm houses the complete
cycle can occur in three
weeks; in cold conditions it
can extend to two years

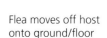

Eggs hatch into larvae
on ground/floor

Flea moves off host
onto ground/floor

Eggs laid in environment
e.g. crevices in house, under
carpets, etc. (*note:* most of
the flea's time is spent in the
environment [the house])

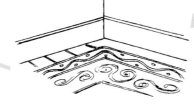

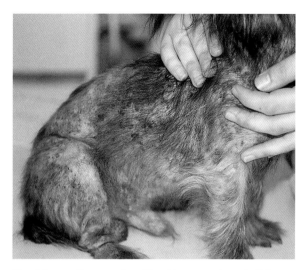

Flea bite reaction on a dog. The skin was extremely itchy.

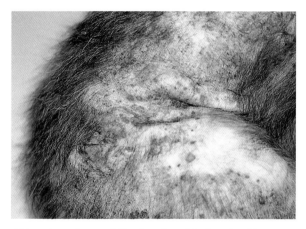

Although no fleas could be found on this dog, the skin problem disappeared when flea treatment was used, indicating that there were fleas at home. A cat was present in the house.

the dog's skin will also be required to assess whether additional treatment for skin reactions or infection is needed, or to control itch. Dogs which have severe rashes caused by fleas will almost certainly require additional medication to alleviate their skin discomfort while the flea control products are working.

Although flea products may be purchased 'over the counter', these may not be as effective as prescription products, nor as simple to use, and long term costs could be higher if they prove ineffective. Veterinary prescribed products come in the form of sprays, or drops, and also tablets to prevent future outbreaks by

No fleas, no flea dirt...

Sometimes fleas can still be the problem! As mentioned earlier, dogs which are hypersensitive to fleas only require a few bites to trigger off a severe reaction. Minute traces of flea dirt can be very difficult to find in long-haired dogs, though grooming dogs while they are standing over a sheet of white paper may help identify it.

Dogs which have been recently bathed may have had all the flea dirt washed out of their coats and appear free of signs of fleas in the veterinary clinic – but an army of the parasites could be waiting for the dog at home.

Dogs may also groom out small amounts of flea dirt themselves.

Tips to help eliminate fleas

- *All* dogs and cats in the house must be treated, even if only one is showing symptoms as the other animals could be acting as reservoirs of infestation. Each animal requires the correct product and dose for its species, age and weight.

- The house and car must also be treated using appropriate products designed to kill fleas and the developing flea larvae. Follow all product instructions to the letter.

- Vacuum the house shortly after insecticide has been applied and dispose of the vacuum bag immediately.

- Thoroughly wash the dog's bedding and spray this with insecticide (air well before use again).

- Prevention of further infestation is possible by carefully combing the dog's coat regularly and re-treating at the first signs of fleas or flea dirt; alternatively, flea prevention products can be given to the dog and/or the house intermittently sprayed.

prevention of flea breeding cycles. Since fleas act as intermediate hosts for the dog tapeworm *Dipylidium* (see page 119), the veterinary surgeon may recommend routine tapeworm treatment if the dog has not been wormed for some time.

OUTLOOK The outlook is good provided veterinary advice is sought and all instructions carefully followed. Even when the dog has suffered from a heavy infestation, improvement in the skin will occur although it may take several months before all signs of the damage have disappeared.

SARCOPTIC MANGE (SCABIES)

CAUSE This disease is caused by a microscopic mite which lives permanently within the top layers of the skin (unlike the flea which only visits the host to feed, spending the rest of the time in carpets, crevices etc). Sarcoptic mange is highly contagious and is easily transferred between dogs. The mite burrows through tunnels created in the upper layers of the skin, where it deposits its eggs.

> ### ⚠ Risk to people
>
> Sarcoptic mange can be transferred to people and owners of affected dogs quite often have symptoms. Small circular areas on the skin are red and intensely itchy. Medical advice should be sought for any itchy skin condition when the dog is also affected. The veterinary surgeon can provide any necessary information for the family doctor.
>
>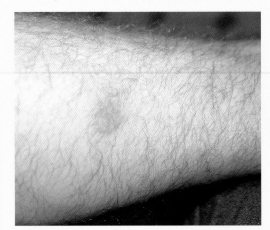
>
> *Sarcoptic mange (scabies) on the arm of an owner whose dog was affected. The area was very itchy but cleared up rapidly with treatment from the doctor.*

SYMPTOMS Sarcoptic mange produces a particularly intense itch caused by a hypersensitivity reaction to the secretions which are produced by the mite. Affected dogs can damage their skin quite badly by relentless scratching and rubbing. Often, the ear tips, elbows and hocks are the areas most affected initially but if neglected symptoms can spread over the entire body surface.

Dogs can become debilitated by this unpleasant disease. Weight loss and listlessness may be seen and secondary skin infections can develop. The condition is often seen in young dogs that have been neglected but any age group can potentially become infected.

DIAGNOSIS This requires a skin scraping, in which adult mites or their eggs can be seen. It is usual to take several scrapings from different areas. Sometimes, although no mites or eggs have been found, the dog may be treated for the condition if the symptoms fit, as locating mites or eggs may be difficult.

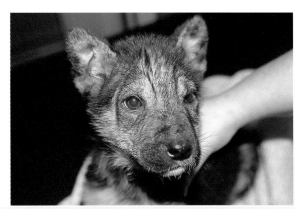

This puppy tested positive for sarcoptic mange.

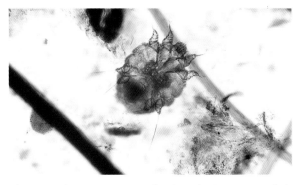

The cause of sarcoptic mange, the tiny mite Sarcoptes scabei.

TREATMENT The condition usually clears up once drugs are given which kill off the mites, though it can take many weeks for severe hair loss and skin thickening to settle down. Some dogs also have bacterial skin infections which will require separate treatment. Treatment of the house may also be recommended, though this less important with mites than with fleas.

OUTLOOK The outlook is good provided treatment recommendations are adhered to.

HARVEST MITES AND 'WALKING DANDRUFF'

CAUSE Two less serious mites can also cause itching in dogs. These are non-burrowing mites, living on the skin surface and feeding on skin cell debris. Harvest mites (berry bugs) are common in certain parts of the country in late summer. With these creatures, it is only the developing larval stages which are parasitic; the adults do not feed on animals. The scientific name for this mite is *Neotrombicula autumnalis*, which describes the time of year in which it is prevalent.

'Walking dandruff' is the common name given to the condition caused by one of three mites affecting dogs, cats and rabbits. Their correct family name is *Cheyletiella*.

SYMPTOMS Harvest mites can cause an intense itch, usually on the feet or underside of the abdomen. 'Walking dandruff' causes a scaly coat that is somewhat itchy. Some dogs don't seem to find this condition itchy, others do.

DIAGNOSIS In affected areas, the seasonal occurrence of harvest mite is very predictable. The condition is also well known among gardeners; after a spell in the garden in late summer/early autumn an itch on the legs or waist area is felt. The larval mites can often be seen between the toes of affected dogs or in the skin folds at the edges of the ear flaps: they are tiny orange dots, just visible to the naked eye, often appearing as clusters.

With 'walking dandruff', the pale mites are sometimes seen to move across a dark surface if they are brushed onto this (hence the name). More often, they are diagnosed using a sticky tape technique: the veterinary surgeon applies clear sticky tape to the coat and then examines this for adults or eggs under the microscope. Note that these mites can also cause irritation to owners, often on the arm areas.

TREATMENT Veterinary insecticidal preparations are effective against both of these parasites. Harvest mites quickly disappear after the first frost in September. With 'walking dandruff', it is also helpful to vacuum the house and use an insecticidal house spray sold for flea prevention, as these mites can live off the host for a short time.

OUTLOOK The outlook is good with both of these parasites.

DEMODECTIC MANGE

CAUSE This potentially serious form of mange is caused by *Demodex canis*, an elongated cigar-shaped mite that lives deep within the hair follicles in dogs' skin.

All dogs have *Demodex* mites within their hair follicles, transmission having occurred from the dam at the time of suckling. They cause no symptoms when their numbers are small. It is not yet fully understood why some dogs develop increased numbers of *Demodex* mites and show symptoms. This may be related to functioning of the immune system, and could be in part a hereditary phenomenon.

SYMPTOMS Symptoms can be restricted to small areas of skin, or be widespread. Localised symptoms are seen most in young dogs, less than a year of age, and generally cause hair loss and skin reddening on the face and front legs. Unlike sarcoptic mange, the condition is not particularly itchy. Widespread symptoms cause general skin disease with hair loss, reddening, crusty skin areas and severe dermatitis. Dogs affected can become depressed, and may run a high temperature and be reluctant to eat. Severe swellings and ulcers on the feet may develop and secondary skin infections are common.

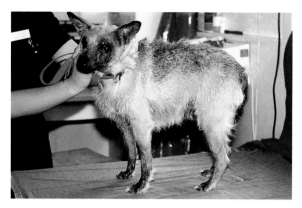

Dog with demodectic mange. This condition is less itchy than scabies.

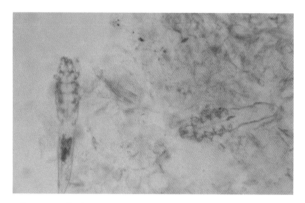

The mite which causes demodectic mange, Demodex canis, *seen here in a skin scraping from an affected dog.*

DIAGNOSIS Skin scrapings are taken to identify the mites. Sometimes biopsies are also used. Tests for severe skin infections may also be called for.

TREATMENT Most cases of localised infection clear up on their own accord after several weeks and treatment may or may not be carried out on these cases. A few dogs which have local symptoms, however, can worsen into the generalised form. Treatment of generalised demodectic mange is a major undertaking and may involve medicated baths or repeated injections of drugs to kill the mites. Additional treatments for severe bacterial skin infections may also be required.

If baths are used, affected dogs may need to be completely clipped of hair and then undergo weekly dips in special preparations designed to penetrate the skin and kill the mites.

For all treatment types, repeated skin scrapings are taken to check progress and treatment is continued for a number of weeks after improvement is seen to try to ensure a complete cure. Treatment may need to be continued for several months in total.

OUTLOOK This is a serious disease of dogs and worst affected patients may require on-going treatment. In some cases the outlook can be very poor and euthanasia may be required on humane grounds.

 Prevention

Dogs with severe demodectic mange should not be used for breeding as there is some suggestion that the tendency to the disease may be inherited.

LICE

CAUSE Two forms of lice affect dogs: biting lice and sucking lice. Biting lice are commoner. Unlike fleas (but like mites) lice spend all of their life on their chosen host. Lice are also very host-specific parasites, i.e. each species of louse tends to stick to the host it has adapted to live on and rarely goes onto another animal. The dog louse stays on the dog and the cat louse stays on the cat. The human body louse is also restricted to people.

Lice get transferred when animals brush against each other or by using grooming utensils which are contaminated with hairs bearing eggs (nits).

SYMPTOMS Lice cause fairly varied symptoms, from almost no irritation to quite severe scratching and skin disease and, in very heavy infestations, even anaemia from loss of blood by the host. This is commoner in neglected puppies.

DIAGNOSIS Examining plucked hairs with a magnifying lens may reveal the eggs (nits) which are cemented onto the shaft of the hair, or else adult lice may be seen.

TREATMENT Lice are easily treated using veterinary insecticides or shampoos prescribed by the veterinary surgeon.

OUTLOOK The outlook is good and a complete cure can be expected after diagnosis.

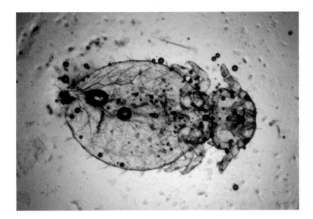

The dog louse lives on the coat surface, unlike mites which bury into the top layers of the skin.

RINGWORM

CAUSE Despite the name, these parasites are fungi, not worms. Several species are found on dogs. Ringworm is more often seen in young animals (with developing immune systems) or in old, sick or debilitated animals where resistance to infection is lowered.

SYMPTOMS Symptoms are areas of hair loss and reddness/inflammation with skin flakes. This does not always have to be in a 'ring' pattern, but usually the edges of the affected area are clear-cut. The affected areas gradually get larger. Itchiness can be present.

Jack Russell Terriers can be affected by a species of ringworm commonly found on hedgehogs. This causes severe inflammation and crusting around the face and muzzle areas, and possibly elsewhere on the body.

DIAGNOSIS Hair samples are taken for examination and culture and if ringworm is grown, a positive

> **⚠ Risk to people**
>
> Ringworm on pets can affect people, and medical advice should be sought if you or any family members have skin symptoms at the same time as your dog.

diagnosis can be made. Some ringworm species show fluorescence under ultraviolet light, so performing this test on a suspect dog may aid in the diagnosis.

TREATMENT Clipping of the hair may be carried out and, in severe infections, a complete body clip may be required. Treatments are either applied onto individual areas of the skin when these are few in number, or else given as tablets in more serious cases. Treatment often needs to be carried on for many weeks as ringworm can be a difficult condition to cure completely.

OUTLOOK Most cases can be cleared up but lengthy treatment is required. Repeat tests are usually necessary to confirm that the condition has in fact gone. Certain ringworm treatments cannot be given to pregnant animals.

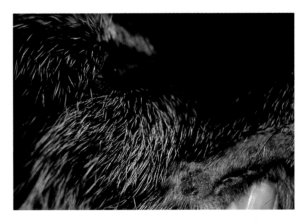

Small itchy area of ringworm on the face of a dog.

TICKS

CAUSE Ticks are small blood-sucking parasites which attach themselves onto the dog, grow in size as they commence feeding over several days, and then eventually drop off to complete their life cycle. A variety of different species can be found on dogs throughout the world. The sheep tick is common in dogs in the UK that are walked in the countryside and several may be found on a dog at once, quite often around the muzzle, neck and shoulders area.

SYMPTOMS Often, the dog seems unaware that a tick is present but they can also cause some irritation and reddening around the attachment site. A reactive area can sometimes be seen where a tick has been removed: the dog develops an immune reaction to substances in the tick's saliva which result in the formation of a nodule.

DIAGNOSIS Diagnosis is usually quite simple. Sometimes, owners think their dog has developed a 'skin growth' when the problem is in fact a large engorged tick.

TREATMENT Ticks should be removed when they are seen. They should be gently pulled using gloved fingers; forceps or tweezers applied near the head area can also be used. Alternatively, insecticidal products from the veterinary practice can be applied. The ticks will then drop off once these products have taken effect.

Many owners prefer to let their veterinary surgeon or nurse remove the tick, however simple tick removal

The sheep tick

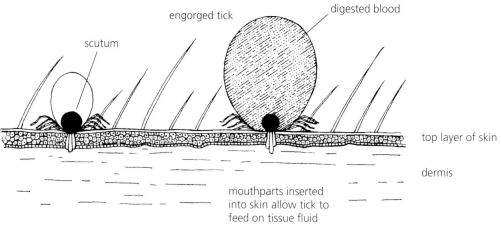

engorged tick

digested blood

scutum

top layer of skin

dermis

mouthparts inserted into skin allow tick to feed on tissue fluid

Ticks are often found in areas where there are sheep. They attach firmly to the skin and drop off once they have engorged themselves with blood (usually after 1-2 weeks).

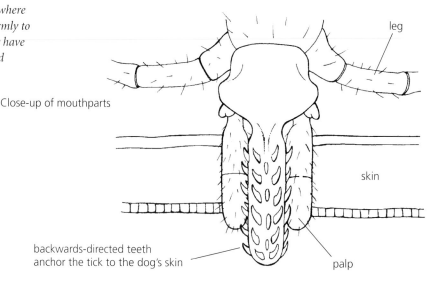

Close-up of mouthparts

leg

skin

palp

backwards-directed teeth anchor the tick to the dog's skin

devices are now available which make extraction of the tick straightforward and painless.

PREVENTION Several veterinary preparations provide good protection against ticks and can be applied before the period of exposure to ensure no ticks will attach themselves onto your dog.

Hazards of ticks and their removal

As can be seen in the diagram opposite, ticks lodge themselves very securely onto the skin via their mouthparts. This means they are not easily dislodged whilst feeding on the host.

On attempting removal, it is theoretically possible that the body is pulled off and the mouthparts remain under the skin, forming an abscess, and this is often mentioned as a hazard of tick removal. In fact, it doesn't occur very often at all if reasonable care is used. The small nodule that may form after removal is more likely to be a reaction to the tick's saliva than to retained mouthparts.

A more serious hazard is the potential that ticks have to transmit blood-borne diseases. Several diseases are transmitted in this way, including Lyme disease, which causes high temperature, lameness and lethargy in affected dogs. The disease is usually treatable with antibiotics and should be suspected if symptoms are present around the time of tick exposure. The risk of Lyme disease is a good reason to remove ticks whenever they are seen and to take preventive action (see above) if going to a place where ticks are likely.

INSECT STINGS AND BITES

CAUSE Bites or stings by other insects, e.g. midges, bees, wasps, etc.

SYMPTOMS In dogs, usually the face/muzzle area and forelimbs are affected. Soft swellings develop; if near the eyes, the eyelids may become involved and the eye may be held closed.

DIAGNOSIS The symptoms are fairly characteristic, allowing a diagnosis to be made even if an insect is not seen to sting or bite the dog. Quite similar symptoms can arise after contact with plants to which the dog develops an allergic reaction (urticaria), and the treatment is similar.

TREATMENT Anti-inflammatory drugs are often given to reduce the swelling. Cold compresses also help.

Several helpful homoeopathic remedies for stings are given in Chapter 18.

OUTLOOK Good. The only risk is if the sting occurs within the mouth/throat area, in which case veterinary attention should be sought immediately and care taken to ensure that breathing is not restricted (see Chapter 18). Rarely, a severe anaphylactic reaction may develop after an insect sting, as in people.

HOOKWORM

CAUSE This is a fairly uncommon condition resulting in dermatitis on the feet caused by the larvae of an intestinal parasite. The larvae, if present in large numbers on the ground, can cause skin irritation, hence the condition is usually only seen in permanently kennelled dogs where run hygiene is poor. (Dermatitis on the feet of pet dogs is more likely to be caused by problems such as skin allergy, foreign bodies or infections in the skin between the toes. See Feet problems, page 98).

SYMPTOMS Reddening and thickening of the skin on the feet is seen and abnormalities in nail growth may occur.

DIAGNOSIS The diagnosis is strongly suggested by dermatitis on the feet of dogs that are housed together in runs, especially if sanitation is poor.

TREATMENT Improvements in run hygiene are required with prompt removal of faeces. Additionally, all dogs should be wormed with a preparation suitable for hookworms.

OUTLOOK Good provided management is improved and all dogs are treated with wormers.

Non-Parasitic Diseases

SKIN ALLERGY

CAUSE The commonest form of skin allergy is called atopic disease or atopy. This term means 'strange disease'. It is common in dogs and is a similar disease to hay fever in people. The allergy causes skin, ear, feet and occasionally other symptoms. Dogs are thought to breathe in the substances to which they become allergic or else the tiny particles suspended in the air are absorbed into the skin directly. Many substances may trigger the disease, including a huge variety of pollens from environmental plants.

Skin allergies can also be caused by foodstuffs and by contact with certain materials which the dog may become allergic to (e.g. wool). Contact allergies are rare in dogs however.

SYMPTOMS Symptoms of atopic disease are first seen in young dogs under three years of age and the main one is itching/scratching. Sometimes only the ears or feet may be affected, i.e. there is little scratching on the body itself. Some breeds are especially prone to atopy.

Breeds prone to atopic skin disease

- West Highland White Terrier
- Staffordshire Bull Terrier
- Golden Retriever
- Labrador Retriever
- Boxer
- Cross-breeds are also affected

Constant scratching/rubbing leads to reddening and thickening of the skin with loss of hair. Severe cases may show black discolouration of the skin. A severe otitis (ear inflammation) or pedal dermatitis (foot inflammation) may occur.

Dermatitis caused by food allergy shows similar symptoms to the above. This can occur in any dog. When contact allergy occurs, the symptoms are worst in those areas of the dog's body that have been in touch with the offending material (i.e. usually the underside of the abdomen and the paws). Skin reddening occurs, with itchiness.

DIAGNOSIS Often, the symptoms will suggest allergic disease, together with the high incidence in certain breeds. Veterinary surgeons may confirm the diagnosis by performing intradermal skin tests. In this procedure, multiple small injections of potentially allergic substances are injected into the top layers of the skin. If the dog is allergic to any of these, a characteristic reaction develops. It is common to find that several substances elicit reactions in dogs tested.

Skin problems caused by food are investigated in the same way as food intolerances causing diarrhoea (see page 115), i.e. an exclusion diet is fed. Diagnosis is not easy, but if food is the main cause of the skin symptoms, or plays an important part, correcting this can mean that treatment of the overall condition becomes more straightforward.

Contact allergies have to be investigated by trying to find out what it is that the dog has been lying on that is triggering the disease. Any changes in carpeting, bedding, washing powder or daily routine may be relevant here.

TREATMENT Skin allergies can sometimes be difficult to treat. They are not life-threatening diseases but do cause significant irritation. Cases definitely caused by foods or contact with allergic surfaces can be cured by avoiding these things. Unfortunately, these causes are the minority: most dogs are allergic to inhaled allergens, usually pollens, and avoidance of these is more difficult unless it is very obvious where they are coming from.

In most cases, good control of symptoms can be obtained using various treatments but complete cures are not possible. Note however that some dogs, especially early in the course of the disease, improve markedly during autumn and winter when there are fewer pollens around. Treatment can be stopped at this time and resumed in the spring and summer if

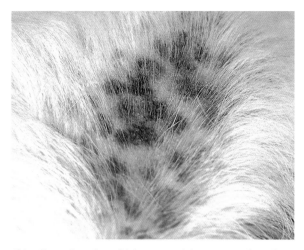

Skin allergy in a dog which was sensitive to a number of grass and tree pollens.

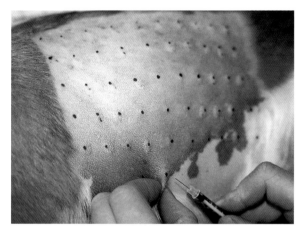

Intra-dermal skin allergy test being performed. Numerous extracts are injected into the skin. If the dog is sensitive to any, an area of local swelling develops. This information can be used to make up desensitising injections to try to limit symptoms.

necessary. Unfortunately, as the dog gets older, symptoms tend to be present all year round.

Various drugs are used to suppress the itchiness, including glucocorticoids (steroids), antihistamines and supplements of essential fatty acids. It is desirable that only the lowest dose of steroid is used, and many dogs can be well controlled on lower doses if other treatments are also employed. Some dogs only require intermittent short courses when discomfort is greatest. Veterinary surgeons tailor the dose to each individual dog as there is no standard treatment for this disease.

In dogs which have received allergic skin testing, it may be possible to give desensitising injections over a period of 6 months to a year to try to reduce the response to the allergic substances. This does not work in all cases but may well result in a lessening of symptoms which can mean that fewer drugs are needed.

OUTLOOK Allergic skin disease is not life-threatening, however symptoms require repeated treatment in most cases.

SKIN FOLD PROBLEMS

CAUSE Skin folds occurring in various parts of the body can lead to dermatitis where skin contacts skin closely, rubs against itself or results in a warm humid environment. The commonest areas affected are:

1. The lip areas (e.g. Spaniels)

2. The face area (e.g. Bulldogs, Pekinese)

3. The vulva area (e.g. obese dogs)

4. The tail area (e.g. Pugs, Bulldogs)

5. The body area (e.g. Sharpeis)

SYMPTOMS The symptoms are of dermatitis. Skin becomes inflamed, reddened, sore and moist. Secretions build up and infection sets in. Ulceration may occur in severe cases and a foul smell may be present.

DIAGNOSIS This is usually obvious upon veterinary examination.

TREATMENT Temporary alleviation of symptoms is possible using anti-bacterial shampoos and washes and various creams, as well as antibiotics. Usually it is beneficial to clip away affected hair to allow the treatments to penetrate better.

Permanent treatment requires surgery to eliminate the pockets of skin which harbour infection. In obese dogs surgery may not be needed if effective weight loss is undertaken.

OUTLOOK The condition is likely to recur if surgery is not performed. Note that surgery may result in changes in appearance which can affect dogs used for showing purposes.

CANINE ACNE

CAUSE The cause of canine acne is not fully understood however the disease causes abnormalities in the hair follicles especially around the chin and muzzle. Larger, short coated breeds are affected most, e.g. Great Dane, Doberman Pinscher, Rottweiler, etc. and acne is seen first in young adult animals.

SYMPTOMS Spots and raised reddened plaques develop on the chin area. These may weep fluid and develop into ulcerated patches. The area is not particularly itchy – most dogs appear to feel no discomfort from the condition.

DIAGNOSIS Skin scrapings are occasionally taken, however the diagnosis is often made on the basis of the age of the animal and the typical symptoms. If skin problems are also present elsewhere on the animal, then acne may not be the cause and further tests would be necessary, e.g. for skin mites.

TREATMENT Usually, medicated shampoos and washes are prescribed. Severe cases, with infection, may be treated using antibiotics. In most cases, the condition clears up over several weeks to months.

OUTLOOK Most dogs eventually 'grow out' of the condition but a few may have repeated bouts throughout their lives.

SKIN TUMOURS/GROWTHS

CAUSE Lumps appearing on or under the skin surface are quite common in dogs and are, understandably, a frequent source of anxiety for owners. They are often noticed incidentally or during grooming, and should always be checked out by the veterinary surgeon soon after they are discovered. Various things can cause swellings: abscesses, foreign bodies (e.g. air gun pellets) and cysts as well as benign and malignant tumours. Lumps arising in the tail and anal area are discussed on page 97. Lumps in the mammary (breast) area are discussed on page 214.

SYMPTOMS Usually there are no symptoms, but sometimes the surface of a skin growth may become red, ulcerated or infected, or the top may be accidentally knocked off, causing bleeding.

DIAGNOSIS It is impossible to say with absolute certainty what a lump is simply by examining it, although simple warts often have a very characteristic appearance in the older dog. Taken together with a dog's clinical history and the rest of a full general examination, informed decisions can be made about how best to approach the problem of an unidentified skin lump.

Many superficial skin growths or those arising under the skin surface are quite harmless and, in older dogs, a decision may be made to simply monitor the lump for a few weeks to see if it is enlarging or changing in any way. This is often the approach used for lumps which the veterinary surgeon considers to be benign or fatty. Often, older dogs have several lipomas (growths of fatty tissue) which do not cause problems and which stay the same for years or enlarge only slowly. Removal of these may not be necessary as they are not life-threatening; also, over time other similar lumps may appear elsewhere.

The problem rests in detecting those growths which are potentially more serious and which require diagnosis or removal. For this reason, you may find that tests or removal and analysis are recommended, to be on the safe side. Tests usually involve biopsies (sometimes using a fine needle and requiring only a mild sedative) or complete removal and analysis, requiring general anaesthesia and surgery.

Occasionally, X-rays and blood tests may also be required to follow up cases suspected of being more serious.

TREATMENT This ranges from simple observation and reporting of any changes in size or appearance, to early surgical removal of a mass suspected of being malignant and dangerous. Whenever a lump is removed, analysis of the tissue by a specialist pathologist is helpful unless it is clear that the growth is harmless (e.g. entirely consisting of fat).

Note that it is common for veterinary surgeons to remove lumps using 'safe surgical margins'. In other words, a wide area around the lump is removed to try to ensure no cells are left behind which could re-grow, so don't be surprised if a relatively small lump results in quite a large surgical wound. In fact, large wounds heal at the same rate as small ones.

Is it a skin tumour and can it be treated?

The words 'tumour' or 'cancer' simply mean a growth of cells, which may or may not be malignant. A large variety of different types of tumour is possible, affecting virtually any cell in the body. Not all of them are dangerous or life-threatening.

Even if a tumour is malignant, it may be potentially treatable if spread to other organs has not occurred. There are also degrees of malignancy, e.g. some tumours are malignant but are slow to spread to other organs. Obviously, these tumours are potentially more treatable than a malignant tumour which spreads to other organs very early in the course of the disease.

Sometimes, however, even a benign tumour may have to be removed quickly if it is near an important area, such as the eye, or if it is constantly getting knocked and damaged or is otherwise causing the dog irritation or discomfort. All such decisions are made on veterinary advice, taking into account individual circumstances. The safest course of action is to assume that any lump is potentially serious, and get it checked out.

Monitoring a skin lump

If a veterinary surgeon decides that a skin lump needs to be monitored over a few weeks or months, you may be asked to keep a check on its size and report back. This can be quite difficult to do objectively, especially if you are worried and tend to check the lump very frequently.

Frequent checks can mean that slow changes in size are not noticed or, alternatively, due to anxiety, you imagine the lump is growing when it is not.

The best way is to measure the lump using a ruler or tape measure in order to put a figure to its dimensions. You can also sketch its outline shape, noting any features on the surface of the lump. Then only check it every few days or every week, and refer to your notes to see if it has changed. Another simple method is to take a photograph of the mass for future reference. You may find that similar records are kept by the veterinary practice.

Most cases of lumps like these turn out to be benign; if the veterinary surgeon suspected something more serious, tests or removal would have been carried out at an early stage. However if monitored lumps appear to be growing, most veterinary surgeons will opt to remove them unless anaesthesia poses special risks for the individual patient.

Some features of benign tumours	Some features of malignant tumours
Appear and grow slowly	May appear and grow more quickly
Loose and moveable	Fixed to underlying or surrounding tissues
Appearance stays the same	Change in appearance
Well demarcated edges	Poorly demarcated edges
Do not spread other than locally	Can spread to distant sites of body and cause disease there
Do not re-grow after surgical removal	May re-grow after surgical removal

CALLUS

CAUSE A callus is an area of very thickened skin which appears immediately over underlying bone; the most usual site for callus in dogs is on the elbow area. In this place the skin thickens because of pressure and friction occurring between the underlying bone, the skin and a hard surface which the dog has been lying on.

SYMPTOMS On the outside of the elbow there is a hairless area of thickened and rough skin (like elephant hide) which may be darkly pigmented. It can resemble a tumour. Callus can also occur in other sites where underlying bone is very close to the surface of the skin, e.g. the hock and chin areas. Dogs lying on hard surfaces are especially prone to the problem.

DIAGNOSIS Although callus can resemble a skin tumour, the characteristic appearance and history usually allow the veterinary surgeon to make the diagnosis without requiring skin biopsies, etc.

TREATMENT The dog's sleeping habits must be changed to ensure a deeply padded bed area is used. Bean bags can be tried, otherwise extra layers of foam padding should be provided. Treatment may be given to reduce the size of the callus and treat any infection present but reduction and size and eventual disappearance usually takes several months.

HAIR LOSS (ALOPECIA) OR POOR HAIR GROWTH

CAUSE Anything which damages the skin may cause hair loss, hence several of the conditions described in this chapter may lead on to this, particularly if they are severe or chronic. Hair loss can be temporary, as it usually is when due to parasites and excessive scratching, or permanent, e.g. after severe burns which obliterate hair follicles. The medical term for hair loss is alopecia.

Dogs may suffer alopecia without any other obvious signs of skin disease, i.e. there has been no skin damage and there is no scratching. In these cases, the loss of hair may be due to underlying hormonal imbalances. Sometimes dogs with these conditions develop symmetrical patches of hair loss on either side of their body on the flanks, or on the tail.

SYMPTOMS Other symptoms of skin disease may be present if skin parasites or infection are present. Hormonal causes of skin disease may have a range of additional general medical symptoms present (see box), but sometimes the hair loss is the only symptom which is easily recognised.

A number of dogs show poor hair growth after clipping (e.g. for an operation). Long after the hair should have re-grown, the outline of the clipped area is visible. In these cases, an undiagnosed condition may be present (e.g. one of the disorders mentioned

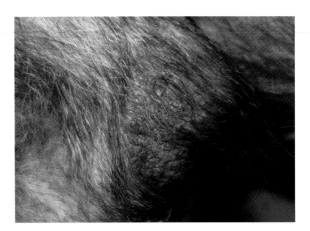

Callus on the elbow caused by lying on a hard, unpadded surface. These areas can be difficult to clear up completely.

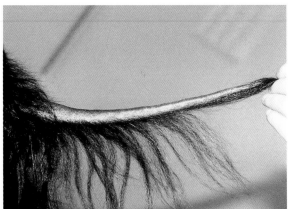

Loss of hair on the tail ('rat tail') in a dog with an underactive thyroid gland.

Some diseases that can cause hair loss with other medical symptoms

Disease	Other possible symptoms
Under-active thyroid gland (hypothyroidism)	Lack of energy; constantly seek warm places; weight gain; 'sad' facial expression
Cushing's disease (involves the adrenal glands)	Drinking to excess and passing excess urine; increased appetite; abdominal swelling; thinning of skin on abdomen; infections
Testicular cancer	Attraction to other male dogs; prostate problems; tail gland enlargement; growths in the anal area
Other hormone-related disorders	A number of other hormonal conditions are suspected to cause hair loss but they are not well understood at present. Several of these conditions may improve after neutering of the dog, but there can be no guarantee that this will occur

above) but sometimes these conditions can be ruled out and the hair growth is still extremely slow. The reason is not fully understood but may be related to a cooling effect on the skin. In most dogs, the hair does eventually thicken again but this can take up to a year.

DIAGNOSIS Diagnosis of hormonal causes of skin disease is not always easy, mainly because there is a wide range of symptoms possible and different constellations of these may appear in different dogs. Most diagnoses are made after specialised blood tests and sometimes skin biopsies.

TREATMENT Several problems are potentially treatable but in some cases this can mean medication for life. Castration of male dogs with testicular cancer or other hormonal cause of hair loss provides a complete cure but it can take several months for symptoms to entirely disappear.

OUTLOOK This varies between the diseases. Improvements in the coat may be slow to occur even when specific treatment is possible.

LOSS OF SKIN OR COAT COLOUR

CAUSE The medical name for this condition is vitiligo. The condition results in loss of pigment within the skin which causes changes to the colouration of the skin itself and the hair coat. The exact cause is not known but it is thought that the body destroys the natural pigment-producing cells for some reason.

SYMPTOMS Loss of pigment is usually seen around the face and muzzle. Normal pigmentation may be lost from the lips and they then appear pink where they had previously been dark. The nose may also be affected (breeders call this 'snow nose'). If the hair coat is affected patches of white or paler hair are seen dispersed throughout the rest of the coat. There are no other symptoms associated with the loss of pigmentation, i.e. the skin is neither itchy nor sore.

DIAGNOSIS This is usually obvious when loss of colour/pigment is seen without any other symptoms of skin disease. Young dogs tend to be affected.

TREATMENT No treatment is effective in reversing vitiligo, but in some dogs the condition disappears on its own.

OUTLOOK In most cases the loss of colour in the skin or coat will be permanent but the condition is painless and causes no problems to the dog.

SKIN BURNS

CAUSE Burns can be caused by hot liquids, fires or electrical appliances. Dogs are protected from minor burns to some extent by their hair coat but even so, all skin burns are potentially very serious – and extremely painful.

Chemical burns (e.g. from acids) can also occur. A particular danger here is that a dog's natural reaction to a burn of this type (e.g. on the paws) will be to lick off the offending substance – thereby causing severe problems in the mouth and oesophagus when the chemical is swallowed.

SYMPTOMS Immediately after the burn, symptoms may not be obvious, especially if masked by the hair coat and if singeing has not occurred (e.g. hot liquid or a caustic chemical has fallen on the dog). Skin damage takes some time to become noticeable, though intense pain will be present from the start. Often, the extent of damage is large and is only properly appreciated once the top skin layers begin to slough (die off). This may take several days.

DIAGNOSIS If a clear history of a burn is not available, close examination of the skin can often suggest that this is what has happened.

TREATMENT Treatment varies depending on severity. Hospitalisation for intravenous fluids (drips) and pain control using potent analgesics is required in severe cases. Sedation is often needed for dressing changes, which in the initial stages may be required twice daily.

Shock is an ever-present threat in badly burned animals, as they are susceptible to dehydration and loss of protein through the damaged skin areas.

Later, once the extent of the damage has been evaluated and initial treatments started, surgery may be required to reconstruct areas of skin loss in order to avoid severe scarring, which can interfere with function around crucial areas (e.g. the eyes, joints, etc).

Treatment of severe burns is often protracted, stretching over many weeks to months, and several operations/courses of treatment may be necessary, as in human burn patients.

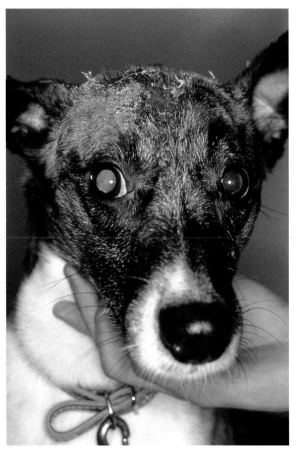

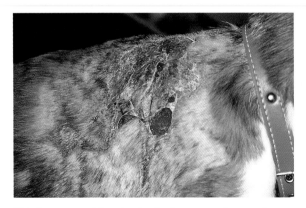

Skin burn caused by a hot kettle. Burns are often much more extensive than they first appear.

Healing burns on the head area.

Burns – vital first aid action to take

- **Chemical burns on body or feet** – Ensure that the dog cannot lick the affected areas. Apply an Elizabethan collar if one is available, otherwise, someone must stay with the dog at all times to ensure it does not lick itself. (This could cause severe permanent damage to the mouth or oesophagus and could also result in liver, kidney or other internal organ damage once the substance is swallowed/absorbed.) Repeatedly drench the contact areas in water to dilute the chemical. Seek veterinary help immediately, preferably with details of the compound concerned, e.g. label from container or other information.

- **Liquid burns** – e.g. hot kettle. Immediately dowse the dog in cool water from a shower head or by gently pouring water over the scalded area. Seek veterinary advice. While transporting the dog, cover the area with cold wet towels and ice packs (e.g. ice cubes or bags of frozen food from freezer).

- **Fire and electrical burns** – Ensure your own safety and that of any other people involved in the incident first. Phone for help. Apply basic breathing and wound first aid to the injured dog (see Chapter 18).

OUTLOOK This clearly depends on the severity of the damage caused. One advantage in dogs is that they have plenty of loose skin, which means that it is usually possible to shift skin from one location to another without too many problems. Thus even quite large areas of skin loss can be repaired, but only once initial treatments have been completed to stabilise wounds and make them healthy. Any skin grafting or 'plastic surgery' procedure always carries some risk of graft failure/rejection and is normally performed 1–2 weeks after the initial injury.

The overall aim is to restore normal function; cosmetic appearance is often helped too but it is not the primary concern. Fortunately, the dog's hair coat often means that acceptable cosmetic results can be achieved as any scars are hidden beneath hair.

SIMPLE SKIN WOUNDS

CAUSE Common causes are bites and injuries caused while the dog is exercising, e.g. from getting caught up on wire. It is also quite common for owners to accidentally injure their dogs while trying to cut off dense mats of hair that are closely adherent to the skin.

SYMPTOMS Most superficial tears are obvious as they will bleed, at least initially. However deep puncture wounds such as bites may not bleed much and, as the entry point is very small, may be surprisingly difficult to detect. Puncture wounds can be important because infection may be introduced and, due to poor drainage from the wound, eventually result in an abscess underneath the skin or in the layers of muscle.

Puncture wounds

Puncture wounds to the chest area should always be considered emergencies as there is a risk the chest wall and lungs could be seriously damaged.

DIAGNOSIS This is usually easy but if multiple puncture wounds are suspected (e.g. after a dog fight), hair may need to be clipped off to reveal the injuries. There is usually considerable bruising surrounding the small puncture wounds.

TREATMENT Larger wounds are normally stitched (sutured) provided they are not too infected. Infected wounds are usually left unsutured to heal more slowly by granulation. If a potentially infected wound is sutured, the veterinary surgeon may insert a drainage device into the wound to protect against build up of infection underneath the stitches. This is normally removed after two to three days. Antibiotics are often used where infection is present or suspected, but are not needed in 'clean' wounds.

OUTLOOK Most healthy dogs heal very quickly, within 7–10 days, but bear in mind that severely infected wounds will take longer and occasionally complications such as wound 'break-down' occur,

Basic first aid for simple skin wounds

1. Don't panic. Most skin wounds are fairly superficial even although they seem to bleed profusely. Only severe major arterial bleeding is likely to threaten a dog's life immediately and this would require major trauma.

2. Slow the bleeding by applying direct firm pressure over the wound for 5–10 minutes. Ideally, cover the wound with a sterile dressing first but in outdoor situations a folded handkerchief or wad of tissue paper will suffice. If there is severe bright bleeding which spurts in pulses and starts up again as soon as you release the wound, maintain hard pressure on the area or apply a firm dressing while you take your dog to the veterinary surgery. A larger blood vessel may have been damaged.

3. Other minor wounds are best covered while you take your dog home or to the veterinary clinic. Wounds on the feet/legs can be covered with a sock or improvised dressing. Those on the body can be covered by a bandage, tee-shirt, etc to prevent further contamination and to help stem bleeding.

4. Very small clean wounds with no gaping skin edges (i.e. 2–5 mm in size) do not require specific veterinary treatment. These can be bathed in saline solution 2–3 times daily and monitored over the next few days while they heal naturally. It is unnecessary to apply antiseptic creams/ointments etc. Anything larger or which appears infected should be seen by the veterinary surgeon as it may benefit from a stitch to close over the edges, or perhaps some antibiotics.

5. Wounds on the foot pads (e.g. caused by glass) are often quite large. These should be checked by the veterinary surgeon as material such as glass fragments may still be present in the wound. These wounds are often sutured and dressings will also be required to protect the area while it heals. Healing of the tough pad takes slightly longer than skin, usually about 10–14 days. Exercise must be severely restricted during this time to avoid stressing the wound while it is healing.

requiring further treatment. Problematic wounds may take many weeks to heal completely. Fortunately, the hair coat of the dog means that unsightly scars are not a significant problem as they are well hidden by the overlying coat.

LICK GRANULOMAS AND PSYCHOGENIC LICKING

CAUSE In this condition dogs continually lick an area of skin in the absence of any known problem in the skin itself. The cause is thought to be an abnormal compulsive activity caused by behavioural/psychological factors. It is possible however that some dogs are suffering from nerve pain, which cannot be readily diagnosed in animals. Similarly, some dogs will lick the skin overlying a painful joint – treatment of the joint pain will often stop the skin licking in these cases.

When as many other factors as possible have been ruled out, the diagnosis of lick granuloma or psychogenic licking may be made, and the cause assumed to be boredom, anxiety or obsessive-compulsive behaviour. Certain breeds seem prone to this problem, and larger numbers of Doberman Pinschers, German Shepherds, Labradors and Great Danes are affected compared to smaller breeds.

SYMPTOMS The usual affected area is the skin on the lower forelimbs in dogs. The area becomes bald, stained, thickened and inflamed and may eventually ulcerate.

DIAGNOSIS Other possible diagnoses will be ruled out first before arriving at this cause. This may entail taking skin scrapes/biopsies and X-rays (to rule out joint or bone pain).

TREATMENT This entails trying to pin-point a source of stress/anxiety, and a wide variety of causes is possible. Many cases are related to changes in routine, to additions or reductions in the household (both animal and human), and to boredom in intelligent dogs. Altering these aspects may improve symptoms.

Otherwise, in obsessive-compulsive disorders, recourse to drug therapy may be required, and this is tailored to individual cases and may possibly need specialist input from veterinary surgeons particularly interested in this type of problem.

OUTLOOK This is a complex disorder and it may prove difficult to isolate a definite cause in every dog. Several different forms of treatment may need to be tried to assess which is the most helpful.

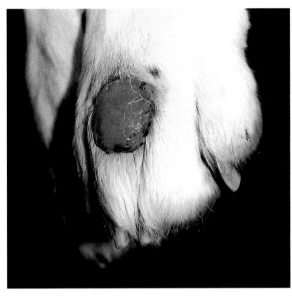

Area of dermatitis caused by excessive licking on the forepaw.

The Tail Area and Feet

ANAL GLAND PROBLEMS

CAUSE The anal glands or anal sacs are two scent glands located under the skin on either side of the dog's anal area, at approximately the 4 and 8 o'clock positions. The small openings for these glands lie internally just inside the anus. Normally, the glands are expressed by the pressure of faeces as these move past the gland openings during defaecation. If this normal emptying of the glands does not occur for any reason, the glands become prone to problems of impaction and infection – a common source of irritation for many dogs.

A diagram illustrating the position of the anal glands is shown on page 72.

SYMPTOMS Irritation and pain at the anal or perineal area is the commonest symptom. Many dogs will sit down and drag their bottom along the ground – a condition veterinary surgeons call 'scooting' and one which is very characteristic of anal sac disease (though many owners think it means their dog needs worming). Excessive licking at the perineal area may also be seen. Simple impaction is the commonest problem and gives rise to these frequently-seen symptoms.

Infections or abscesses in the anal sacs are extremely uncomfortable for the unfortunate dog. Affected animals may 'scoot' as above, but are also likely to be miserable, may yelp whenever the hindquarters are approached or touched and may even be uncharacteristically aggressive to their owners. Odd periods of hyperexcitability may be seen in some dogs if the discomfort becomes too much to bear, resulting in potentially confusing symptoms, but the reason is simply the intense pain and discomfort caused by the infection or abscess which the dog can do nothing to relieve.

DIAGNOSIS This is usually very straightforward but in dogs with severe pain, sedation may be required to allow full examination and treatment.

TREATMENT Simple impaction is treated by manually expressing the glands – a procedure which brings instant relief but also results in a foul smell (the secretion from the glands) being produced.

Infections/abscesses require expression of the glands (usually under sedation or anaesthesia) and specific treatment for the abscess and/or infection itself. This may involve irrigation/flushing of the affected gland under anaesthesia and a course of antibiotics, as well as painkillers in the initial period.

Sometimes, the abscess in the affected gland

Why are some dogs prone to anal gland problems?

The usual causes are:

- Incorrect diet resulting in poor faeces and inadequate natural emptying of the glands. Correcting the diet, e.g. by improving fibre content to promote a bulkier stool, may help. Many 'select' pate-type foods designed for small dogs have a low fibre content and could contribute to anal gland problems.

- Bowel diseases causing diarrhoea or loose-formed faeces. When these conditions are treated or controlled, anal gland function normally improves.

- Obesity: overweight dogs are prone to anal gland disease. Weight loss will help.

- Anatomical problems with the duct of the gland, which mean that normal emptying is interfered with.

- Unknown: some dogs just seem prone to impaction without any obvious underlying cause. Most routine cases probably fall into this category.

Simple impaction, though a nuisance to the dog and owner periodically, is not a serious disease. The usual course of action is to arrange to have the glands expressed whenever symptoms such as 'scooting' are seen. It is a very common problem in pet dogs.

---

ruptures before treatment can be started or completed. Although this results in a lessening of the pain, continued treatment is required to prevent the infection re-establishing. In these cases, gentle bathing of the area and warm compresses are very helpful and are usually well-tolerated by the dog. The ruptured abscess area is allowed to heal naturally without stitches.

In dogs prone to frequent and severe anal gland disease, removal of the glands may be advised. Most dogs however are not in this category.

OUTLOOK Simple impaction tends to be a recurring problem in many dogs, requiring periodic expression of the glands. Some owners are able to perform this task if shown by the veterinary surgeon, but many do not feel confident about it or have no wish to do it.

Dogs prone to diarrhoea or loose faeces (e.g. dogs with colitis, see page 112) tend to acquire full anal sacs since the normal bulk of faeces is not present to encourage natural expression of the glands. The glands require to be emptied but function usually returns to normal once the diarrhoea is improved.

Increasing the fibre content of the diet (e.g. by adding in some unrefined bran or giving the dog raw vegetables) may help the glands to express normally as faeces are passed, though it has to be said this does not seem effective in all dogs.

ANAL FURUNCULOSIS

CAUSE This is an unpleasant condition seen most in German Shepherd dogs. It results in painful ulceration and skin infection under the tail and around the anus. The precise cause of furunculosis is uncertain; several factors may result in an increased tendency to develop the condition. The characteristic low tail carriage of German Shepherds may lead to poor ventilation of the area and thus a higher risk of skin infections developing. Immune system problems may also be involved.

SYMPTOMS Discomfort during defaecation is seen, together with lethargy and signs of pain. On examination, the skin under the tail area is found to be inflamed, ulcerated and sore. A foul discharge may be present.

DIAGNOSIS The condition is easily diagnosed from the symptoms, although sometimes tumours in the area may appear in a similar way. The condition can be so painful that sedation is required for proper assessment.

TREATMENT Various surgical techniques are usually employed including cryotherapy (freezing) and surgical excision of all ulcerated and infected tissue. Usually the anal glands (see above) are removed at the same time. Sometimes amputation of the tail is advocated to increase the ventilation and air flow in the area. This helps limit the humid warm conditions which tend to promote further infection.

OUTLOOK This is a very difficult condition to manage and relapses often occur, even after extensive treatment. Any recurrences should be dealt with promptly.

First aid/home nursing

Twice daily showering of the area with tepid water for 20 minutes at a time can be extremely beneficial and helps promote the development of healthier tissue. A fairly strong water pressure should be used if the dog will tolerate this. Showering several times a week may help prevent future recurrences. Always check with the veterinary surgeon first before commencing showering.

GROWTHS IN THE ANAL AREA

CAUSE Anal growths most commonly arise in response to hormonal influences in older, un-neutered male dogs. Most are benign (adenomas), but malignancy is a possibility. Occasionally, female dogs are affected.

SYMPTOMS Growths are seen in the skin of the anal area under the tail. If these become inflamed and ulcerated they may resemble furunculosis (see above). Bleeding may occur during defaecation or at other times and the dog may experience pain when straining.

DIAGNOSIS This is usually straightforward upon examination of the anal area. Often, anal growths of this type are associated with other, related, problems:

- Enlargement of the tail gland (see opposite)

- Enlargement of the prostate gland (see page 198)

- Testicular tumours (see page 197).

For this reason, additional tests to investigate these possibilities may be recommended.

TREATMENT Small benign growths not causing problems in very old animals may simply be monitored, although in general castration or hormone therapy is the usual treatment and is employed in most cases.

Larger growths causing problems of bleeding or pain on defaecation can be removed surgically provided not too large an area is involved. Castration is usually performed at the same time since this helps prevent recurrences and leads to shrinkage of any unremoved growths.

Removal of very large, deeply embedded growths may carry some risk of incontinence post-operatively.

OUTLOOK Most cases are managed successfully by castration/hormone treatment, but the outlook for malignant tumours in this region is very poor.

ENLARGEMENT OF THE TAIL GLAND

CAUSE This is a common problem, often existing alongside anal adenomas/ growths (see above), and is caused by an excess of male hormones in older un-neutered dogs. It may occur in association with testicular cancer (see page 197). It is occasionally seen in bitches and castrated male dogs, when it may indicate a problem with the adrenal gland.

SYMPTOMS The skin on the top surface of the tail loses its hair and becomes thickened and swollen. The surface of the swollen area may be greasy to touch. There is not usually any pain present.

DIAGNOSIS This is usually straightforward although the veterinary surgeon may also want to examine the testicles, for possible tumours, and the prostate gland (see page 198) in male dogs.

TREATMENT Although hormone injections can be given, castration is the best treatment and will anyway be required if testicular cancer is suspected. Sometimes, shampoos may be prescribed to treat skin problems around the enlarged tail gland if the skin here is particularly greasy and/or infected.

OUTLOOK This is favourable, even when testicular cancer is present, since testicular tumours do not tend to spread early on in the course of the disease. Castration therefore provides a cure in most cases.

FEET PROBLEMS

CAUSE Problems affecting the feet and nails are fairly common in dogs. These may be very simple conditions, such as a torn nail, or else they may reflect more general skin diseases. Common causes of foot problems are:

1. **Parasitic problems**, e.g. harvest mite, demodectic mange, hookworms – these parasites are discussed in detail earlier. Symptoms may be restricted to the feet.

2. **Allergic or irritant dermatitis**. Dogs with allergic skin disease frequently have symptoms on the feet and ears as well as the body generally. Any irritant substance accidentally walked through (e.g. chemicals, salt on roads) may also set up dermatitis or pad irritation.

3. **Infections**. The skin between the toes may become infected, causing reddness and itch/pain. Abscesses can appear. These may be associated with 'foreign bodies', e.g. grass seeds, glass or other objects lodged in the pads or skin. Small wounds can also become infected.

4. **Interdigital cysts** are seen in certain breeds. These appear as swellings between the toes and can rupture and become infected.

5. **Nail problems** may occur due to bacterial or fungal invasion. These can be difficult to clear up, requiring very lengthy courses of treatment.

6. **Immune system diseases**. Some rarer immune system problems show up initially as disease of the nails or the nail/skin junction.

7. **Overgrown** or **broken** nails are a very common and straightforward cause of foot problems in dogs.

8. **Tumours** may appear on the feet. Some foot tumours are highly malignant and spread to underlying bone and elsewhere in the body.

SYMPTOMS Foot pain or tenderness is caused by most of the disorders listed above. The dog may be lame and may frequently lick or bite at the affected foot. The exact cause requires close examination of the foot and, sometimes, the rest of the dog's skin if the problem is a generalised one.

DIAGNOSIS As with skin conditions elsewhere on the body, diagnosis may require tests such as skin scrapes or biopsies. X-rays may be used if a foot tumour or foreign body is suspected. Simple wounds or nail injuries, however, are usually readily apparent and easily managed.

TREATMENT Whenever possible, treatment is directed towards a specific cause of the foot problem. Treatment may be applied locally (in the form of shampoos and washes to the feet) or systemically, i.e. via tablets. Tumours and cysts may require surgery, so too might foreign bodies which have become lodged deep within tissues – grass seeds, in particular, are prone to migrate through tissues from their point of entry and need an operation to try to locate and remove them.

 First aid treatment for the foot

- Always keep foot bandages completely dry. Restrict your dog's exercise to short lead walks and cover the bandage with a plastic bag when out of doors. (Remove the bag when inside again).

- If shampoos/washes are prescribed, make sure they are used thoroughly. In particular ensure that the product reaches all the affected areas between the toes and that the contact time is as given on the directions.

- Excessive licking and chewing at the feet can be prevented using an Elizabethan collar.

- Keep all re-check appointments. Some foot problems require lengthy courses of treatment which are continued for some time after the problem has apparently cleared up in order to prevent early recurrences.

CHAPTER 6

The Digestive System

Common symptoms of digestive system disease
• Vomiting • Diarrhoea • Poor or abnormal appetite
• Weight loss • Constipation/straining • Swollen abdomen

Structure and Function

Many diseases affect the digestive system. Of all symptoms which vets see in dogs, two of the most frequent relate to the digestive (or gastrointestinal) system: vomiting and diarrhoea. Confusingly, these symptoms can be caused by both very mild and self-limiting diseases, but also by some serious and life-threatening ones. Additionally, vomiting can be caused by diseases of other body systems – a common cause of vomiting in old dogs, for example, is kidney disease. Recognition of the potential seriousness of each condition is therefore a major consideration when the vet tries to establish a diagnosis.

Dogs have evolved as meat-eating and scavenging animals and their digestive system is designed to cope with these food sources. Diseases affecting the mouth and teeth are discussed in Chapter 2. This chapter takes up the story from the point at which the chewed food is swallowed. Swallowed food passes through the digestive system in an orderly way, subjected at each stage to the actions of digestive processes, which release nutrients from the food and allow their absorption into the body's metabolism.

General anatomy of the digestive system
(see also chart opposite)

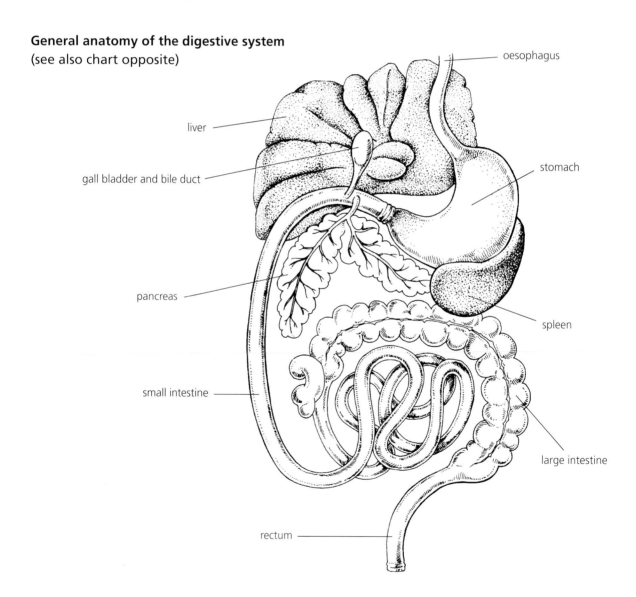

oesophagus

liver

gall bladder and bile duct

stomach

pancreas

spleen

small intestine

large intestine

rectum

Digestive organ	Function	Potential problems (see later sections)
Oesophagus (gullet)	Conveys food from the mouth to the stomach	• Food items (e.g. bones) may become stuck • Inflammation (oesophagitis) can occur if the oesophagus is damaged • Perforation of the oesophagus is life-threatening • Some dogs have swallowing disorders meaning that food does not enter or pass down the oesophagus properly
Stomach	Stores food and starts digestion	• Minor irritations/inflammations • Swallowed objects (e.g. stones, toys) may get stuck • Severe distension and torsion (twisting) occurs in larger breed dogs and is life-threatening • Ulcers, stomach cancer and severe inflammatory diseases • Problems with incoordinated emptying of the stomach
Small intestine	Continues digestion and absorbs nutrients	• Inflammatory disease/enteritis • Swallowed objects may get stuck • Bowel cancer • Worms • Intussusception in puppies
Large intestine	Absorbs water and minerals; stores faeces	• Inflammatory disease/enteritis • Bowel cancer • Constipation/diarrhoea • Perineal hernia
Pancreas	Important in digestion and metabolism	• Digestive diseases • Pancreatitis (inflammation) • Diabetes • Pancreatic cancer
Liver	Vital organ important in digestion and metabolism	• Liver failure – various causes • Hepatitis (inflammation) • Liver cancer

Vomiting and diarrhoea, the two commonest symptoms in digestive diseases, can be caused by problems in most areas of the gastrointestinal tract; they are not in themselves very specific symptoms and vets have to rely on additional information to make the diagnosis in most cases.

Feeding the Dog

Can my dog be a vegetarian?

Unlike cats, dogs can exist on a purely vegetarian diet provided it is properly balanced with respect to essential vitamins, minerals, protein content and fat. If you wish to feed your dog a vegetarian diet, the best method is to buy a complete vegetarian dog food in order to ensure that all the dietary requirements are being met.

Vegetarian or not, probably the safest and most convenient way to feed pet dogs is by using a properly formulated pet food from a reputable manufacturer. Many such foods are available and your veterinary practice can advise on which would be suitable for your dog's age, type and any medical condition, if present.

It is quite possible to feed home-prepared diets, but care must be taken to ensure all nutritional requirements are being met; most pet owners would find this less convenient and if improperly carried out problems could be caused.

Tinned versus dried food

Tinned and dried foods are essentially the same, except that the dried variety has had water removed. Some advantages and disadvantages of both are given in the table below.

A constant source of clean water is required for all dogs but dogs fed on dried food will drink much more than those fed from tins. Note that once a suitable dog food is chosen, it is best not to change around too much between brands and flavours. In many dogs this can promote minor digestive upsets, with vomiting and diarrhoea.

Titbits and treats: to give or not to give?

Owners often enjoy treating their dogs with occasional titbits of human food or dog treats. This only becomes a problem when it interferes with normal eating and dietary balance. Unfortunately, this often becomes the case with small breeds, who very easily learn to manipulate their diet so that they eat almost exclusively human foods or only selected brands and flavours of tinned foods (often small tins of pâté-like meat or cat food).

	Advantages	Disadvantages
Tinned food	Some dogs find it more palatable	Less convenient; more expensive
	Can be mixed with biscuit to give a more 'interesting' meal	May go 'off' in warm weather unless kept in fridge
		Not so good for teeth unless hard biscuit also fed
Dried food	Cheaper; more convenient	Small dogs in particular may not like dried foods
	Better for teeth	Possibly 'boring' to eat
	Easily kept and stored	

Is grass eating abnormal?

Many dogs eat grass occasionally. It is not considered abnormal or signs of a major dietary deficiency, nor is it accurate to say that the dog is 'trying to make himself sick'. It's true that some dogs will retch after consuming grass or tough stems, but by no means all do.

Wild dog relatives also eat grass and other vegetation; they will frequently eat the vegetable material present in the stomachs of their prey animals as well as nibble at growing grass and plants. The reason is thought to be a natural desire to obtain indigestible fibre (which is required for normal bowel function) in animals which, like dogs, are mainly carnivorous.

Feeding raw vegetables (e.g. carrots) occasionally may reduce the frequency of grass eating in some dogs which seem particularly keen on it.

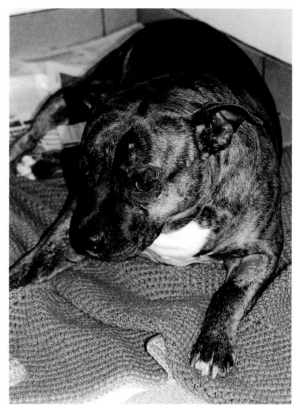

A very overweight Staffordshire Bull Terrier. She dislocated one elbow after falling down a step and then had problems supporting her excessive weight on the remaining three legs.

Even an exclusive diet of good quality human food, such as cooked chicken, is not ideal as though this will be an excellent source of high quality protein, other essential dietary ingredients are missing – fibre and carbohydrate, for example, and certain vitamins. Any single source of meat like this can potentially lead on to dietary or digestive problems.

Dogs which are reliable eaters of normal dog food need not be denied occasional table scraps or titbits within reason, but dogs prone to fussiness may need to be more stringently confined to their own food in order to ensure a balanced overall food intake.

Note that some dogs with specific digestive diseases need to be kept to a very strict diet of special foods. In these animals, even the occasional mouthful of another food may have an adverse effect.

- Early arthritis and mobility problems

- Respiratory and heart disorders

- Diabetes

- Urinary incontinence

- Skin infections

- Increased risks should anaesthesia and surgery be needed for any problem

Overweight dogs should be put on to a carefully controlled diet to ensure a gradual return to optimum weight. This can be achieved by simply feeding less food, or replacing part of the normal food with cooked or raw vegetables. This should ideally be done under veterinary supervision, when guidance as to quantities fed can be given. Cross-breed dogs should

Obesity

Although not strictly a 'disease', obesity (or being overweight) can have serious consequences for dogs, and yet it is very common. Many of the vital body systems suffer when a dog is too heavy for its size, and common problems include:

weigh approximately the same as a pure breed of similar size and stature.

Many food manufacturers produce reducing diets for dogs. These have the advantage of supplying all the essential nutrients whilst still allowing controlled weight loss. Many of these diets have added fibre so that the dog feels satisfied after eating. One of the problems with simply feeding less of a pet's normal food is that the dog may still feel and appear hungry after the meal has been consumed, and may resort to scavenging or bin-raiding.

Veterinary Diagnosis and Treatment

A very important aid to diagnosing digestive system diseases is the information provided by the dog owner concerning their pet's illness. This can often help narrow down a large list of possible diagnoses. It can also mean that further tests are chosen more selectively, saving both time and money.

Important basic questions, which you should try to supply the answers to, are listed in the box.

As with other diseases, a basic examination will be carried out and then decisions made about any further tests. A wide variety of tests are possible

with diseases of the gastrointestinal system, including:

- Blood tests

- X-rays, possibly including barium meals or enemas

- Ultrasound

- Endoscopy and biopsies

- Exploratory surgery

Each of these can reveal the cause in selected diseases, or at least narrow down the range of options to consider.

Cost and prognosis in digestive diseases

Simple gastrointestinal upsets are by far the commonest problem seen in dogs, and they are usually very easily treated. A complete cure is normal and this usually occurs within a few days, requiring no further treatment.

More complicated diseases require further investigation, and this can be expensive because of the complex nature of the gastrointestinal tract and the many places where things can go wrong. A number of these diseases require special management or drugs to

---

 Helping the veterinary surgeon: 10 basic questions

1. When did the symptoms start: days, weeks or months ago?

2. Has your dog encountered the problem before, or has there been any other related problem?

3. Are the symptoms present all the time or only occasionally?

4. Has the diet been altered recently? Have bones been fed or is there a chance an object has been swallowed?

5. Is there any weight loss?

6. Has the dog accidentally or deliberately been given any tablets, e.g. aspirin, paracetamol?

7. Is water intake normal, reduced or increased?

8. Has there been any change in the dog's elmination behaviour (e.g. straining, passing faeces more often/diarrhoea, constipation)?

9. Is there blood in the vomit or faeces?

10. Are any in-contact dogs or people suffering from gastrointestinal disease?

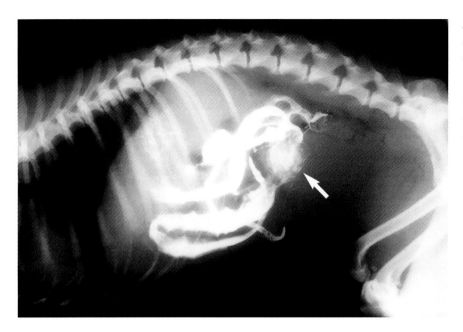

An X-ray combined with a barium meal used to diagnose a dangerous intestinal obstruction. In this case, a peach stone was removed from the dog's small intestine. The arrow shows where the stone was found.

keep them under control, meaning that on-going costs will be involved.

Surgical operations can be expensive but, when successful, can mean that no further treatment is required. Most pet insurance policies would cover this type of treatment and the necessary tests leading up to it.

As with all other body systems, a few diseases are very serious and difficult to cure or even control and some, such as gastric dilation (see page 109), present as life-threatening emergencies. These conditions carry a poorer outlook overall.

Commonest Digestive System Diseases in Dogs

VOMITING/RETCHING

CAUSE Many digestive disorders cause this symptom, from the commonest and mildest to the most severe problems. A variety of diseases which mainly affect other body systems also have vomiting as a sign (e.g. kidney disease, pyometra, poisonings).

Dogs vomit easily; in digestive diseases the cause is usually irritation or inflammation of the lining of the stomach or bowel, or else obstruction to normal passage of food through the bowel. It is important to assess the urgency of vomiting in dogs. In general, vomiting is viewed slightly more seriously than diarrhoea, in that deterioration can occur more quickly, sometimes in dogs that initially appeared very bright.

Is it vomiting, regurgitation or retching?

It is helpful if you are able to distinguish between three similar symptoms: vomiting, regurgitation and retching, as this can often provide valuable clues to the diagnosis.

- **Vomiting**: Semi-digested food is produced a variable time after eating. If the dog has not eaten recently, yellow (bile) stained fluid may be produced. Vomiting occurs when the dog adopts a head-down position and undergoes repeated powerful contraction of the abdominal muscles, eventually culminating in the production of the vomit.

- **Regurgitation**: The food has never reached the stomach. It is brought up soon after swallowing, often in a 'tube' shape, and looks completely undigested. Regurgitation occurs with very little effort or warning, unlike vomiting.

Assessing the severity of vomiting

Mild vomiting

Seek a routine appointment with any of these signs:

- Sporadic vomiting/retching (once or twice daily)

- Gradual onset

- Dog behaves much as normal

- Swallows saliva normally

- Abdomen normal size

- Eats as normal

Severe vomiting

Seek immediate attention with any of these signs:

- Frequent vomiting/retching (more than 4 times daily)

- Sudden onset

- Dog depressed and subdued

- Swallowing problems; drooling saliva

- Abdominal distension

- Will not eat

- **Retching**: Coughing/gagging occurs and some fluid or saliva can be produced. Retching may follow a bout of coughing. It can also indicate a problem in the throat area, as well as disease of the oesophagus and stomach. It may be difficult to distinguish retching from vomiting but no digested or undigested food appears with retching.

This information will greatly help your vet, along with the details discussed on page 104.

SYMPTOMS These are as described in the box. Often, dogs will show agitation just before vomiting, which is probably due to intense nausea. Simple vomiting from mild gastritis/gastroenteritis may be accompanied by diarrhoea.

DIAGNOSIS Simple cases of gastritis (stomach inflammation) and related disorders may need no special tests other than normal clinical examination and checking of the temperature. More serious disorders may require full 'work-up' including blood tests, X-rays, etc.

TREATMENT See under individual conditions. This can range from no treatment other than dietary rest (as described under Diarrhoea), to major surgery.

OUTLOOK Simple vomiting due to gastritis has an excellent outlook. Other conditions are detailed later in this chapter.

DIARRHOEA

CAUSE The most frequent cause is mild dietary upset, perhaps caused by a sudden change of food, raiding the bin, eating rubbish when out for a walk, or receiving too many treats, e.g. at Christmas time. In this case the diarrhoea may be accompanied by occasional vomiting.

More serious causes include inflammatory bowel diseases, problems with absorbing certain foods in the bowel or intolerances to them, infectious causes of diarrhoea (especially parvovirus) and bowel cancers.

SYMPTOMS Affected dogs require to pass faeces more frequently. They may only pass small quantities at a time, despite much straining, and may repeatedly ask to go out, or else soil in the house if they are unattended or overnight.

Mucus (clear jelly-like substance) may be present in the faeces passed and often there is also a small trace of blood.

In bowel cancer alteration between periods of diarrhoea and constipation may be seen, usually also with signs of chronic weight loss.

DIAGNOSIS Details provided by the owner together with clinical examination usually allow a preliminary diagnosis to be made. Further tests, used in serious or chronic cases, may include blood samples, X-rays, examination of stool samples and biopsies.

Simple diarrhoea in the healthy dog

- Withhold food for 12 hours, but allow full access to water (not milk)

- Start feeding with small meals (2–3 tablespoons) of a bland diet, e.g. cooked chicken/ boiled rice, fish/boiled rice, scrambled egg/boiled rice, or a bland prescription diet from your veterinary practice

- Give a small meal every 3–4 hours, gradually increasing the quantity fed and increasing the time between meals

- After 2 days mix a little of your dog's normal food into the bland diet, gradually replacing the bland food with dog food over the next few days

Avoid: milk, raw eggs, uncooked meats, other human foods, dog treats

- *Large quantities of blood, or faeces that appear to consist solely of blood, should be considered emergency situations. Phone the veterinary clinic for advice.*

TREATMENT Uncomplicated cases are normally treated by dietary rest, followed by the feeding of a bland, easily digested food for several days before weaning back onto the normal diet again. Most cases fall into this category. Antibiotics and other drugs are only used if there if a possibility of infection. Severe cases may require hospitalisation for intravenous fluids (a 'drip') and further tests.

OUTLOOK The outlook for simple diarrhoea is excellent.

CONSTIPATION/STRAINING

CAUSE Various problems can lead to constipation and straining in the dog. Note that dogs with diarrhoea also frequently strain to pass small quantities of liquid faeces with mucus present. In constipation, straining is generally unproductive and if severe can be exhausting.

Possible reasons for constipation/straining:

- Impacted dry faeces/bony material in colon

- Change of diet or routine

- Obesity/lack of exercise

- Enlarged prostate gland in male dogs (see page 198)

- Anal gland irritation (see page 95)

- Perineal hernia (see page 115)

- Bone or joint problems which make squatting painful

- Dehydration

SYMPTOMS Dogs attempt to pass faeces with little or no effect. In cases of bony material in the colon or anal gland disease, the dog may yelp as it attempts to pass the faeces. Severely constipated dogs feel miserable and become depressed and lethargic. Chronic constipation can lead to toxaemia and other symptoms such as vomiting.

DIAGNOSIS The impacted colon can usually be felt when the veterinary surgeon palpates the abdomen. Sometimes X-rays are taken. Finding an underlying cause may require additional tests and detective work.

TREATMENT Initial relief is obtained by administration of an enema. Long term control involves treating any underlying causes (e.g. enlarged prostate gland in male dogs) or modifying the diet to promote normal bowel function.

Occasionally the cause of the constipation is something quite unrelated to the digestive system: painful hips may mean that an older dog cannot squat properly to pass faeces, and constipation arises due to lack of regularity in emptying the bowel. Painkillers may cure the constipation in these cases.

Behavioural problems also occasionally may lead to constipation if the dog's elimination behaviour is upset.

> ### Simple first aid for constipation
>
> 1. Adding several tablespoons of liquid paraffin to the food daily may help to relieve symptoms.
>
> 2. Adding bran to the food (1–2 heaped tablespoons daily) may help by increasing roughage and promoting a softer stool.
>
> 3. The veterinary practice may be able to advise on other products which can be administered to promote bowel function and a normal stool.

OUTLOOK This depends on the underlying cause. Constipation caused by incorrect diet normally responds well when a suitable diet is found – this can vary between individual dogs; in many cases, a higher fibre diet is fed. Sometimes allowing these dogs limited access to milk (which can be a laxative in dogs) helps control symptoms.

Constipation arising from other causes may not clear up until the underlying problem is treated.

OESOPHAGEAL DISORDERS

CAUSE These diseases are fairly rare in dogs. The commonest problems include bones (especially chop bones) which have become stuck in the oesophagus, oesophagitis (inflammation) and, occasionally, problems in young dogs where the oesophagus cannot function properly due to abnormal development of large blood vessels in the chest, which prevent the oesophagus from accommodating solid food.

A variety of rarer diseases of the oesophagus are also seen, including hiatal hernia and diseases which cause the oesophagus to dilate to enormous proportions without transmitting food into the stomach (mega-oesophagus). Cancer of the oesphagus is not often seen in dogs.

SYMPTOMS Oesophageal foreign bodies such as bones, and oesophageal inflammation, are intensely painful. Common symptoms include pain, retching blood-tinged saliva, reluctance to eat or drink and a high temperature. Affected dogs look and feel miserable.

Oesophageal problems in puppies are not usually painful but the affected pups regurgitate solid food when they attempt to eat. Poor weight gain may be seen. Regurgitation can be seen in adult dogs with nervous system problems which affect the oesophagus and prevent it functioning normally.

DIAGNOSIS X-rays and endoscopy are the main diagnostic methods in oesophageal diseases.

TREATMENT Oesophageal foreign bodies must be removed, either with the use of an endoscope or, if this is not possible, by means of major surgery.

Oesophagitis can be a problematic disease; it is extremely unpleasant for the animal and hospitalisation for intensive treatment may be required. Treatment may be prolonged and in severe cases permanent damage may result from scar tissue.

Problems caused by abnormal blood vessels constricting the oesophagus in puppies can be treated successfully if caught early enough. Major surgery is required.

OUTLOOK If the oesophagus becomes perforated (e.g. by a bone or other swallowed objects) the outlook can be poor, as animals often rapidly deteriorate from chest complications. Intensive treatment and major surgery is likely to be required and even then, a successful outcome cannot be guaranteed.

STOMACH DISORDERS

CAUSE Stomach disorders are common in dogs and simple gastritis is by far the most frequent one seen. It is caused by mild inflammation of the stomach lining, often triggered by eating unsuitable foods or scavenging.

More serious or chronic forms of gastritis are also encountered; in these, the inflammation can lead onto ulceration, with severe illness resulting. There are various causes including infections, immune system problems and in response to certain drugs (especially drugs related to aspirin).

Foreign objects are frequently found in the stomach of dogs, e.g. bony material, stones, chewed plastic etc. Always alert the veterinary surgeon if you suspect something unusual may have been swallowed.

Some dogs have problems which interfere with normal emptying of the stomach into the small intestine; these are known as gastric motility disorders. There are a variety of causes of this type of disorder and careful diagnosis using specialised X-ray techniques is often employed.

Gastric dilation and volvulus is an emergency condition in which the stomach distends with gas and then twists on itself, causing severe and life-threatening complications. It is seen oftener in large, deep-chested dogs.

Stomach cancer can also be diagnosed in dogs.

SYMPTOMS See also Vomiting on page 105. Most stomach diseases have vomiting as a symptom. The nature and frequency of the vomiting may vary, and other signs may also be present, e.g. the dog with simple gastritis due to dietary upset may vomit several times but otherwise be alert, active and keen to eat, play etc.; whereas a dog with a severe ulcer or tumour will be depressed, lethargic, with a poor appetite and possibly signs of blood in the vomit – these symptoms are likely to have developed over days, weeks or months and will often occur with signs of chronic disease such as poor coat, weight loss, etc.

Dogs with foreign bodies in their stomachs may show no obvious signs unless the object starts to block the exit from the stomach, when repeated vomiting, nausea and weakness will be seen. Sometimes, objects are discovered in dogs' stomachs when they are being X-rayed for quite different reasons, but the potential for an obstruction is always there.

Dogs which have stomach emptying problems can show patterns of vomiting related to food intake – sometimes the dogs vomit partially digested food many hours after feeding, when the food would normally be expected to have passed on into the small intestine. Careful observation and timing by the owner can help considerably in pin-pointing these disorders, which usually develop over a period of weeks to months.

Dilation of the stomach: important signs

- It is seen more frequently in larger and deep-chested breeds of dog, e.g. German Shepherd, Doberman, but smaller breeds can also be affected

- Large meals of dried food or exercise soon after feeding may make the condition more likely

- Repeated retching is seen but no vomit of food occurs; some fluid and saliva may be produced. It often seems as if the dog is unsuccessfully trying to bring up excess gas

- The abdomen swells and becomes tense and drum-like; gurgling noises are heard

- Respirations are shallow, rapid or irregular

- The dog becomes anxious, restless or even collapses

- The dog's condition can deteriorate quickly

Always seek veterinary advice immediately if you suspect this condition.

DIAGNOSIS This depends very much on what your veterinary surgeon suspects may be causing the disorder. Any of the tests listed on page 104 may be used. The most frequent ones are X-rays, endoscopy and blood tests. Sometimes, a substance called barium is used in combination with X-rays (as a barium meal, swallow or enema). Barium shows up very well on X-rays and can be used to outline diseased areas inside the dog more clearly.

More chronic diseases (developed over weeks to months) are rarely immediately life-threatening and a planned sequence of tests may be worked through over a period of a few days to a few weeks before diagnosis is made.

TREATMENT Simple gastritis may only require the sorts of dietary recommendations given on page 107, whereas gastric dilation will necessitate an emergency admission to the hospital and intensive treatment to stabilise and then operate on the patient.

Exploratory surgery may be indicated for other gastric diseases: this allows the surgeon to inspect all areas of the stomach and remove samples for biopsy if required. Surgery is also needed to retrieve foreign bodies from the stomach.

OUTLOOK The outlook is good for simple gastritis and foreign bodies that can be successfully removed. Gastric dilation is an extremely serious condition and few veterinary surgeons will make definite predictions of success when treating this disease as individual cases vary greatly in the extent of damage caused to the stomach, spleen and other organs.

Other disorders have variable outlooks, depending on the duration and extent of disease, but treatment (medical or surgical) is available for most of them.

INTESTINAL DISORDERS – GENERAL

Individual diseases are discussed in following sections.

CAUSE A large variety of diseases can affect the small and large intestine and interfere with the digestion and absorption of food or the normal passage of food through the bowel. Some of these are infectious (e.g. parvovirus), inflammatory (e.g. inflammatory bowel diseases/colitis) or obstructive (e.g. stuck foreign bodies or tumours). In most pet dogs, worms do not often cause serious intestinal disease thanks to regular worming, but occasionally in young dogs or strays a heavy worm burden is seen and can produce severe symptoms.

SYMPTOMS The commonest symptom of intestinal diseases is diarrhoea (see page 106) but vomiting can also occur, and vomiting with diarrhoea is typical of mild gastro-enteritis associated with scavenging or eating unsuitable foods. Chronic small intestinal diseases lead to weight loss and poor overall condition, whereas severe acute diseases can lead to rapid dehydration and death if serious.

DIAGNOSIS Clinical examination, X-rays with barium, endoscopy and exploratory operations may all be used. Blood tests are often also indicated.

TREATMENT General treatment for moderate to severe small intestinal disease usually involves hospitalisation and intravenous fluids (a 'drip') to correct dehydration, while awaiting the results of further tests to get to the root of the problem. Mild gastro-enteritis, a common condition in dogs, is usually treated by dietary measures for simple diarrhoea (see page 107); drugs are not often required.

INTESTINAL 'FOREIGN BODY' OBSTRUCTION

CAUSE These are objects that have successfully negotiated the throat, oesophagus and stomach but which become lodged in the relatively small diameter of the small intestine. Balls, bones, corn cobs, fruit stones, plastic materials and many other items have all been removed. A frequent and serious cause of obstruction is linear material such as string or cassette tape, which causes the bowel to concertina on itself, forming severe obstruction and damage.

SYMPTOMS At first, dogs may just appear slightly off colour. There is usually a rapid deterioration, however, with vomiting, reluctance to eat or drink, straining to pass faeces (sometimes blood is seen) and progressive illness from dehydration. Abdominal pain is likely. Some dogs may simply appear extremely subdued with tenderness in the abdomen area and a tendency to stand or sit in unusual positions to try to alleviate the abdominal pain they are experiencing. If the intestine ruptures or perforates, severe deterioration due to peritonitis is seen and death can quickly follow.

DIAGNOSIS Quite often, the veterinary surgeon may be able to diagnose the obstruction by feeling (palpating) the abdomen, though if the dog is in a lot of pain muscle spasm may prevent this. Most obstructions can be diagnosed by X-ray; sometimes barium is used to help outline the object.

TREATMENT Surgery is indicated to remove the object. If possible, dehydration is corrected with an intravenous drip beforehand. If the bowel is extensively damaged, a section of it may need to be removed otherwise peritonitis could follow. Removal of even very large sections of small intestine causes no problems for dogs.

Obstructions are slightly rarer in the large intestine (due to its bigger diameter) but they do occasionally occur.

OUTLOOK Many dogs recover well following bowel surgery for obstructions, but there are occasional fatalities due to severe damage and peritonitis.

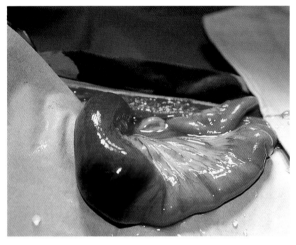

Segment of small intestine suffering from bowel obstruction in a dog which had been vomiting for 4 days.

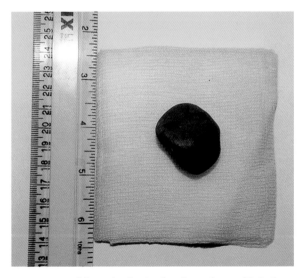

Stone removed from the dog in the photo above. If left, the dog would eventually have died from complications and peritonitis.

 Protruding foreign bodies

Never be tempted to pull on linear foreign bodies (e.g. string, cassette tape, fishing line) you see protruding from the mouth or anal area. Severe, life-threatening internal damage can be done. Always contact a veterinary surgeon first – it is likely that hospitalisation will be required.

PERITONITIS

CAUSE The cause is the introduction of infection or irritation to the lining of the abdomen, caused by rupture of an abdominal organ (e.g. stomach, intestine) or by a penetrating injury from the outside (e.g. airgun pellet). Peritonitis is also a potential major complication following abdominal surgery.

SYMPTOMS The symptoms are of severe illness with abdominal pain, vomiting and depression/collapse. Irregular breathing due to pain may be seen.

DIAGNOSIS In the early stages this isn't always easy. Usually the diagnosis is made by taking into account the dog's recent medical history and is aided by X-rays, blood tests and tests on fluid removed from the abdomen.

TREATMENT Intensive treatment may be required, including further surgery, lengthy hospitalisation and antibiotics, intravenous drips, etc.

OUTLOOK The outlook is always serious with peritonitis of any cause as this is a condition which tends to pursue a relentless course in many patients. However recovery is possible.

INTUSSUSCEPTION

CAUSE This is a problem mainly seen in puppies or young dogs, when it can follow a bout of diarrhoea. The intestine becomes hyperactive and part of it telescopes into another section, causing an obstruction.

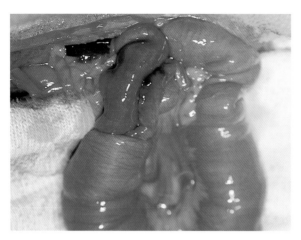

Intussusception in a young dog. One segment of bowel has telescoped into the other, causing severe illness, pain and vomiting.

SYMPTOMS Initial symptoms are of vomiting, followed by listlessness and abdominal pain. Small amounts of faeces with blood may be passed, or else the vomit may be blood-flecked. Dehydration quickly sets in and can be rapidly fatal in young puppies.

DIAGNOSIS It is easy to feel the bowels in small puppies as their abdominal wall is thin, and intussusceptions are often diagnosed in this way: the vet feels the abnormally thickened portion of intestine through the abdominal wall. X-rays may also be used.

TREATMENT If caught early, all of the bowel may be able to be saved; but if severe damage has occurred a section may need to be removed (this does not cause any future problems as dogs can survive normally when even very large amounts of bowel are removed). Usually, preventive measures are taken to try to avoid another intussusception developing after surgery by securing the intestine to itself. Hospitalisation for intravenous drips will also be required.

OUTLOOK As long as this is caught and treated early, the outlook is usually favourable, but it is still major surgery for such a young animal, with more risks than normal. Some puppies die from dehydration and complications before surgery can be performed.

INFLAMMATORY BOWEL DISEASES

CAUSE A range of disorders featuring inflammation without infection are found in dogs, with some breeds such as the German Shepherd being particularly affected. Stress may play a role in triggering attacks. (See also Colitis, and Infectious causes of enteritis below.)

SYMPTOMS Recurrent diarrhoea is the typical symptom, sometimes with blood present. During attacks, dogs may be subdued and uncomfortable.

DIAGNOSIS Normally, quite extensive tests are required, including biopsy, in order to categorise the problem so that similar diseases can be separated in order to choose the most effective treatment.

TREATMENT Most dogs' symptoms can be controlled using drug treatments and possibly diet once a diagnosis has been made.

OUTLOOK A complete cure may not be possible, but many dogs have extended periods without symptoms, requiring medication only during flare-ups. These dogs may however need to be kept to a carefully controlled prescription diet. Some patients require continuous low-dose drug treatment to keep symptoms at bay.

COLITIS

CAUSE Colitis is a form of enteritis which affects the large intestine/colon. The commonest form is a frequent cause of diarrhoea in dogs. Rarer forms may affect both small and large intestine and require biopsies for diagnosis. One type of ulcerative colitis is seen particularly in Boxer dogs and Bulldogs. Colitis, like enteritis, can also be caused by bacteria and protozoa and heavy worm burdens may also occasionally produce symptoms.

SYMPTOMS Diarrhoea is seen. Affected dogs have to pass faeces more frequently and often at short notice.

The faeces may be very liquid and a transparent slimy substance (mucus) is often passed. Traces of blood may be present. Very small quantities of faeces may be passed at a time, despite much straining.

Most dogs with colitis are not seriously ill, remaining bright and alert with a normal appetite. Occasionally, in bacterial infection, a high temperature and listlessness are seen.

DIAGNOSIS Simple colitis caused by dietary upset is usually diagnosed by clinical examination alone. More chronic cases may require examination of a faeces sample and tests such as X-rays or biopsies, which will also usually be carried out if the animal appears generally ill.

TREATMENT Dietary colitis responds to the treatment described on page 107 for simple diarrhoea. Inflammatory or infectious colitis may require specific drug therapy depending on the cause in each case. Sometimes diet manipulation can help to limit the episodes of symptoms in chronic cases.

OUTLOOK The outlook is good in most cases, which are of the simple dietary type of colitis. Inflammatory disease may require continuous medication, or short medication courses whenever a relapse occurs.

INFECTIOUS CAUSES OF ENTERITIS

CAUSE Inflammation of the intestine can also be caused by infections. The most well-known of these is parvovirus – a highly infectious cause of life-threatening enteritis in dogs, especially young dogs. Symptoms can also be seen with distemper, another potentially fatal viral illness of dogs which affects the intestine as well as other areas. Milder diarrhoea is thought to be caused by certain other viruses; in these cases, diarrhoea is usually the only symptom and these mild infections usually clear up after several days. They are commoner in kennelled dogs.

Certain bacteria and protozoa can also cause diarrhoea in dogs. In several of these, the dog

Infections passed between dogs and people

Always inform your veterinary surgeon and doctor if you or another family member has diarrhoea at the same time as your dog. A few infections can be passed between dogs and people.

remains bright and alert, but with persistent diarrhoea. Salmonella is possible in dogs, though quite rare. Usually the cause is another form of bacteria or a protozoa.

SYMPTOMS Parvovirus is a severe illness which causes marked symptoms of diarrhoea with blood, vomiting and severe depression. The pattern varies between individual dogs, with some succumbing quickly whereas others seem to fight the infection better, only to suddenly deteriorate later on. (Parvovirus and distemper are also discussed in Chapter 1).

In less serious infections, diarrhoea may be the only symptom, with the dog otherwise remaining well with a good appetite and normal energy levels.

TREATMENT Only supportive treatment is possible for viral illnesses. Antibiotics may be given, but these are to prevent secondary infections and are not useful against the virus itself. Intravenous drips are commonly used since severe diarrhoea quickly produces dehydration.

Diarrhoea caused principally by bacteria and protozoa can be treated using drugs specifically directed against these organisms. Tests may be required initially to determine the best drug to use and you may be asked to collect a faeces sample from your dog.

OUTLOOK Parvovirus and distemper are potentially fatal illnesses and unvaccinated dogs may die despite intensive treatment. Recovery is possible but sometimes permanent damage to the bowel or other organs may result. Milder bacterial, viral and protozoal infections usually clear up quickly given appropriate treatment.

Prevention

All dogs should be vaccinated against the major infectious diseases, and dogs kept together should be managed under hygienic conditions with proper disposal of waste material.

HAEMORRHAGIC ENTERITIS

CAUSE This is a further form of enteritis usually seen in smaller breeds of dog. The cause is not known, but a type of allergic reaction is suspected.

SYMPTOMS The disease produces a severe diarrhoea with blood present, very similar to that produced by parvovirus on initial appearance. Dogs frequently also vomit and this too may be blood-tinged.

DIAGNOSIS If the dog is vaccinated, parvovirus can be ruled out. X-rays may be taken to rule out obstructions.

TREATMENT Intravenous fluids are usually given to counteract the shock caused by blood loss in severe cases, and precautionary antibiotics may be administered. Hospitalisation and observation is necessary in most cases.

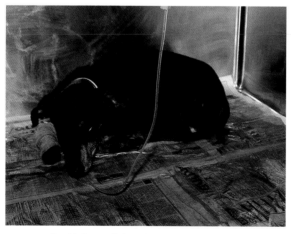

A 6-month-old dog suffering from haemorrhagic enteritis. As the dog was not vaccinated, parvovirus was suspected.

OUTLOOK Most dogs recover well if severe shock is avoided. Unfortunately, the problem can sometimes recur, in which case early treatment is needed again.

BOWEL CANCER

CAUSE Cancer can affect the small or large intestine. The exact cause, as with people, is not known. A problem in diagnosis is that tumours can grow to some size before symptoms appear, at which stage they may be beyond treatment.

SYMPTOMS Diarrhoea, sometimes alternating with constipation, is a frequent finding. Other symptoms of chronic disease may be seen, e.g. weight loss, poor coat, general debility. Tumours may cause signs of obstruction, with vomiting, once they are large enough to interfere with normal bowel movements and food passage. Tumours may also spread to other organs such as the bones or lungs, and cause symptoms here.

DIAGNOSIS Often the diagnosis is made after exploratory surgery, when other tests have provided inconclusive results. Occasionally the diagnosis is strongly suspected from palpating the abdomen in the relaxed or anaesthetised dog.

TREATMENT Not every tumour is malignant and sometimes removal of a single growth is possible. Usually samples will be sent for analysis to discover exactly what type the tumour is; this information can then be used to predict future survival.

In some instances when an extensive tumour is discovered at surgery, the veterinary surgeon will suggest that the dog is not allowed to recover from anaesthesia, and that painless euthanasia is carried out at this time. If this suggestion is made, it is wise to follow it as dogs with extensive carcinoma are not likely to recover well from abdominal surgery when nothing can be done to alleviate the condition.

OUTLOOK Good for benign tumours, poor for malignant ones.

PERINEAL HERNIA

CAUSE The perineum is the area around the tail base and anus. A perineal hernia results when the muscles in this area become weakened and even break down, causing underlying structures to move into an incorrect position (a hernia). The condition is commoner in male dogs.

SYMPTOMS The symptoms may be of constipation and straining. A swelling in the area around the anus is often visible. Affected dogs have difficulty in passing faeces. Occasionally, the bladder becomes trapped in the hernia, causing severe problems which can rapidly become life-threatening.

DIAGNOSIS The condition is usually readily identified by the veterinary surgeon. Sometimes associated problems are also present (e.g. enlargement of the prostate in male dogs). This condition (see page 198) can itself produce straining which eventually weakens the muscles of the perineum and causes the hernia to form.

TREATMENT Initial treatment consists of relieving the obstruction caused by the impacted faeces and assessing how severe the hernia is. If the bladder is involved, blood tests, hospitalisation and intravenous drips may be required to stabilise the dog.

Symptoms can often be improved somewhat by altering the diet to change the consistency of the faeces, and this may be the approach used in very old dogs. Simple first aid measures for constipation are mentioned on page 108. Generally, surgery is required to correct the muscle weaknesses that caused the hernia and carries much better results.

OUTLOOK Some complications are possible following surgery, including recurrence of the hernia. It is a difficult area in which to operate and infection is obviously a risk. Many dogs do well, however, provided they have not suffered severe problems due to trapping of the bladder beforehand.

FOOD SENSITIVITIES

CAUSE A number of food constituents are suspected to cause diarrhoea in dogs. These can be difficult to prove, however evidence suggests that several different problems exist and some Irish Setters are known to be sensitive to gluten. Golden Retrievers may be prone to food sensitivities also.

SYMPTOMS Diarrhoea is the main sign. Skin disorders may also occur.

DIAGNOSIS Diagnosis is not easy. More common disorders may need to be ruled out first. Usually, if this problem is suspected, the dog is placed on an exclusion diet. This consists of one single protein and one carbohydrate foodstuff which must be fed for anything up to 10 weeks. No other foods, treats ot tit-bits should be given otherwise the test may be spoiled.

If the symptoms improve, the dog is then put back onto its previous diet. If this causes a relapse of symptoms, and that relapse is reversed by going back onto the exclusion diet again, then it can be assumed that something in the original diet is indeed causing the problem. Efforts can be made to identify this ingredient so that a diet which does not contain it can be devised.

Typical exclusion diets used in dogs

- **Protein sources**: chicken *or* fish *or* egg *or* cottage cheese

- **Carbohydrate sources**: rice *or* potato

Commercially prepared exclusion diets are also available from veterinary practices but the above are alternatives. Do not swap between alternatives: choose one protein and one carbohydrate and stick to those for the duration of the dietary test. All exclusion diets must be carried out under veterinary advice.

TREATMENT This relies on being able to find or devise a diet which avoids the ingredient causing the sensitivity.

Be strict

Make sure everyone involved with the dog understands the importance of sticking to the exclusion diet for the full duration. One person giving treats or alternative foods could spoil the test and render the results confusing in positive cases.

Outlook It may take some time to conclusively prove that a diet ingredient is the cause in any particular dog, but if other conditions have been ruled out, it is worth the effort.

ROUNDWORMS

Cause Several species of roundworm infect dogs. The commonest is called *Toxocara canis*; the other types, known as hookworms and whipworms, may be seen less frequently.

Symptoms Common roundworms may be observed in the faeces or occasionally in the vomit of affected dogs. They are seen most often in puppies and young dogs and resemble strands of thin spaghetti. Most dogs show few symptoms with worms unless they are heavily infected, in which case poor growth, poor coat quality and bouts of vomiting and diarrhoea may occur. Rarely, worms may cause an intestinal obstruction in young puppies which can be life-threatening.

Diagnosis Diagnosis can be made when worms (sometimes still alive) are seen in faeces or are occasionally vomited up. Alternatively, checking a faeces sample under the microscope may allow the veterinary surgeon to detect worm eggs.

Treatment Modern worming preparations from your veterinary practice effectively destroy roundworms. Note however that pregnant bitches must be repeatedly wormed during pregnancy, on veterinary advice, in order to limit the infestation of puppies developing in the uterus.

Life cycle of the roundworm, *Toxocara canis*

While living in the intestine of their host (dog), the adult worms produce thousands of eggs which pass out in the faeces. The eggs are not immediately infective for other dogs: it takes around three weeks for a worm larva to develop within each egg. After this stage, they are ready to infect another dog.

These eggs with larvae within them are extremely durable, and survive on the ground long after the faeces they were passed in has disappeared. Once accidentally eaten by another dog, the worm larva undergoes a complex migration, passing through various body tissues before finally settling in the gut wall in younger dogs. Severe infections may result in a cough as the larvae migrate through lung tissue on their way to the gut.

In older dogs, rather than taking up residence in the gut, most worm larve migrate into other tissues (especially muscle) where they form tiny cysts. These cysts do not cause any problems, and remain for life, but in pregnant female dogs the cysts can re-activate. When this happens (in response to the hormone changes of pregnancy) the larvae now move towards the uterus, where they infect the developing puppies. Thus, nearly all puppies are born with worms even when the dam herself has no worms in her own gut, because the parasites have come from the tissue cysts which are present in all dogs.

Further infection may be acquired as the puppies suckle because some of the re-activated larvae migrate to the mammary gland and are present in the milk which the suckling puppies drink. The roundworm therefore has an ingenious and complex way of continuing its life cycle which depends on the infection of female dogs. See diagram opposite.

Hookworms and whipworms

These worms are rarer and mainly confined to kennelled dogs, especially if hygiene is not maintained at a high level. Symptoms, when they occur, are of diarrhoea. These parasites are killed by modern worming drugs.

Life cycle of the roundworm

thick shell

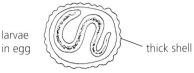

larvae
in egg

thick shell

eggs are now infective,
with a larva inside

3–4 weeks on
the ground

eggs passed in faeces
of infected dog
(especially young dogs)

can survive on the
ground for many
months due to
thick shell

larvae settle in dog's
intestines, mature into
adults and produce eggs

eggs and larvae accidentally
eaten by another dog

young dogs, up to
6 months

dog becomes infected
and larvae migrate
through dog's tissues

older dogs, over
6 months

larvae settle in
muscle and form
harmless cysts

no further problems
usually caused

male dogs

pregnant
female dogs

cysts re-activate and larvae
migrate to uterus and mammary
glands to infect puppies directly
and through suckling

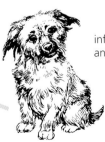

infected puppies
and young dogs

What is the risk to people?

The dog roundworm can cause a condition called 'larva migrans' in man. This term describes the migration of the larva that takes place when this occurs in the wrong host (i.e. a human being rather than a dog). The larva may migrate to various tissues, including the eye. This is a very rare disease in people but it still needs to be taken seriously. Part of the problem is the lengthy time for which eggs may remain infectious on the ground (this can be for several years). For these reasons, dog owners should remove faeces their dogs have passed in public places and dispose of them carefully. The faeces are not infectious when passed, but would be after several weeks if left on the ground.

In fact the risk from adult dogs is small: the most risk comes from puppies, young dogs and pregnant or lactating bitches. Sensible precautions regarding hand-washing and disposal of waste material should be taken in these cases, particularly when children may come into contact with the bitch or her litter. Additionally, a worming regime should be discussed with your veterinary surgeon before mating, and throughout pregnancy and lactation of the bitch. Puppies should also be wormed appropriately.

Adult dog roundworms cannot live in the intestine of people. Any worms noticed in children, therefore, will be human parasitic worms, not dog ones.

Tapeworms
Rare causes of human illness can be caused by the tapeworm *Echinococcus* (see page 120). Other species may very occasionally infect people; these are less serious and would be likely to cause abdominal pain.

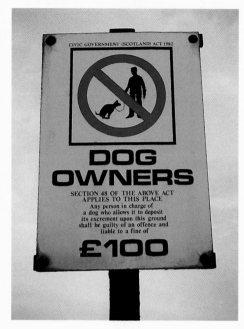

In urban areas, responsible dog owners clean up after their pets.

 ## Prevention

Most pet dogs are routinely wormed whether or not any signs of parasites have been noticed. The frequency is normally two to four times per year. Careful collection and disposal of dog faeces will prevent roundworm transmission. Immediately after passing, the faeces are not infective (see the box on page 117 describing life cycle).

TAPEWORMS

CAUSE Tapeworms are so named because of their flattened appearance. They attach themselves to the intestinal wall via tiny spikes in the head area. From here they absorb nutrients and grow by the addition of segments.

There are several different species of tapeworm and in order to complete their life-cycle they must all spend some time in another animal, known as an intermediate host (see the box opposite). For certain of these species, dogs which catch and eat rabbits or other wild animals, or which are fed raw meat, are at a higher risk of infestation as the animals eaten can act as intermediate hosts for the tapeworm. Cooking destroys the infectious stages present in the flesh of any intermediate host.

SYMPTOMS Symptoms are not often seen with tapeworm infestation as the adults cause very little damage to the host unless they are present in huge numbers. The intermediate stages, however, can cause

The ingenious alliance of fleas, lice and tapeworms

Dipylidium caninum

This is the commonest tapeworm in dogs. Very occasionally, it may also infect people when it would cause abdominal pain/cramps. The adults, living in the gut and absorbing some of the dog's food, cause no disease, even when present in very large numbers. When segments break off, they move actively out of the anus on to the surrounding hair and may cause irritation and excess grooming. Each segment contains 20 or so eggs. As the segment dries up, the eggs are released.

Flea larvae and lice now play their part by eating the eggs, which develop into cysts in the body of these parasites. After 1–3 months the developing tapeworm, inside the flea or louse, is ready to infect another dog. It can do so when the dog grooms itself and accidentally swallows an infected flea or louse which has been causing it minor skin irritation. The dog has now also taken in a developing tapeworm which, once inside the dog, soon latches onto the intestine and begins feeding.

continued on page 120 ▶

**The tapeworm and
its life-cycle**

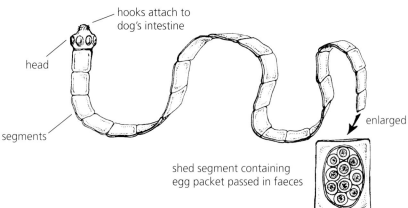

hooks attach to
dog's intestine

head

segments

enlarged

shed segment containing
egg packet passed in faeces

egg packet

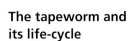

segments are shed from the
tapeworm and passed in the
dog's faeces. These segments are
mobile, resemble rice grains, and
may be seen moving around the
tail area of the dog

eggs are released by
the active segment
when it disintegrates

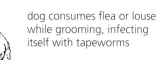

dog consumes flea or louse
while grooming, infecting
itself with tapeworms

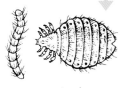

eggs are eaten by an
intermediate host,
usually a flea larva
or a louse

tapeworm eggs
develop in the
flea or louse

The ingenious alliance of fleas, lice and tapeworms (continued from page 119)

After this, is takes about 3 weeks before the tapeworm is ready to shed segments with eggs and start the life-cycle all over again. Therefore to treat tapeworms effectively, fleas (and lice if present) must also be controlled. Fleas, lice and other parasites are discussed in Chapter 5.

Other tapeworms

The other tapeworms use mammals, instead of fleas and lice, as intermediate hosts and usually depend on the dog eating the raw flesh of the mammal to complete the life-cycle. The adult tapeworms are successful parasites in that they cause few problems for their host; but the intermediate stages can cause disease in the animals concerned (sheep, cattle, rabbits, hares, pigs, etc.)

Taenia is a long tapeworm (unlike *Dipylidium*). It can grow to several feet in length. In order to become infected, dogs must eat raw meat or catch and eat wild mammals.

Echinococcus, in contrast, is tiny – it only measures a few millimetres. It causes few problems for the dog but can sometimes cause disease in the intermediate host. Occasionally, human beings can act as the intermediate host for this tapeworm, when it can cause serious disease due to the formation of a 'hydatid cyst' in human tissues.

---

problems for the intermediate host animals in which they occur.

DIAGNOSIS Tapeworm segments of some species may be seen moving around the tail area. They are small whitish objects which quite quickly dry up to resemble rice grains.

TREATMENT Modern anti-parasitic drugs are used to treat both roundworms and tapeworms. Note that flea treatment is always necessary when the *Dipylidium* species of tapeworm is being treated, as these two parasites' life-cycles are closely related.

PREVENTION Dogs which regularly consume raw meat or wild mammals should be treated for tapeworms frequently. Cooking the meat eliminates the chance of infection.

DISEASES OF THE PANCREAS

CAUSE The pancreas is an important organ of digestion which lies close to the start of the small intestine. It is involved in the digestion of proteins, fats and carbohydrates through the production of digestive enzymes and it also produces hormones which have widespread effects on all body cells: the best known of these is insulin.

Several disorders can cause pancreatic disease, including pancreatitis (inflammation), pancreatic enzyme deficiency, diabetes ('sugar diabetes') and pancreatic tumours.

SYMPTOMS **Diabetes** is discussed on page 219.
Pancreatitis is a very unpleasant condition which causes severe abdominal pain, vomiting and dehydration. Diarrhoea may also occur. Severely affected dogs are miserable. In order to alleviate internal pain they may adopt unusual crouching postures while sitting.

Pancreatic enzyme deficiencies can follow repeated bouts of severe inflammation, but the condition is commonly seen without inflammation and it occurs more frequently in German Shepherd dogs. Symptoms are usually diarrhoea, weight loss and a ravenous appetite, which do not respond to simpler treatments such as worming, dietary rest, etc. The cause for the enzyme deficiency in German Shepherds and other dogs which have not suffered bouts of pancreatitis is unknown, but the glands that produce the digestive enzymes somehow reduce in size and number, until deficiency sets in.

Pancreatic tumours cause signs of general illness, weight loss, vomiting and poor appetite. Jaundice may be seen.

DIAGNOSIS Pancreatic problems can be difficult to diagnose. There is no single test that identifies pancreatitis, but suspicion of this disease is often raised by results from several investigations and from careful observation of the patient. X-rays, ultrasound and blood tests may all be employed.

Enzyme deficiences can be identified by blood and faeces tests in most cases. Pancreatic tumours present in various ways, sometimes mimicking pancreatitis. X-rays and ultrasound are used frequently in an attempt to diagnose them.

TREATMENT For pancreatitis, this usually entails hospitalisation, nil by mouth, and intravenous drips to reverse dehydration. Painkillers, antibiotics and drugs to reduce vomiting are frequently given. Often, all food needs to be witheld for two days in order to completely rest the pancreas. Animals which have had pancreatitis are usually put onto a low fat diet once they recover, as fats in the diet require the pancreas to work harder. Recurrences can occur.

Enzyme deficiency problems are treated by feeding replacement enzymes mixed into the food. This usually brings about remission of the symptoms: dogs start to pass normal faeces and gain weight. These dogs will need continued enzyme replacement throughout their lives, as they are unable to manufacture the enzymes for themselves. Usually, veterinary surgeons will try to maintain dogs on the lowest dose of enzyme which keeps symptoms at bay in order to limit long term costs to the owner.

Pancreatic tumours are notoriously malignant and, unfortunately, at the time of diagnosis most tumours will have spread extensively.

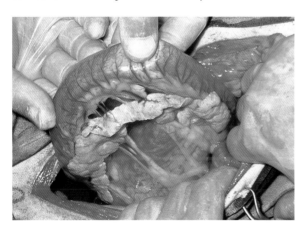

The pancreas as seen during exploratory surgery in a dog.

OUTLOOK Very poor for pancreatic tumours; enzyme deficiencies can usually be kept under control but no complete cure is available; pancreatitis usually resolves with treatment but a few dogs have further attacks and some may develop chronic problems from this.

LIVER DISEASE

CAUSE The liver is a complex organ which is vital to life. It receives a large blood supply and performs many different functions. It is central to normal digestion and metabolism; it also manufactures blood proteins and stores a wide variety of essential nutrients. It is responsible for detoxifying any substance that might be harmful to the body (including medical drugs) – a role which can result in the liver itself being injured.

SYMPTOMS The liver has tremendous powers of regeneration. Up to 80% of the organ can be damaged or lost before any adverse effects are seen. This fact means that whenever symptoms due to liver disease are present, much damage has already occurred. In an important sense, symptoms only appear when the

Symptoms suggestive of liver disease

Many liver symptoms are vague in nature, and could be caused by any serious disease. Commoner ones include:

- Poor energy levels
- Reluctant appetite
- Drinking to excess and passing more urine than normal
- Vomiting/diarrhoea
- Weight loss
- Jaundice: a yellowish tinge to the white of the eye (sclera) or the gums/lining of the mouth
- Swelling of the abdomen due to fluid accumulation
- Mental confusion and incoordination

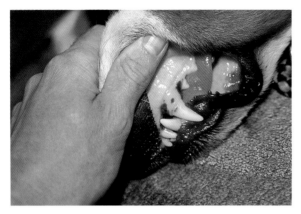

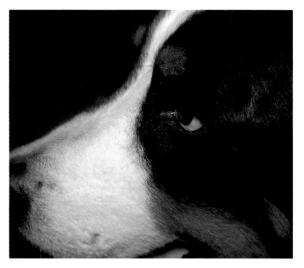

Jaundice in a dog with liver disease. There is severe yellowing of the mucous membranes and of the white of the eye (sclera).

liver can no longer cope and is almost beyond repair. This means that liver diseases can be very difficult to treat effectively.

DIAGNOSIS The diagnosis of liver disease frequently involves numerous tests including blood tests, X-rays, ultrasound and biopsy. Quite often, exactly what caused the original damage will remain unknown. The important thing to determine is whether the remaining liver is able to cope and function adequately.

TREATMENT Treatment is often supportive, in other words the function of the liver is helped and its workload eased, while hopefully allowing it to heal using its considerable powers of regeneration. Common treatments used are intravenous fluids (drips), antibiotics and sometimes anti-inflammatory drugs.

Diet plays an important part in supporting the injured liver and specially formulated diets containing high quality proteins and enriched with certain vitamins and minerals may be prescribed. Some dogs are fed chicken and pasta/rice-based diets initially, but long term maintenance on a prescription diet may be required.

Young dogs with abnormal blood vessel development, which leads to blood by-passing the liver through shunts, may be treatable by surgery. If successful, symptoms may be well controlled or even removed after the operation.

Some causes of liver disease in dogs

- Infectious canine hepatitis } both of these diseases are preventable by vaccination
- Leptospirosis
- Poisoning by toxic compounds
- Abnormal blood vessel development (in young dogs)
- Copper accumulation – a disease found in Bedlington Terriers and possibly several other breeds
- Liver tumours or spread of tumours from elsewhere to the liver
- Diseases of the gall bladder or bile duct, e.g. infections
- Cirrhosis – this term refers to a scarred liver which has been damaged by some other process
- Hepatitis (acute or chronic) – this term refers to inflammation arising in the liver, whether this happens suddenly (acute) or becomes a long-standing problem (chronic)

OUTLOOK It is always a serious sign when the liver shows signs of disease or failure, precisely because it copes so well with most damage. The aim is to maximise what resources remain and to treat any causes of on-going liver damage which can be identified.

CHAPTER 7

The Heart and Respiratory System

Common symptoms of heart and respiratory disease
• Coughing • Choking/wheezing • Irregular, heavy or
rapid breathing • Reluctance to exercise • Tires easily
• Collapse or fainting • Weight loss • Abdominal swelling

Structure and Function

Taken together, the heart and respiratory system are responsible for delivering oxygen to all the tissues of the body and removing the 'waste gas', carbon dioxide. This vital exchange of gases allows all the various body organs (brain, liver, kidney, etc) to function normally. This is obviously a crucial role and any disease which seriously affects the heart or lungs is potentially fatal. Without a steady supply of oxygen and removal of carbon dioxide, life quickly ceases.

The process of respiration involves the transfer of oxygen from the inhaled air to the blood circulating through the lungs. During expiration, carbon dioxide generated from tissue metabolism in the body is 'blown off' in the exhaled breath. There is still quite a lot of oxygen left in the exhaled breath, which is why artificial respiration (Chapter 18) can save an animal's (or human's) life when properly applied.

Throughout a dog's life, breathing (respiratory) rate and heart (pulse) rate are controlled within fairly narrow limits. There are alterations, of course, especially during exercise or during periods of panting – the dog's main means of losing excess heat from the body. But after these periods, the respiratory and heart rates quite quickly return to the normal, or resting, values.

The chest

The heart and lungs are protected within the chest. The chest wall in the dog is made up of thirteen pairs of ribs, with the bony sternum underneath and vertebral column above. Dogs' chests are compressed from right side to left side, unlike human chests which are compressed from in front to behind. The diaphragm is a muscular sheet which is important in breathing and which divides the chest and abdomen internally.

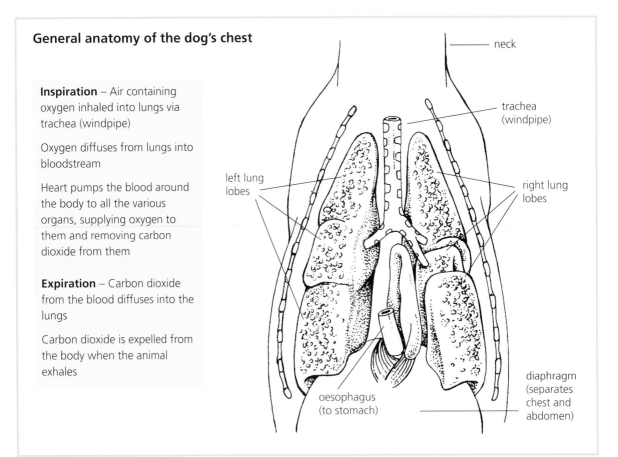

General anatomy of the dog's chest

Inspiration – Air containing oxygen inhaled into lungs via trachea (windpipe)

Oxygen diffuses from lungs into bloodstream

Heart pumps the blood around the body to all the various organs, supplying oxygen to them and removing carbon dioxide from them

Expiration – Carbon dioxide from the blood diffuses into the lungs

Carbon dioxide is expelled from the body when the animal exhales

neck

trachea (windpipe)

left lung lobes

right lung lobes

oesophagus (to stomach)

diaphragm (separates chest and abdomen)

What is my dog's normal (resting) heart and respiratory rate?

- Normal respiratory rates for dogs are 15–30 breaths per minute.

- Normal heart rates for dogs are 60–120 beats per minute.

There is some variation: small dogs tend to have rates towards the upper ends of these ranges and larger dogs have rates towards the lower ends. Stress or excitement (e.g. attending the veterinary surgery) may elevate the heart and respiratory rate and, of course, dogs frequently pant on hot days. Diseases can also alter the normal rates and rhythms.

In some occasions, it can be useful for owners to monitor heart and respiratory rate in the relaxed dog at home. This is especially valuable in dogs on treatment for heart disease, when alterations in heart rate may necessitate changes in medication. Although vets will use a stethoscope and listen carefully to the heart sounds in the clinic, sometimes the heart rate is falsely high at these times due to fear or excitement, therefore knowing the readings at home can occasionally be helpful in fine-tuning drug treatments.

Taking the respiratory rate

This is straightforward and involves watching the breathing movements of the chest wall or abdomen.

One complete breath is made up of (**1**) an inhalation, (**2**) an exhalation and then (**3**) usually a short *pause* before the next inhalation. Count the number of breaths per minute while your dog is relaxed and quiet. It is best to do several counts and then take an average.

- Any changes in the *pattern* of breathing will be of interest to your vet, e.g. does the dog seem to use more effort to breathe, with exaggerated movements of the abdomen? Or are the breathing movements themselves uneven or irregular?

Taking the heart rate

With practice, this can be done by placing your flattened palms over the area of the heart, just behind the dog's elbows on both sides of the chest (this is impossible in dogs that are seriously overweight however). Alternatively, your vet or nurse may show you how to take the femoral (hind leg) pulse if they would like you to monitor heart rate at home. Many owners can become proficient at this and are able to detect rhythm irregularities in their dog's heart beat.

(Note that young healthy dogs often have an irregular heart rhythm which slows down and speeds up in time with breathing. It is a predictable and constant alteration in the rhythm, unlike pathological heart rhythm irregularities. No treatment is needed.)

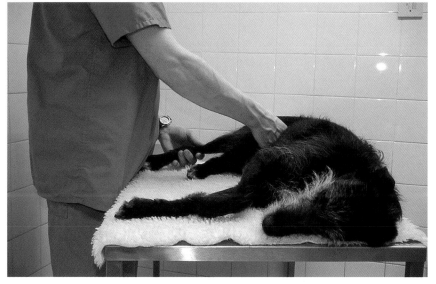

In dogs, the pulse is normally taken from the femoral artery, which is situated in the inner thigh area.

The oesophagus (gullet) and major blood vessels pass through the diaphragm. The diaphragm can become injured – it may rupture, most often after traumatic accidents, producing the serious condition of diaphragmatic hernia (see page 136), which requires major surgery for correction.

The heart

The heart is composed of specialised muscle which has a remarkable ability to contract rhythmically throughout the duration of an animal's life. The rate and force of contraction is subject to fine control exerted by the nervous and hormone systems. There is also an area within the heart (the pacemaker) which sets a basic heart rate, which can then be altered by

other control systems as circumstances dictate (e.g. a sudden fright causes the heart rate to increase above the basic rate due to release of the 'flight or fight' hormone, adrenaline). Certain heart conditions in the dog are responsive to artificial pacemaker implantation. Pacemakers that have been taken out to be replaced in people can be adapted for use in dogs and function very well.

Heart valves and heart murmurs

The heart valves ensure a one-way flow of blood through the heart and onwards to the rest of the body. Anything which interferes with the smooth operation of these valves and the smooth flow of blood creates turbulence within the heart – this turbulence can be heard and diagnosed as a heart murmur through a

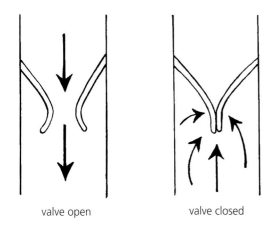

valve open   valve closed

normal heart valve only allows flow of blood in one direction

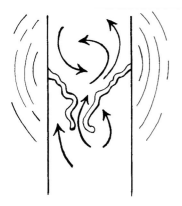

leaky or distorted valve allows backwards flow of blood, creating turbulence which is heard as a heart murmur

The structure of a heart valve and the creation of murmurs when valves become 'leaky'.

> ### Are all heart murmurs dangerous?
>
> The normal heart does not produce murmurs, but this does not mean that every heart murmur is immediately life-threatening. In particular, murmurs are often picked up incidentally in middle-aged to older dogs (often at vaccination time); these dogs may have no outward symptoms of heart disease. The decision of when, or whether, to begin treatment in these cases depends on various factors and your vet will advise accordingly.
>
> Many times, the cause is partial leakage or back-flow of blood through a heart valve that is not closing properly. This type of murmur is common in pet dogs of all breeds, and especially in Cavalier King Charles Spaniels, when it can appear even in young adults. The condition does tend to progress as the dog gets older and symptoms such as cough or reluctance to exercise will usually appear. Fortunately, current treatments can greatly help off-set these symptoms, and a good quality of life can be achieved in most cases if treatments are adhered to.
>
> Murmurs in young puppies should be investigated if they persist, as this can indicate congenital heart problems which may be serious.
>
> Certain more serious problems in specific breeds may present with a heart murmur. Diagnostic tests, as described on below, are often employed.

stethoscope. In severe cases, it can even be felt on the dog's chest wall as a steady vibration or 'thrill'.

Other, rarer, causes of turbulence and murmurs include 'holes' in the heart (allowing direct communication between heart chambers) or abnormal connections between major blood vessels in the chest area.

The lungs

The lungs function rather like a very sophisticated pair of bellows. They accommodate the air that is breathed in and, thanks to a network of tiny blood vessels in their walls, oxygen can pass from the inhaled air into the bloodstream and carbion dioxide can pass from the bloodstream into the exhaled air. This exhange of gases is the basis of respiration and is necessary for normal life. If it becomes inadequate for any reason, health suffers.

The trachea, or windpipe, is the tube that transfers air from the throat area to the chest.

Veterinary Diagnosis and Treatment

Examination of the heart and lungs usually involves use of the stethoscope. When the vet uses this instrument, he or she is listening to the heart rate, heart rhythm and whether or not any murmurs are present. The function of the lungs is also assessed since, to the trained ear, lung problems cause altered breath

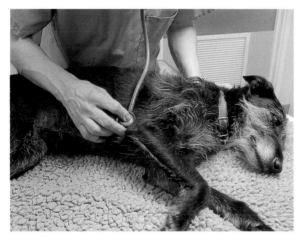

Using the stethoscope to check the heart rate and rhythm and to listen for murmurs.

sounds in the chest. The abnormal chest may sound 'harsh', 'crackly' or, in cases of pneumonia, fluid sounds may be heard.

Other circulatory tests used include taking the pulse (see page 125) and checking the colour of the mucous membranes or gums (see page 30). These should be a salmon-pink colour and, when pressed and then released, their colour should return promptly, indicating a healthy circulation. This test, known as the capillary refill time, can be abnormal in dogs with heart or respiratory problems or in those which have suffered severe internal or external bleeding (haemorrhage).

The vet may wish to perform an 'exercise tolerance test' – in other words, he or she may ask you to run with the dog, or perhaps negotiate a flight of stairs, to see if this provokes signs of heart or respiratory disease.

 Signs of poor exercise tolerance

- Breathlessness
- Coughing
- Refusing to move, e.g. sitting down
- Fainting/collapse

It is useful if you can explain any changes you may have noticed in your dog's symptoms or behaviour, such as when symptoms began, when they seem worst, what effect exercise seems to have, and so on. These may provide valuable clues to the diagnosis.

X-rays

X-rays are very important in chest diseases – both to diagnose disease initially and also to monitor its progress. Often, several different views are taken to ensure that the heart and lungs are adequately evaluated.

One of the problems in severely ill dogs is the risk of anaesthesia or sedation for X-rays. Normally, to position dogs accurately for X-rays, they are sedated or anaesthetised as, unlike adult humans, cooperation is not guaranteed!

Sedation or anaesthesia allows a good X-ray to be

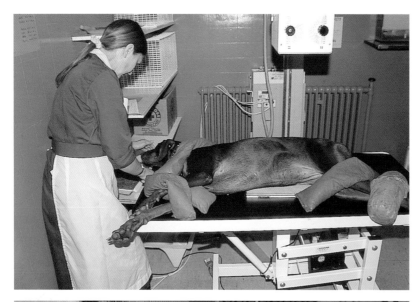

Unsedated dog lying for a chest X-ray. Many dogs will lie quietly with gentle restraint using sandbags and reassurance.

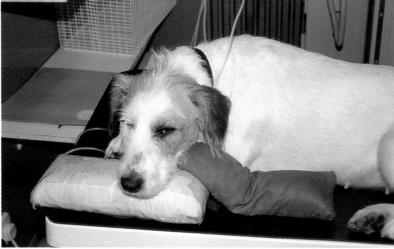

Sedation may be needed to get a diagnostic X-ray in nervous dogs or in cases where very accurate positioning is required. This dog has been given a mild sedative and is perfectly cooperative and relaxed for his X-rays.

safely taken. However, in chest diseases, this may carry an increased risk. Vets assess each case on its merits, balancing the need for a diagnostic X-ray with any dangers to the patient. Many dogs will lie still enough without sedation for some basic X-rays to be taken; treatment can then be started and further X-rays delayed until the patient is more stable.

ECG (electrocardiograph)

As the heart beats, tiny electrical signals are given off. These can be captured and recorded by an ECG machine, allowing important measurements to be made. An ECG evaluates the rhythm and rate of the heart and provides some information on the size of the four different heart chambers.

Most dogs with irregular heart rhythms will have an ECG taken at some stage unless the diagnosis is obvious.

Cardiac ultrasound

This test is carried out in more complex heart disorders, or in order to confirm or refine a diagnosis. It is a very sensitive, advanced test and provides much useful information. In order for this procedure to be carried out, referral to a specialist vet or hospital may be required.

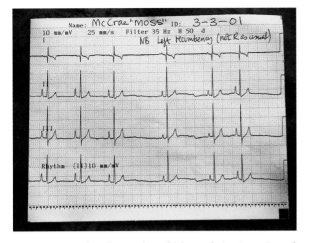

ECG tracing taken from a dog which was being investigated for intermittent collapsing while exercising.

Quality of life is always an important assessment to be made, but a wide variety of conditions can be successfully managed using modern drugs and hence quality of life can remain good over a long period of time. Many pet dogs are very successfully treated for chronic heart failure, for example.

Insurance policies are likely to help in the initial stages of many of these conditions but if life-long treatment becomes necessary, the condition may be excluded from the insurance policy. Although this is sometimes cited as a reason not to take up insurance, it has to be borne in mind that the initial diagnostic investigations may be the most expensive part; a reputable insurance policy would cover this aspect, as well an initial courses of treatment.

CT scans and MRI scans

These advanced techniques, used widely in human medicine, are gradually becoming available for use in pets. Some veterinary colleges or referral hospitals have their own units; in other places, arrangements can be made to use the facilities in human hospitals. CT and MRI scans are powerful diagnostic tools which help pin-point diseases and aid in their management.

Cost and prognosis in heart and respiratory diseases

Many different diseases are possible with these body systems, from simple, easily curable conditions such as 'kennel cough' to complex cardiac and respiratory diseases requiring surgery or life-long medical treatment.

For the more serious conditions, fairly extensive tests may be needed to reach a diagnosis. Whilst some treatments (e.g. certain surgical operations) may be 'one-off' expenses, other conditions, such as chronic heart failure due to heart valve leakage (which is common in dogs), require on-going treatment and periodic tests to check progress throughout the dog's life. Additional or alternative drugs may be prescribed, depending on progress, and special diets may be recommended.

Commonest Heart and Respiratory Diseases in Dogs

 First aid resuscitation

See the 'ABC' guide to saving a collapsed dog's life in Chapter 18.

Heart Diseases

CONGENITAL PROBLEMS IN PUPPIES

CAUSE A variety of heart diseases may be diagnosed in puppies. Exactly how these are inherited is not always fully understood. In general, male puppies are more often affected than females. Overall, congenital heart problems are seen infrequently in dogs compared to acquired heart problems, i.e. those which develop *after* birth.

SYMPTOMS Affected puppies are likely to grow poorly and be less active than their litter mates. Sometimes sudden death may be the only indication that a heart problem has been present. Other puppies may show breathing irregularities and coughing, becoming more noticeable as they grow older and start to move around actively. Swelling of the abdomen (due to fluid accumulation) can be a sign of congenital heart disease in puppies, as can bluish gums or mucous membranes.

A heart murmur, indicating turbulent blood flow within the heart, may be detected when the puppy is presented for its vaccination and may be the first sign that a heart abnormality is present.

Puppies with regurgitation of food at weaning may have a persistent aortic arch – a blood vessel abnormality which compresses the oesophagus (gullet) and prevents solid food from reaching the stomach. This can be remedied by surgery but swallowing problems may remain even after surgical correction due to permanent damage to the oesophagus having occurred.

DIAGNOSIS A full diagnosis, which may be essential in order to predict future problems, may require extensive tests, including X-rays, ECGs and cardiac ultrasound.

TREATMENT Treatment, if possible, rests on an accurate diagnosis. Many conditions are potentially treatable with either surgery or medications. Treatment may need to be continued throughout the animal's life, although some surgical treatments if used early enough can bring about complete cure.

OUTLOOK Congenital heart diseases are serious conditions and the outlook may not be good for normal life. However a few congenital disorders are relatively harmless and do not require any specific treatment once they have been accurately diagnosed, e.g. small 'holes in the heart' can be lived with, without any obvious symptoms.

HEART VALVE DISEASE AND CHRONIC HEART FAILURE

CAUSE This is the commonest heart problem in dogs, seen most in middle to old aged animals. Cavalier King Charles Spaniels are particularly prone to heart valve degeneration, but the disease is encountered frequently in many other small breeds, e.g. Poodles, Chihuahuas, and less frequently in larger

dogs. Heart disease of this type is important in canine medicine – around 10% of all dogs acquire heart disease, and in most of these the problem is associated with the heart valves.

SYMPTOMS A heart murmur is heard during examination with a stethoscope. The murmur is caused by turbulent blood flow around the distorted heart valve. The presence of the murmur does not always mean that the dog will show symptoms of heart disease; it is well known that some dogs may have a heart murmur and never go on to show signs of chronic heart failure. Many murmurs are picked up incidentally during the yearly health examination before booster vaccination. If other symptoms are present, treatment will normally be started.

Symptoms of heart failure include coughing, breathlessness, reduced ability or inclincation to exercise, abdominal swelling and, in severe cases, fainting/collapse. The defective heart valves mean that the heart functions less efficiently as a blood pump. Blood therefore 'dams back' into the chest, where it causes fluid accumulation (hence the cough and breathlessness), and also the abdomen, where it results in abdominal swelling (ascites).

Early signs of chronic heart failure

- Stopping while out on walks
- Coughing during or after excitement or exercise
- Laboured breathing
- Restless at night

DIAGNOSIS The symptoms of this form of heart disease are very characteristic. Nevertheless, because some chest diseases can give similar symptoms, tests are usually carried out – most frequently X-rays and ECG examination. Cardiac ultrasound may also be suggested.

TREATMENT The disease cannot be cured; however it can usually be successfully managed during the earlier stages using drugs which are designed to ease the work load on the heart and prevent fluid accumulation in the chest. Many dogs live a number of years of good quality life with heart failure which is being well controlled by drugs and careful management at home.

Progression of the disease is treated by adjusting dosage rates and possibly adding new drugs to the treatment, as well as altering lifestyle factors such as weight, amount of exercise and possibly diet. Periodic chest X-rays, ECGs and blood tests (e.g. to check that the kidneys are working effectively) are also usually required.

Severe disease or severe deteriorations in condition may require hospitalisation for cage rest, oxygen and additional drugs in an attempt to 'rescue' the failing heart and allow the dog to regain a steady state again.

OUTLOOK The rate of deterioration varies quite a lot between dogs. Some patients seem to stabilise and remain just the same for years; others follow a faster downhill course. Any dog with heart failure needs a lot of care: medication must be given reliably and care taken to avoid undue stresses such as heat, fear and excitement. A constant daily routine is best. Stresses such as kennelling should be avoided if at all possible since this can sometimes precipitate a decline in condition.

Most dogs under treatment do well with a good quality of life for a significant period of time. The expense of continuous medication and periodic tests has to be taken into account also.

CARDIOMYOPATHY

CAUSE This is a disease of the heart muscle (rather than the valves). It also differs from the above in that young to middle aged dogs are mainly affected (rather than older ones). Most affected dogs are of large, pure breeds – again in contrast to heart valve disease, which affects smaller breeds more frequently.

The cause of cardiomyopathy is not yet fully understood but the high incidence in certain breeds (e.g. Dobermans, Boxers and giant breeds such as the Great Dane and Newfoundland) suggest that it may be inherited.

SYMPTOMS It is thought that the condition, though present, remains 'silent' for months or years before severe disease strikes. It may be picked up at an early stage if the dog was to receive an ECG or heart scan, but unless screening is carried out, such testing does not usually happen. Occasionally, signs of cardiomyopathy may be picked up via the stethoscope when the dog is undergoing routine examination.

When symptoms start, the gradual progression seen in chronic heart failure does not occur: cardiomyopathy is much more likely to be acute and severe and can cause sudden death.

Symptoms shown could include coughing, breathing problems and inability to exercise or even stand. Abnormal heart rhythms are often seen. The most severe signs are seen in Dobermans and Boxers.

DIAGNOSIS X-rays, ECGs and cardiac ultrasound are all used to confirm the suspected diagnosis of cardiomyopathy.

TREATMENT Some dogs respond to treatment for developing heart failure and symptoms can be kept at bay for months or even years with frequent assessment. Unfortunately, individual dogs (and many Dobermans) do not respond well and deteriorate quickly despite treatment.

OUTLOOK Cardiomyopathy is a serious disease which can lead to sudden death in dogs. Certain forms of it are more amenable to treatment, but once signs of heart failure appear, deterioration is usually much more rapid than with heart valve disease.

HEART RHYTHM PROBLEMS

CAUSE Abnormalities of heart rhythm have a variety of causes. They may be temporary or permanent. Sometimes they can arise as a result of disease or injury elsewhere, and will disappear when that is treated; at other times they are a sign of worsening of an existing heart condition.

The rhythm may be slower or faster than normal, or else irregular and episodic, possibly coming in 'bursts'. All abnormal rhythms are potentially serious.

Sinus arrythmia

Note that healthy young dogs often show alterations in heart rhythm which correspond with breathing. Owners sometimes notice this when the dogs are lying resting and a heart beat is visible or felt in the chest area. This is a normal rhythm and no treatment is required. If you have any doubts at all, then get your dog checked, but in a young otherwise healthy dog, sinus arrythmia may well be the cause.

SYMPTOMS There may be symptoms of an underlying heart disease, such as cough and poor exercising ability. Fainting may be seen, along with general weakness. Some medical conditions which primarily affect other organs may result in abnormal heart rhythms as a (serious) complication, e.g. gastric dilation and torsion (see page 109). Any injury to the chest wall can potentially result in heart rhythm irregularities.

DIAGNOSIS ECGs are used to diagnose abnormal heart rhythms. Other tests such as X-rays and cardiac ultrasound may also be required.

TREATMENT For abnormally slow rhythms, pacemakers, as used in humans, can be employed to regulate the heart rate. Drugs are also available to control both fast and slow rhythms. Adjustment of existing medication may be required in dogs with known heart disease. When the cause is due to a problem elsewhere in the body, this should be diagnosed and treated.

OUTLOOK This depends very much on the exact cause of the irregularity, and whether it will be responsive to treatment.

HEARTWORM

CAUSE The cause is a parasitic worm (not found in the United Kingdom) which lives in the heart or large blood vessels in the chest. Transmission requires the presence of mosquitos which, when they bite the infected dog, take in minute larvae which the worms

have released into the bloodstream. The mosquito then bites another dog and passes the larvae onto the new host. The larvae pass in the blood to the heart and large blood vessels and take up the adult position there.

SYMPTOMS Heartworms can cause heart failure if there is a heavy infestation, so signs of coughing and poor exercising ability may be seen.

DIAGNOSIS This requires a blood test or blood examination.

TREATMENT This is not an easy condition to treat effectively since very powerful drugs (with potential side-effects) need to be used.

Prevention

In countries where heartworm is found, it is usual to give regular preventative medicine to stop an infestation occurring in the first place.

Respiratory/Lung Diseases

COUGHING; SNEEZING

CAUSE Coughing is a strong reflex response to anything which might endanger an animal's airway, thus interfering with respiration. Receptors are present throughout an animal's throat, trachea (windpipe) and lungs and whenever they are stimulated, a cough results. Coughing therefore does not have one single cause – many things can trigger it, from smoke inhalation to pneumonia. Sneezing is similar, though less common in dogs.

SYMPTOMS Coughing is a very forceful expiration of breath. Pressure in the chest area is made to build up and then this is suddenly released. The rapid rush of air is designed to dislodge and expel the irritation, whether this is a bacterium/virus, an accumulation of phlegm or mucus, or an inhaled object such as a grass

Useful information for your vet

- When did the cough start? Did it come on suddenly or gradually?

- Has your dog been in contact with other dogs recently, e.g. kennels, dog shows?

- When is the cough worst – morning, evening, or no real pattern?

- Is your dog able to exercise as normal?

- Is your dog sleeping or resting more?

- Are any other symptoms present?

First aid for the dog in respiratory distress

Try to keep calm. Follow the guidelines in Chapter 18, if the dog is collapsed or you suspect something is lodged in the throat. If the temperature is hot and you suspect hyperthermia/heatstroke, immediately begin cooling the dog down using cool water, fans etc. Overheating is quite a common problem in warmer months, especially in dogs suffering from laryngeal paralysis (see page 137) and in overweight dogs.

seed. It is a very effective mechanism indeed and when it is absent for any reason, the animal is at high risk of developing respiratory infections or accumulation of mucus; these can be extremely dangerous.

Coughing may occur as a single isolated episode or it may be a chain or paroxysm of coughs. At the end of the cough or coughs, material may be expelled (or swallowed). In human medicine, coughs are often labelled 'productive' or 'non-productive' but this is generally less useful in dogs.

DIAGNOSIS Clinical examination and X-rays are commonly used. Further tests may then be indicated to follow up lines of diagnosis.

TREATMENT A specific cause must be found, as the treatment varies. Many coughs are caused by heart disease; others may be caused by infections, bronchitis, tumours, allergies or inhaled objects.

OUTLOOK This depends on the cause. See other diseases on following pages for some of the commoner problems encountered in the dog.

BREATHING PROBLEMS; WHEEZING

CAUSE As with coughing, there are various causes of breathing difficulty or wheezing and many dogs with

respiratory or heart disease show both coughing and breathing problems/wheezing.

SYMPTOMS The respiratory rate may be abnormal. Usually, breathing is more rapid than normal, with shallower breaths. Sometimes, the pattern of breathing may be altered: the dog may put more effort into breathing, using the muscles of the abdomen to a large degree and forcefully expanding the chest wall as air is drawn in.

High pitched wheezing/whistling sounds may be heard and occasionally crackles. The dog may pant more than usual.

DIAGNOSIS Clinical examination and X-rays is the usual starting point, with further tests as indicated.

TREATMENT Again, this depends on the precise cause, as with coughing. Some of the commoner causes are discussed in the sections below.

KENNEL COUGH

This common infectious cough is discussed on page 24.

TRACHEAL COLLAPSE

CAUSE The trachea (windpipe) carries air from the throat to the lungs. Narrowing of the trachea from any cause (e.g. an object lodged inside it, or something from outside pressing against it) interferes with the flow of air and affects respiration.

Tracheal collapse is a condition where the walls of the trachea lose their shape, resulting in narrowing of the airway and breathing problems. The rings of cartilage which normally hold the trachea apart are insufficiently rigid to maintain the normal open tube. The disease is commoner in small breeds of dogs, with a high incidence in Yorskhire Terriers. Symptoms usually begin in middle age.

SYMPTOMS A characteristic cough is heard (often described as 'honking'). This can be very persistent and cause severe respiratory distress as the disease progresses with increasing age.

DIAGNOSIS X-rays and endoscopy may be used, although the diagnosis is often suggested by the breed, age and symptoms.

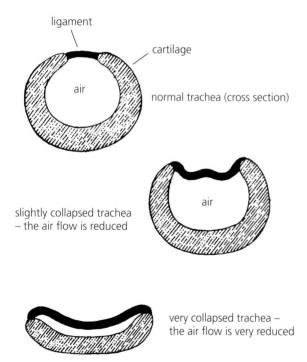

Diagram to illustrate tracheal collapse. The interior of the trachea is gradually lost as the structure collapses rather like a squashed straw. The problem is common in Yorkshire Terriers and other small breeds.

TREATMENT Milder cases are treated by weight control (overweight dogs have much worse symptoms), and drugs for any chest and heart problems that may also be present. Over-excitement should be avoided as this invariably makes symptoms worse. Severe cases may be treated surgically in an attempt to alter the shape of the collapsed trachea.

OUTLOOK This can be a difficult disease to cure completely. Many dogs are successfully managed without surgery, but they will show symptoms to a greater or lesser degree no matter which drug treatments they are on. Temperament plays an important role, with more excitable dogs exacerbating their symptoms. Surgery can sometimes help, but it is not a guarantee of success in every case. For very severe chronic cases, the outlook is not good.

BRONCHITIS

CAUSE Bronchitis means inflammation of the air passages in the lungs. Acute bronchitis is caused by such things as smoke inhalation, infections (e.g. kennel cough) and allergic responses.The symptoms are usually of short duration and are responsive to treatment.

Chronic bronchitis is of longer standing duration. It is seen quite frequently in small dogs of terrier breeds. The condition can complicate other problems such as tracheal collapse and heart disease. Severe damage may be caused to the airways, such that they never return to absolutely normal structure and function.

SYMPTOMS Coughing is the main symptom; during severe periods the animal may be ill, with a high temperature and poor energy levels. Breathing irregularities may be present and exercising ability will be reduced.

DIAGNOSIS X-rays, blood tests and endoscopy are all used, depending on the case.

TREATMENT Drug treatments usually include antibiotics when infection is present or likely and anti-inflammatory drugs and dilators, which help improve breathing efficiency.

Physiotherapy

Chest physiotherapy can be helpful. 'Coupage' (firm patting/drumming of the chest wall) can be carried out on either side several times a day to help dislodge and expel mucus adhering in the airways. Steam inhalation also helps in moving airway secretions. Having the dog in the bathroom while taking a bath or shower can be a useful method of steam inhalation, which most dogs will tolerate well!

OUTLOOK Bronchitis can be a serious disease if it is progressive and respiratory failure sets in. Most patients are helped considerably by treatments if these are followed carefully.

PNEUMONIA

CAUSE Pneumonia has a number of causes. Diseases such as distemper, adenovirus and parainfluenza virus (all preventable by vaccination) can cause pneumonia, as can kennel cough in old or debilitated dogs. Various other organisms/bacteria can lead to pneumonia and several diseases, especially those which affect swallowing or produce severe vomiting or regurgitation, carry a high risk of pneumonia as a complication.

SYMPTOMS There is usually a cough, though not nearly as loud as that produced by kennel cough. The cough of pneumonia is quieter and sounds moist. A nasal discharge may be present and severely affected animals are normally very ill, with a high temperature and reluctance to eat or move.

DIAGNOSIS X-rays, blood tests and endoscopy may all be used to diagnose pneumonia.

TREATMENT Antibiotics are given. Some animals require hospitalisation for oxygen provision and intravenous fluids (a 'drip') or intravenous antibiotics. Long courses of antibiotics are likely.

OUTLOOK Localised pneumonias usually respond well to treatment. The worst cases are general pneumonias of sudden, severe onset, and these can be fatal or result in permanent lung damage.

Prevention

Vaccination against the infectious diseases of dogs will prevent this source of pneumonia (see Chapter 1).

LUNG CANCER

CAUSE This disease is detected less frequently in dogs than in people. Often, the cause is a tumour elsewhere in the body which has spread to the lungs. This tends to be a disease of older dogs.

SYMPTOMS Cough with weight loss over a period of a few weeks to a few months is seen in some cases; in other cases few symptoms are noticed until the disease becomes very advanced, when irregular breathing and poor exercising ability is seen. These dogs are likely to be subdued with a poor appetite. Blood may be produced on coughing.

DIAGNOSIS Chest X-rays are used. It is often necessary to check other areas of the body too since tumours in the chest may have originally come from the mammary (breast) area in female dogs, prostate in male dogs or from the bones or other organs. Biopsies confirm the diagnosis.

TREATMENT For single tumours in a localised area of the lung, excision by removal of the lung lobe may be possible. There is always the possibility that spread to other areas has occurred however, and surgery will therefore not effect a complete cure, but it may extend life in certain cases.

For tumours which have already spread to the lungs and affect many places within it, anti-inflammatory drugs and pain relief can sometimes help. Euthanasia will eventually be required however once quality of life deteriorates.

OUTLOOK The outlook for all forms of lung cancer is poor.

BROKEN RIBS

CAUSE Broken ribs can result from road traffic accidents or other severe trauma (e.g. a kick) or, in smaller dogs, from crushing injuries to the chest inflicted by larger dogs during a fight. Puppies dropped or fallen upon by children may fracture ribs, although this is not that common due to the softer, pliable bones of puppies which tend to spring back readily into shape.

SYMPTOMS Fractured ribs are painful and this may be the main feature whenever the affected area is touched. Breathing may be shallow and 'careful'.

❗ Dangers of chest injuries

Dogs that have injuries on the chest wall should always be suspected of having puncture wounds into the chest cavity. Veterinary attention should be sought immediately, since life-threatening problems can arise if the chest cavity is not air tight.

DIAGNOSIS This is usually by X-ray. One of the dangers is that further damage to underlying organs may also have occurred, e.g. there may be lung tears, allowing air to leak into the chest cavity – a potentially dangerous situation termed pneumothorax. Alternatively, bleeding may have occurred in the chest or the heart muscle may be bruised. These are both more serious conditions than rib fractures; X-rays should help detect them if present.

TREATMENT Single rib fractures heal well. The dog should be rested, perhaps in a cage, while healing takes place. Mutliple fractures may be treated the same way or else a splint may be applied to the chest wall. Sometimes fine pins may be inserted to realign

severely disrupted rib fractures which are very painful and would otherwise take a very long time to heal.

OUTLOOK The outlook is usually good provided more severe damage to the lungs, chest cavity and heart has been avoided.

DIAPHRAGMATIC HERNIA

CAUSE The diaphragm is the muscular sheet which separates the chest from the abdomen. It is important in breathing, when it helps to create the negative pressure which draws air into the chest. A diaphragmatic hernia occurs when severe trauma causes the muscle to split, allowing abdominal organs to slide through into the chest area.

SYMPTOMS The abdominal organs that move into the chest cavity restrict the space available to the lungs, hence breathing is affected. Additional complications can mean that the displaced abdominal organs (e.g. liver, spleen, stomach or intestine) become ensnared in the chest and portions may get strangulated (their circulation is cut off, causing further severe problems).

Animals with diaphragmatic hernias often breathe with more abdominal effort than normal. Alternatively, respirations may be rapid and shallow. In some cases, breathing may be apparently normal and unless X-rays are taken the condition is sometimes not detected. Precautionary chest X-rays are therefore quite often advised in any dog that has suffered trauma in case a diaphragmatic hernia is present but not showing many symptoms.

Dogs may in fact live for many months with a hernia which has become chronic. This is, however, potentially dangerous since entrapment of organs could occur at virtually any time, causing life-threatening complications.

DIAGNOSIS The condition may be suspected in an animal which has suffered trauma and which is experiencing breathing difficulty. Sometimes the abdomen feels or looks emptier than normal – because organs have moved forwards into the chest. Diagnosis is

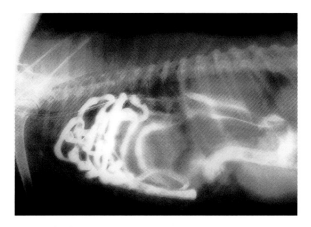

X-ray of a dog which had been hit by a car. The diaphragm has ruptured and a barium fluid swallow (white areas) appears in the chest, showing that abdominal organs have moved forwards out of their normal position. Major surgery is required to treat this life-threatening problem.

confirmed by an X-ray, perhaps involving a barium swallow.

TREATMENT Treatment in most cases is delayed until the dog is stabilised – which may take 24–48 hours. Repair of a diaphragmatic hernia is a major operation, not without some risk, so the dog must be prepared adequately to give the best chance of recovery. Other injuries may also need to be evaluated since any trauma which has caused a diaphragmatic hernia could easily have led to other problems, e.g. lung bleeding or air leakage, fractured bones, etc. Neverthless, the diaphragmatic hernia will be repaired early (before any surgery for broken bones is undertaken, for instance) since it is the more immediately life-threatening.

OUTLOOK Dogs with this injury are high risk patients, and may in addition have further complicating problems arising from major trauma. Surgery carries the best chance of success once the patient is fit for anaesthesia.

LARYNGEAL PARALYSIS

CAUSE Degeneration of the nerves which supply the muscles of the larynx causes this condition in most animals, and symptoms appear in middle to older age. The disease causes the structures of the larynx to collapse inwards, interfering with the normal flow of air.

SYMPTOMS A number of symptoms may appear depending on severity. A change in the tone of the bark is heard in many cases. The dog may not cope well with exercise or excitement (collapse can occur) and coughing is heard. During inspiration, turbulence in the air flow produces a harsh noise. Symptoms are much worse in hot conditions and in overweight dogs, when collapse and heatstroke may be seen.

DIAGNOSIS Most dogs are given a light anaesthetic and their laryngeal movements closely observed. X-rays may be needed to rule out complicating factors. Some dogs have other associated problems such as nostril narrowing (see page 38) and elongation of the soft palate. These contribute to the general breathing problems and may also need to be treated.

TREATMENT The best treatment is a surgical operation to improve the airway by widening it and securing the collapsed cartilage in a new position. Although both sides of the dog's larynx are usually affected by the disease, surgery on one side only is normally sufficient to alleviate the symptoms.

It is a difficult operation and some potential for complications may exist, however advanced laryngeal paralysis is a disease that cannot be well controlled by drugs or other means. Overweight dogs must be placed on a strict diet.

OUTLOOK Successful surgery brings about large improvements in the dog's ability to exercise and breathe normally.

LUNGWORM

CAUSE Lungworm follows the eating of larvae of a parasitic worm; the infection is frequently passed from dam to offspring during the suckling period. Following infection, the adult worms form nodular areas in the trachea and lung airways, which causes inflammation and a harsh cough similar to kennel cough. The condition is diagnosed far less frequently than kennel cough and when it occurs it is usually seen in young dogs housed together.

SYMPTOMS Harsh cough.

DIAGNOSIS X-rays and endoscopy may be used to confirm the diagnosis.

TREATMENT Prescription wormers kill the worms.

OUTLOOK Good; the condition should be cured completely.

FOREIGN BODY/INHALED OBJECT

CAUSE It is fortunately quite rare that foreign objects are inhaled into the chest area: strong protective mechanisms in the pharynx and the cough reflex should prevent this. However, it does occasionally happen, e.g. a dog running through a field of tall grass may inhale a seed head which passes deep into the chest. Sometimes objects, usually larger ones, become jammed in the throat area, completely cutting off the air supply. This is a life threatening situation.

SYMPTOMS Usually a sudden onset of coughing occurs after exercise or after playing with small objects (e.g. small stones thrown for a dog). The situation worsens over a few hours or even days and the dog may become generally ill with bad breath and a reluctance to exercise. Breathing difficulty may be apparent.

If something is stuck in the throat, extreme breathing difficulty and collapse may be seen immediately after the object becomes lodged there.

DIAGNOSIS X-rays and endoscopy are used most frequently for small objects such as grass seeds.

TREATMENT Many objects can be successfully removed from the airways via the endoscope without the need for major chest surgery; but in some patients surgery will be required. Complications such as pneumonia and collapse of the lung are a potential threat.

Emergency first aid for throat obstructions

See Chapter 18 for what to do if a large object, e.g. rubber ball or stone, is lodged in your dog's throat. This action could save your dog's life if carried out promptly as no time may be available for transportation to a veterinary clinic.

OUTLOOK Provided the object can be removed safely and effectively, usually with an endoscope, the outlook may be good. In certain cases however, even after successful removal, some permanent damage may remain. Major chest surgery, if needed, carries significant risks and if complications develop the prognosis is worsened.

CHAPTER 8

The Kidneys and Urinary System

Common symptoms of kidney and urinary disease
• Frequent urination • Blood in urine
• Straining to pass urine • Licking at penis or vulva
• Discharge from penis or vulva • Incontinence
• Excessive thirst • Weight loss or poor appetite
• Vomiting • Bad breath and mouth ulcers

Structure and Function

The paired kidneys receive approximately one quarter of all of the blood output from the heart. This is a large quota, reflecting the vital function these organs play in life. The kidneys are responsible for controlling the precise conditions of the fluid which surrounds every single cell in the body, maintaining the steady chemical state necessary for normal activity. It is a very important role and perhaps this is why nature has supplied two of these organs, when most animals could survive perfectly adequately with only one. The 'extra' kidney may be a safeguard against injury or disease affecting its partner, a case of 'belt and braces'.

By means of elaborate and complex mechanisms, the kidneys regulate the water balance in the body and also the concentration of electrolytes (chemicals) and other substances in the blood and tissue fluids. They are involved in control of the blood pressure and in the production of red blood cells – the vital oxygen-carrying cells which give blood its colour. In their role as a filtration and purifying system, the kidneys ensure that waste products are removed from the blood to be excreted from the body in urine, thus preventing a build up of toxins which would damage and ultimately kill the animal.

Thirst and urine production are carefully regulated to maintain optimum conditions for metabolism and healthy functioning of the body: too much water is excreted before dangerous rises in blood pressure occur; too little water stimulates a series of protective changes (including thirst) to guard against dehydration. This fine balancing act is performed 24 hours a day in the ever-changing conditions of an animal's body.

Loss of kidney function

With so many important activities going on, it is not surprising that loss of kidney function poses a serious threat to life. Paradoxically, however, by the time kidney disease is recognised, it is almost always at a very advanced stage. Like the liver, the kidneys compensate for and 'hide' early signs of disease. It is only when these compensating mechanisms themselves start to fail that signs of kidney disease eventually begin to be shown. This means that kidney diseases can be very difficult to treat effectively – indeed, treatment usually consists of limiting further damage and easing the workload on the kidneys rather than curing them.

General anatomy of the urinary system

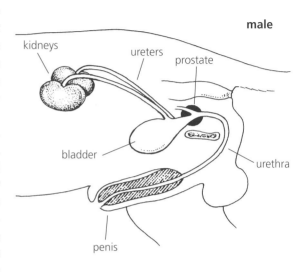

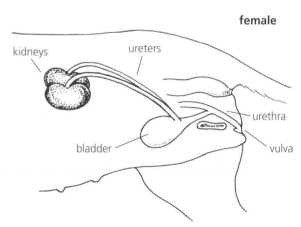

Male and female urinary tracts. The male's uretha is longer and narrower than the female's.

Bladder and urethra

Each kidney is linked to the bladder by a long, slender tube called a ureter. Urine constantly flows slowly through the two ureters to be stored in the bladder and then elmininated from the body by urination at convenient times. To leave the body, urine passes from the bladder into the single urethra, and then to the outside. The urethra is relatively long and narrow in male dogs compared to bitches.

The bladder itself is an elastic organ which alters in size to accommodate urine. When full, it can occupy a large area of the abdomen and is easily felt through the abdominal wall but when empty it is very small indeed and cannot usually be detected by palpation of the abdomen. The act of urination is a complex response governed by voluntary and involuntary controls.

The full bladder acts, via a series of nerve pathways and links, to produce the urge to urinate and thus empty the organ. Inflammation of the bladder can also have this effect, i.e. the animal feels the desire to pass urine even although the bladder itself may be empty. This is a common symptom of cystitis (inflammation affecting the lining of the bladder).

What can go wrong with the urinary system?

Any failure or obstruction in the production or flow of urine is extremely dangerous. This effectively means that toxins cannot be eliminated from the body, hence they accumulate within the body's organs and tissues and damage them. Renal failure, acute or chronic, has this effect because the kidneys lose their ability to concentrate and control the composition of urine.

Physical blockages, such as mineral stones formed in the body and which then become lodged in the relatively narrow ureter or urethra, may result in a build up of pressure above the obstruction, which can also damage organs or even cause rupture. In these circumstances a whole series of dangerous complications can arise.

Like other organs and tissues, the kidneys and urinary system can become infected by organisms (bacteria and viruses) which may cause damage or even organ failure. Traumatic injury, e.g. following a road accident, can also damage or rupture any of the organs of the urinary system, and cancer affecting these organs is also seen, with bladder cancer being commoner than cancer of the kidneys or other structures.

Veterinary Diagnosis and Treatment

Diagnosis of kidney disease usually involves blood and urine tests. Many of the general symptoms of kidney and urinary system disease can be caused by a variety of other illnesses and these need to be ruled out. X-rays or ultrasound technques may be required and, in a few cases, biopsies of the kidney may be indicated.

Blood tests measure the concentration of substances that are normally effectively removed from the blood by the kidneys. If these substances, such as creatinine, are not being removed well, the blood tests will show high results – indicating that the kidneys are not performing adequately. Blood tests like this can be used to monitor how the kidneys are responding to treatment over a period of time and are interpreted in conjunction with other information on the dog's health. Conditions of the ureters, bladder and urethra are often diagnosed using X-ray or ultrasound techniques. Some of these conditions require surgery for treatment.

Special diets are often used in urinary system diseases, e.g. diets designed to spare the workload of the kidneys in chronic renal failure or to reduce the tendency to form mineral stones within the urinary system. These are prescribed under veterinary advice.

Cost and prognosis in kidney and urinary diseases

The commonest kidney problem – chronic renal failure (see page 145) – is an incurable condition, requiring diagnostic tests initially and then on-going treatment hopefully to keep the problem under control so that the dog can have a good quality of life. Periods of hospitalisation may be necessary at the outset since dogs with renal disease often benefit from intravenous fluids (a drip) to help eliminate accumulated toxins and get the kidneys functioning again. Medication may be needed long term, together with special diets in order to support the kidneys. This can mean on-going costs for treatment and periodic check-ups of kidney function.

Sometimes, dogs that have been responding well suffer a set-back, where the kidneys deteriorate

Measuring water intake and urine output

Measurement of both of these provides very useful information for the veterinary surgeon when urinary system disease is suspected.

To measure water intake you must ensure that there is only one source of water available, to which your dog has constant access. It is best to measure the amount taken over several 24 hour periods and then work out an average of, say, 4 occasions. This eliminates day-to-day variations. A useful routine is:

1. Fill a large container/basin with water up to a mark which you can see or have made on it. This should contain more water than your dog is likely to drink in 24 hours.

2. Note the time.

3. 24 hours later measure the amount of water needed to return the water level exactly to the mark. Measure in millilitres/litres.

4. Obviously, other animals drinking from the same source could lead to confusion and account would need to be taken of this.

A healthy dog should not drink more than 100 ml of water per kilogram of body weight per day.

Collecting a urine sample

Simple tests on a urine sample can provide much useful information. The sample should be as fresh as possible when taken to the veterinary clinic as changes can occur if it is allowed to stand.

Any container used to collect a sample must be absolutely clean and dry. Confusion could easily result if, e.g. traces of sugar were present in a bottle or jar. This may lead to the mistaken finding of glucose in the urine (a symptom of diabetes).

Veterinary practices can provide collection bottles which are designed to make it easier to obtain the sample from your dog, but if another container is used it should be washed in hot detergent, rinsed repeatedly and then allowed to dry before it is used for urine.

Try if possible to obtain a 'mid-stream' sample from your dog, i.e. not the very beginning or end of the urine flow. Male dogs are easier to collect from than females. If you have to store the sample, enclose it completely in two plastic bags which are tied and sealed, and keep in the fridge, preferably in an air tight container.

suddenly in function. This can be provoked by a number of factors, e.g. stress, infection, or just the natural progression of the disease. The failing kidneys can sometimes be 'rescued' by a short period of hospital treatment to get the dog back onto an even keel again. Eventually, however, the time may come when quality of life is very poor and little effective kidney function remains. This is the point at which euthanasia may be discussed by the veterinary surgeon.

Bladder diseases, other than cancer of the bladder (which is less common than the other problems), are generally less severe and a cure is often possible. This may entail surgery in certain cases, but on-going treatment may be needed in cases of incontinence and very severe cystitis (see later).

In general, adequate diagnosis and monitoring of urinary system diseases cannot be made without a number of investigations and tests, making this group of diseases more expensive to diagnose than some of the others. Prognosis varies between the conditions

but if the disease cannot be cured it can often be managed for a considerable period of time with a good quality of life resulting for the dog.

Are kidney transplants available for dogs?

Although the operation is technically possible, this procedure is not performed routinely in dogs. There is no system of availability of suitable organs for transplant and the operation requires specialist surgical skills. It may become possible in the future, however there are important ethical questions surrounding its use in pets since dogs donating organs cannot give informed consent.

Renal dialysis, another technique employed in human kidney patients, often those awaiting transplant, is also not used in dogs and is associated with similar ethical and animal welfare considerations.

Commonest Kidney and Urinary Problems in Dogs

CHANGES IN FREQUENCY OR AMOUNT OF URINATION

CAUSE Alterations in the pattern of urination occur frequently in various kidney and urinary diseases. Occasionally, however, the problem lies outwith the kidneys or urinary tract. Excess urination may be caused by diabetes or infection of the womb (pyometra), for example. These are discussed in other chapters.

SYMPTOMS Careful observation of the symptoms will help the veterinary surgeon narrow down the large list of possibilities. Study the box and try to decide which pattern is present in your dog. It is particularly important to distinguish between urinating normal or increased amounts and *unproductive* straining because the latter could indicate the serious condition of urinary obstruction (as well as the less dangerous condition of cystitis).

 Important observations to help the vet

- Is urine being passed more or less frequently than normal?

- Is the amount passed normal, increased or reduced (i.e. very small quantities)?

- Does the dog strain to pass urine?

- Is a steady stream of urine produced?

- Is there any blood present? (Collect a urine sample if possible).

- Is the dog's bedding damp or has the dog been urinating in the house overnight?

- Is this the first occurrence of symptoms? If not, when did they last occur?

- Are there any other symptoms present, e.g. increased thirst, weight loss, poor appetite, vomiting?

DIAGNOSIS This is dealt with under the individual diseases, but is likely to involve blood/urine tests and X-rays or ultrasound scans.

TREATMENT See individual diseases.

OUTLOOK See individual diseases.

BLOOD IN URINE

CAUSE As with alterations in the amount or frequency of urine, this can be a symptom of several different urinary system diseases. Blood arises when areas of the urinary tract are inflamed or damaged. The blood can come from any of the urinary organs: kidneys, ureters, bladder or urethra. Common causes include cystitis and urinary stone formation.

Blood in urine can also come from other organs. Two common examples are from the prostate gland in male dogs and from the uterus in females. In bitches, the blood may be either as a result of the normal oestrus cycle in unspayed dogs, or because there is

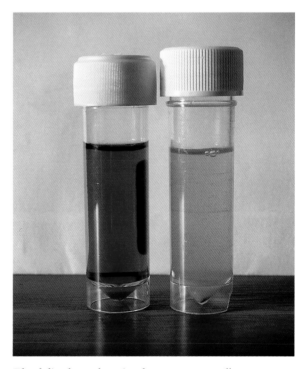

Blood discolours the urine, however very small amounts may not be visible to the naked eye.

inflammation present within the uterus (pyometra). These conditions are discussed Chapters 11 and 12.

SYMPTOMS Large quantities of blood are obvious because they give the urine a red tinge, or else blood droplets may be seen at the prepuce in males or at the vulva in females. Testing a urine sample that looks normal may reveal hidden levels of blood, i.e. small traces invisible to the naked eye. This can be important in monitoring responses to treatment.

DIAGNOSIS It is important to determine where the blood is coming from. Clinical examination, urine/blood tests and X-rays may all be needed to trace the source of the blood.

TREATMENT This is as described under individual conditions.

OUTLOOK Blood in the urine is always a worrying symptom for owners to find but, although it can indicate serious problems, most cases are not life-threatening and will respond to treatment.

ACUTE KIDNEY (RENAL) FAILURE

CAUSE This condition results in an abrupt failure of the normal functions of the kidney. It is less common than chronic renal failure in dogs (see below), but when it occurs must be treated quickly if permanent damage or death is to be avoided. A large variety of causes is possible, including:

- Interruption to the blood flow to the kidneys. A severe haemorrhage or fall in blood pressure can cause this. Without an adequate blood pressure the kidneys cannot filter the blood of toxins and waste products; these therefore accumulate and cause symptoms of renal failure.

- Poisoning with substances which are toxic to the kidney, e.g. antifreeze. Dogs may lick these substances if their feet or coat become contaminated. Dogs which scavenge indiscriminately may take in other poisons such as rat poisons or weed killers, both of which can severely damage the kidneys.

- Infections. Leptospirosis can cause acute kidney failure in unvaccinated dogs. Parvovirus may also cause kidney failure due to secondary infections and severe dehydration from bloody diarrhoea.

- Blockage of urine flow. Mineral stones produced in the urinary system may move into narrow structures such as ureters or the urethra and block them, preventing the flow and elimination of urine. Pressure builds up which can cause damage or rupture of urinary organs and toxins are absorbed from the urine into the body. Bladder paralysis after pelvic or spinal injury can also effectively block normal urination, with similar consequences.

- Traumatic injury to the kidneys or urinary tract. The commonest injuries causing damage to the urinary system are road traffic accidents.

SYMPTOMS Typical signs are vomiting, dehydration, poor appetite and collapse. There is little or no urine production in many cases, in contrast with chronic renal failure where urine production is increased over a period of weeks or months. Other symptoms may be present depending on which of the above problems are present.

DIAGNOSIS This depends on blood tests and also trying to find out if the dog has an underlying disease or has encountered any chemical or injury which might have led on to the acute kidney failure. The underlying cause of the kidney failure needs to be treated as well whenever it can be identified. X-rays and ultrasound pictures of the kidney and urinary system may be taken to check that their structure is intact.

TREATMENT Complications affecting the heart due to potassium build up develop quickly in acute kidney failure. These must be diagnosed and treated promptly. Other abnormalities in body chemicals and dehydration must also be treated, so hospitalisation is required and intravenous drips will be needed. Whenever possible the underlying cause of the kidney failure is also treated, e.g. damaged organs are repaired once the animal is stabilised; antidotes to poisons, if available, are given. The aim is to prevent irreversible changes occurring to the kidneys and to provide good conditions for their recovery.

OUTLOOK The condition is rapidly life-threatening and always carries a guarded outlook. However if caught early dogs can respond well to treatment, after which they may make a full recovery or else go on to develop chronic renal failure (see below), which can usually be controlled, if not cured.

CHRONIC KIDNEY (RENAL) FAILURE

CAUSE This is the commonest kidney disease diagnosed in dogs and is frequently encountered in older animals. However, dogs of all ages may experience chronic renal failure. The term simply describes the situation that arises once the kidney can no longer compensate adequately for damage which has occurred to it.

Chronic kidney failure can follow on from acute failure and any of the causes of that condition but the exact cause of the initial damage to the kidney may not be known in many patients. In old animals, gradual deterioration in association with age is often assumed to be the reason. In younger dogs, inherited disease may be involved and certain breeds seem prone to this. Some of these conditions preferentially affect one sex more than the other. Although born with normal kidneys, renal function steadily deteriorates resulting in symptoms of chronic failure appearing in young adulthood.

SYMPTOMS Chronic renal failure produces symptoms of general illness. Dogs with the disease frequently pass more urine than usual as their kidneys have lost the ability to concentrate urine. As a result, they have to drink more to prevent dehydration. This gives rise to the symptom of 'polyuria/polydipsia' which simply means passing more urine and drinking more than normal.

Other symptoms include weight loss, poor appetite, vomiting, weakness and debility, mouth ulcers and anaemia. Note that very similar symptoms can be caused by a variety of other diseases, which makes diagnostic tests very important in kidney disease.

DIAGNOSIS Blood tests and urine tests are used most frequently. Blood tests allow for the measurement of substances which should normally by efficiently filtered out of the bloodstream by the kidneys. If this is not happening because the kidneys are under-performing, higher than normal levels will be detected. Substances measured include creatinine, urea and phosphate. All of these rise in chronic renal failure (and in acute renal failure).

Urine tests provide additional information on urine infections, loss of protein in the urine and on how well the kidneys are concentrating the urine. X-rays and ultrasound may also be used and kidney biopsies are occasionally undertaken.

TREATMENT There is no treatment to restore kidney function to normal and kidney transplants are not carried out on canine patients, however by easing the workload on the kidneys and treating complications arising from the poor kidney function, the condition can often be successfully managed for long periods of time. New treatments becoming available may lead to further improvements in managing chronic renal failure in dogs.

Generally, treatment involves making certain changes to the diet, treating anaemia and infections and, possibly, treating elevated blood pressure if this is present. Additional drugs may be needed to cope with

Ensure plenty of water

On no account should a dog suffering from chronic renal failure have its water intake restricted, as otherwise dehydration and toxaemia may result. The excess drinking is a necessary compensation for the water that is being lost in the urine and the dog is unable to control this symptom. This can, unfortunately, result in occasional house wetting in certain dogs, but it is important to realise that it is the excess urination that leads to the increased thirst – and *not* the other way round, so that depriving the dog of necessary water is dangerous.

retention of phosphate if this is occurring and causing symptoms. Re-assessment of blood tests at intervals, taken together with the general health of the dog, can show how the patient is responding and may influence the treatment given.

OUTLOOK This depends on the severity at the time of diagnosis and, to some extent, the course that the disease takes in the individual dog. In most cases, improvements in quality of life can be expected as the progress of the disease is slowed or even halted, thereby extending life expectancy.

CYSTITIS

CAUSE Cystitis occurs when the lining of the bladder is inflamed. Two common reasons for this occurring are infections and the formation of crystals or stones in the urine which irritate the lining of the bladder. Urinary crystals and stones are discussed in more detail below.

SYMPTOMS Cystitis results in a frequent urge to urinate. Often only very small amounts of urine are passed at a time and these may contain blood. There are usually no other major symptoms in simple cystitis.

One problem is in distinguishing cystitis from the much more serious condition of urinary obstruction. Urinary obstruction can happen in any animal for a variety of reasons but is seen oftener in males, due to their relatively long and narrow urethra which may trap small stones being passed in the urine. The female urethra is shorter and wider and less prone to obstruction.

Because of the risk of obstruction, all dogs showing straining with poor urine flow should be checked by the veterinary surgeon promptly. Most of the time, and especially in female dogs, it will just be cystitis but if you suspect obstruction (see symptom box opposite) contact the clinic immediately as this is an emergency condition.

DIAGNOSIS If possible collect a urine sample and take this to the veterinary clinic for your appointment as performing a few simple checks on this can help in diagnosing the cause of the cystitis. The veterinary surgeon will perform an examination to try to find the reason, and may recommend further tests such as X-rays. Biopsies may be needed in severe or difficult cases.

TREATMENT Antibiotics are usually given for infections. With cystitis caused by mineral deposits or stones, the treatment is to remove the source of irritation by dissolving the stones using a special diet, or by surgery. Cases of chronic cystitis, when the bladder lining has become very thickened due to long-term inflammation, can be difficult to treat.

OUTLOOK The outlook is good for most cases of cystitis, although antibiotics may be needed for a lengthy time and the full course should always be completed. A few cases of chronic cystitis are difficult to treat and require continuous low-level treatment with antibiotics. Even then, symptoms tend to recur.

URINARY STONES

CAUSE Mineral stones can be formed in various places in the body but they are commonest in the urinary system, when they are known as uroliths. In some dogs, minerals dissolved in the urine coalesce to form crystals. Various things can trigger this, including a tendency to produce more minerals in the urine in certain dog breeds, and also alterations in the acidity of the urine which can promote crystal formation. Infection or other disease may lead to changes in the urine composition such that crystal formation becomes much more likely.

The crystals grow into stones, which can become suprisingly large. Both crystals and stones cause irritation to the lining of the bladder, producing the symptoms mentioned below. Although stones may be found in the kidneys, most problems occur when they develop in the bladder or when smaller stones move into a narrow area such as the urethra of male dogs. This is when the dangerous situation of urinary obstruction may occur.

SYMPTOMS Common symptoms are straining to pass urine, blood in urine and dribbling of urine. With straining, only small quantities of urine are passed at a time. The symptoms are very similar to those of cystitis in uncomplicated cases without obstruction. In severe cases, when obstruction has occurred, symptoms are more severe. A worsening of the condition can occur quickly, leading onto collapse and death from acute renal failure within 12 to 24 hours.

DIAGNOSIS Diagnosis can be made by examining a urine sample for crystals, by feeling larger stones in a dog's bladder, and with the help of X-rays or ultrasound since bigger stones may be visible with these techniques (however some types of stone are invisible

Symptoms of urinary obstruction – an emergency situation

- Abdominal pain, agitation
- Frequent straining to pass urine but only a few drops produced, usually containing blood
- Depression
- Vomiting
- Disorientation and collapse

This condition is most often seen in male dogs when a small urinary stone obtructs the urethra (the narrow tube which carries urine from the bladder to the outside)

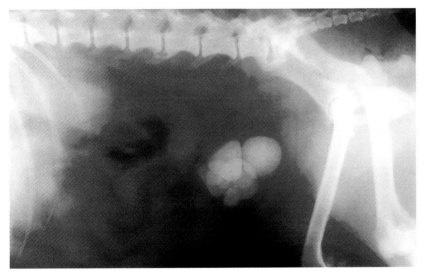

Bladder stones as seen on an X-ray. The dog had been straining to urinate with blood present in the urine.

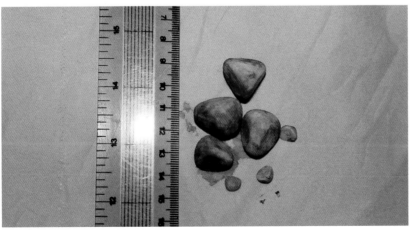

Stones removed from the bladder of the dog shown in the X-ray above.

on X-ray). Dogs which have severe obstruction are emergency cases and need rapid treatment to stabilise their condition.

TREATMENT Once it is understood what the stones are composed of, a means of removing or preventing them is decided upon.

Infection is usually present and must be treated with antibiotics; sometimes long courses are required. If the stones themselves can be dissolved by altering the conditions of the urine, then this can be started after diagnosis and the symptoms should gradually improve. Certain stones respond well to this treatment. For a common type of stone in dogs, the urine is made more acidic in order to dissolve the stones. The dog may need to stay on an acidifying diet long-term to prevent recurrences but this treatment avoids the need for surgery.

Other types of stone can sometimes be dissolved using specific drugs and it is occasionally possible to remove smaller stones via urinary catheters in the anaesthetised dog. Surgery is needed for stones that cannot be dissolved or easily removed by other means. It is also needed when obstruction has taken place and must be relieved. Occasionally, artificial openings for the urethra have to be created when the urethra has become severely damaged after obstruction.

Stones present in the kidney may be dissolved or removed surgically if they are causing symptoms.

OUTLOOK Dogs that have produced crystals or stones once are likely to do so again therefore preventive treatment must be started to avoid future attacks. The treatment used depends on the type of stone being formed in each case.

INCONTINENCE

CAUSE Incontinence means leakage of urine without the dog being aware that this is happening. The dog makes no attempt to squat in order to pass urine normally or else puddles of urine are found, especially after the dog has been lying down. A number of things can cause signs of incontinence:

- In young dogs, congenital problems with the ureters may lead to incontinence. This is occasionally mistaken for poor house training but in fact the dog has no control over its urination, so no amount of training will correct the problem. Various other congenital problems affecting the bladder may also produce incontinence.

- Problems with the position of the bladder and the function of the urethral sphincter can be encountered in middle-aged spayed female dogs, and occasionally in neuetered males. This is a common cause.

- Nerve damage, especially after pelvic fractures or spinal disease, may result in incontinence due to paralysis of the bladder. This condition is usually reversible if the underlying injuries are treated and the bladder has not been damaged irreversibly.

- Disease of the prostate may cause incontinence in males (see page 198).

- Certain diseases of the bladder may cause incontinence, e.g. severe cystitis, bladder cancer.

The commonest cause of incontinence is that affecting middle-aged spayed female dogs due to a pattern of symptoms comprising:

1. Lack of muscle tone in the urethral sphincter

2. A short urethra, and

3. An incorrectly positioned bladder neck.

This group of disorders is known as 'urethral sphincter mechanism incompetence' or USMI. Most affected dogs have been neutered although the precise connection with neutering is currently unclear. Other causes of incontinence are encountered less frequently in comparison.

SYMPTOMS Leakage of urine at inappropriate times is seen. The dog's bedding may be found wet frequently. Urine may flow without the dog being aware of this or the area around the prepuce in male dogs and the vulva in females may be permanently damp with signs of urine staining and an offensive smell caused by urine scald and skin irritation.

Note that dogs with incontinence may also pass urine in the normal way, i.e. with squatting. The leakage occurs at other times, often indoors and during sleep.

DIAGNOSIS This can be quite involved as it important to find out why the incontinence is occurring and where the source of the problem may be. In young dogs, congenital problems are always suspected; both males and females can be affected. Golden Retrievers seem to have an increased incidence of this congenital incontinence. In all cases, a combination of clinical examination, X-ray techniques and trial treatments may be adopted. Examination of the urine and blood tests may also be necessary. Full diagnostic evaluation of incontinence can be lengthy and expensive.

TREATMENT Surgery to correct congenital problems once they have been diagnosed may be used if it is possible to fix the abnormality. The dog should then be free of symptoms for the rest of its life.

For urethral sphincter mechanism incompetence, the commonest cause, either drugs or surgery may be employed. Surgery, if successful, has the advantage that continuous medication is not needed to control the incontinence.

OUTLOOK The outlook is good if the problem is amenable to surgery. For USMI treated by drugs, most dogs respond well but the medication must be kept going otherwise symptoms tend to recur. A few dogs may stop responding to the particular drug used, in which case another approach may need to be tried.

For other causes, the outlook depends on the disease that is causing the problem. Disease of the prostate, for example, can often be treated, and if this was causing incontinence in a male dog, symptoms should be improved. Similarly, bladder paralysis caused by pelvic or spinal injury normally resolves if it is possible to treat the underlying problems which affected the bladder nerves.

TRAUMATIC INJURY

CAUSE In any case of serious injury, such as a road traffic accident, there is always the risk of damage to the urinary system and other important 'soft tissues' such as the liver, spleen and lungs. Bladder rupture can occur, as can damage to the kidneys, ureters or urethra. Seriously injured animals are monitored for the possibility of such important organ damage.

SYMPTOMS Signs of a ruptured bladder include diminished urination (though it is still possible for the animal to pass some urine), blood in urine, abdominal swelling and progressive general illness and weakness leading to poor appetite, vomiting and collapse from renal failure.

DIAGNOSIS This may not be easy in the early stages. X-rays may be used, together with close observation of urinary output and, perhaps, sampling of fluid present in the abdomen to find out whether urine is leaking.

TREATMENT Tiny tears in the bladder seal by themselves but larger injuries require surgical repair. Rupture of a kidney is a serious injury which may require removal of part or all of the damaged organ. Fortunately, dogs can live normally on the one remaining kidney provided it is healthy.

OUTLOOK Most traumatic problems are treatable but it must be remembered that in animals with mutliple injuries, other serious problems may also be present. Therefore the outlook has to be cautious.

KIDNEY INFECTIONS

CAUSE Kidney infections are less common than cystitis. They may be caused by infectious organisms entering the kidney either via its blood supply or via the urine. The latter is often called an 'ascending infection' since it works its way up the urinary tract. Kidney infections may be termed 'pyelonephritis'.

SYMPTOMS Severe symptoms may be produced including fever, reduced appetite, lethargy and abdominal pain. Blood may be seen in the urine.

DIAGNOSIS This depends on urine samples, blood tests and usually X-rays or ultrasound.

TREATMENT Most cases would be admitted to the hospital for an intravenous drip, antibiotics and close monitoring of blood test results.

OUTLOOK A complete recovery is possible, but kidney damage may also occur which, if severe, could lead on to chronic renal failure.

TUMOURS

CAUSE Any of the organs of the urinary system may be affected by cancer, but they are not as common as some of the other conditions mentioned here. Tumours may be benign or malignant. Polyps are benign growths which may be encountered in the bladder wall.

SYMPTOMS Blood in urine is the commonest symptom, with straining also frequently present due to inflammation. These symptoms are very similar to those of cystitis. Indeed it can be difficult to separate cystitis from cancer without a biopsy, but cystitis is certainly commoner.

DIAGNOSIS X-rays of the bladder and other organs (e.g. lungs) are often used, together with biopsies.

TREATMENT Removal of benign or localised malignant tumours can be carried out. A tumour affecting one kidney can be treated by removal of that kidney provided the second one is healthy. Sections of the bladder can be removed without problems if a tumour or polyp is restricted to one area.

OUTLOOK The outlook is best for benign tumours. Malignant tumours carry a poor outlook overall as they frequently spread to other organs.

CHAPTER 9

Bones, Joints and Muscles

Common symptoms of bone, joint and muscle disease
• Lameness – continuous or occasional • Abnormally shaped limb or limbs
• Reluctance to exercise, jump or climb stairs • Pain/discomfort
• Loss of muscle mass

Structure and Function

The 'locomotor' system consists of all the structures which allow normal movement (locomotion) in dogs:

• Bones

• Joints, with associated ligaments

• Muscles, with associated tendons

The nervous system (see Chapter 10) is also very important as all movement is initiated and coordinated here. Some movement problems which might at first seem to involve the bones, joints or muscles actually arise from disturbances within the nervous system.

Bones

Dogs have over 300 bones in their bodies, from the tiny 'ossicles' which are present in the ear to transmit sound waves from the ear drum across the inner ear,

to the long bones of the limbs. The shape of bones varies considerably but a 'typical' bone has a middle portion known as the shaft and two end portions, which articulate with other bones at joints.

For its weight, bone is a very strong material indeed and can withstand great pressure. In the case of the weight-bearing bones of the limbs, the structure resembles a hollow cylinder on cross-section. Bones developed as hollow structures in order to save on weight – if they were solid, they would be extremely heavy to move around and rapid motion would be impossibly tiring. The hollow portion or marrow cavity is where blood cells are produced (bone marrow).

Joints and ligaments

Bones are connected by joints, which allow movement to occur in various planes. Some joints act as simple hinges; others allow complex rotational movements to occur. To work effectively a joint must have a low degree of friction. Within the joint, a lubricating fluid

Skeleton of the dog

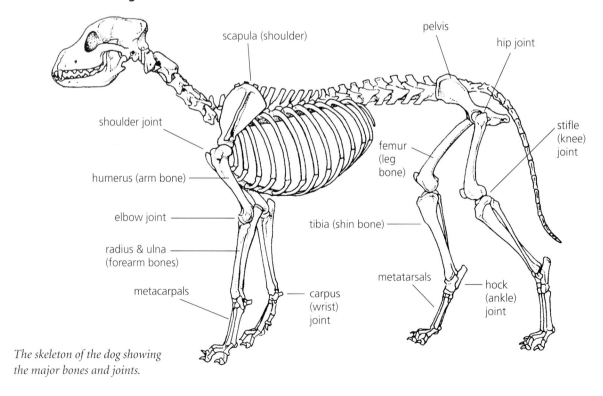

The skeleton of the dog showing the major bones and joints.

known as synovial fluid permits easy movement. The ends of the bones are also covered in cartilage, which is a smooth layer of tissue designed to enable bones to glide effortlessly over each other. The joint is supported by ligaments and a joint capsule – tough, fibrous structures which keep the joint stable and support the surrounding tissues in proper alignment. Most joints have several different ligaments which ensure stability in various directions. If a ligament is torn, instability arises in the joint. This will usually cause lameness.

Muscles and tendons

These structures, working in conjunction with the nervous system, allow voluntary movement to take place. Muscles have the ability to contract (shorten) and when they do so in a coordinated way around bones and joints, movement can occur. There are actually several different types of muscle:

1. Skeletal muscle – this is the muscle that is attached to the skeleton and is concerned with activities of movement.

2. Cardiac muscle – this is the specialised muscle of the heart which pumps blood around the body.

3. Smooth muscle – this muscle is present in the walls of the bowel and bladder and in other places. It is concerned with moving material along hollow tubes or organs.

Tendons are extensions of skeletal muscles and are the structures through which muscles attach to bones. In a dog's limb, most of the major muscles are on the upper part of the limb (above the elbow and stifle joints) – it is the thin but tough tendons of these muscles which extend down into the foot areas. Having muscles themselves down near the foot would result in a bulky and unmanageable limb. When the muscles above contract, the tendons also move and alter the position of joints according to whereabouts the individual tendons are attached. By selectively contracting and relaxing individual muscles, all the complexities of movement of which dogs are capable can occur.

Coordinated movement however is impossible without a functioning nervous system. The brain and nervous system acts as the 'computer' through which all the minute adjustments needed to maintain posture, balance and normal movement are controlled. Many of these adjustments occur automatically (i.e. the dog does not need to 'think' about them).

Veterinary Diagnosis and Treatment

Clinical examination and X-rays are used to diagnose many of the diseases of bones, joints and associated structures. Sometimes biopsies of muscle are taken, but muscle diseases are fairly infrequent in dogs. Joint fluid may be sampled and analysed in cases of joint disease.

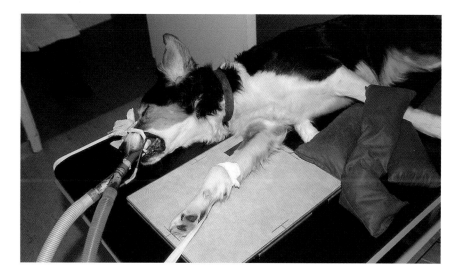

Anaesthetised dog positioned for X-rays of the carpus (wrist). She jumped down from a high wall, overextending and dislocating the joint. It was extremely sore and too painful to X-ray without full general anaesthesia.

Treatment may involve surgery (for broken bones and developmental problems) or drug treatment (e.g. for arthritis and bone infections). Complicated fractures and dislocations may be referred to specialist orthopaedic surgeons for treatment.

Many dogs with fractures have been involved in road traffic accidents and may have additional injuries which need treatment too. If serious, these will normally be tackled before bone fractures are repaired as they are more immediately life-threatening.

Cost and prognosis in bone, joint and muscle diseases

Fractures, dislocations and developmental problems

In general, orthopaedic surgery is one of the most expensive types of treatment carried out on dogs. Operations tend to be long and complex with expensive equipment and implants needed to repair broken bones or correct developmental abnormalities of the leg. Additionally, X-rays will be needed before and after surgery and throughout the healing period. If complications arise during the healing period, further surgery or adjustments may be needed and operations to remove implants such as bone pins or plates may be necessary after the fracture has healed.

The prognosis for most fractures and associated problems treated by specialist surgeons however is very good. A return to normal activity can usually be expected, but this will take time and stringent care from the owner is required in addition to the surgery. It is with treatment like major orthopaedic surgery that the advantages of a good pet medical insurance policy come into their own.

Other bone and joint problems

Ruptured or strained ligaments may be treated by rest or surgery, mostly with a good outcome, although secondary arthritis can occasionally cause problems.

Arthritis is a degenerative disease of joints which cannot be cured, but most dogs respond to drugs given to alleviate the symptoms. On-going or intermittent treatment is required depending on the severity.

Bone infections are very serious indeed and can jeopardise successful repair of a fracture. They must be treated very thoroughly. This can be a lengthy and expensive process.

Bone tumours generally carry a poor outlook in dogs but sometimes amputation is possible to prolong life. Most dogs cope very well with three legs should this operation become necessary.

First aid

First aid treatment for suspected fractures and dislocations is covered in Chapter 18.

Commonest Bone, Joint and Muscle Problems in Dogs

LAMENESS

CAUSE Lameness is usually caused by pain but non-painful lameness may also occur. Two examples of non-painful lamenesses are 'mechanical lameness', when limb movement is restricted but pain-free (see Luxating patella page 165), and neurological lameness, which usually means paralysis of a limb or part of a limb.

Apart from non-painful lameness, anything which hurts the dog will cause it to limp. Usual causes are:

- Sprains and strains
- Arthritis
- Fractures
- Dislocations
- Bone inflammation or infection
- Developmental problems in young dogs
- Spinal or neck injuries
- Bone tumour.

A simple and common cause of lameness in dogs is 'foreign bodies' (e.g. glass) lodged in the foot pad.

Which leg is the sore one?

Make sure you refer to the correct leg when describing a lameness to the veterinary surgeon, especially if it is a slight or intermittent lameness that may not be demonstrated well when the dog is trotted up at the clinic. When using the terms 'right' and 'left' make sure you are referring to the *dog's* right or left, and not *your* right or left when you are facing your dog head on – otherwise confusion can arise!

Front leg lameness

The dog needs to be trotted towards the observer as lameness is harder to detect while walking unless it is very severe. Trot the dog slowly in a straight line on a relaxed lead. If your dog scrabbles, pulls or leans to the side it can be impossible to see the lameness clearly. Good basic training helps here.

The dog favours the sore leg by taking less weight on it. The impression given is that the dog nods downwards with its head *on the good leg*. The sore leg is the opposite one to the one which is nodded on.

Hind leg lameness

Here, the dog should be trotted slowly away from the observer. The dog favours the sore leg by taking less weight on it. The impression given is that the hindquarter on the *good* side moves down more – the dog seems to fall onto it. The sore leg is the other leg.

Lameness in more than one leg

This can be harder to detect! The dog may seem to be generally sore and adopt a 'paddling' or 'pussy-footing' gait. More weight may seem to be taken on the front or hind legs, or on one or other side of the body. Two-limb lameness may only be able to be detected by the veterinary surgeon.

'Shifting' lameness is when all the legs are sore, either at once or at different times. This can be a characteristic of bone inflammation in younger dogs (see Panosteitis page 168) or certain other rarer conditions.

The foot should always be examined carefully in a limping dog, but sometimes it may be very difficult to detect a tiny piece of glass or metal, etc. because the tough digital pad may close over above the entry hole.

SYMPTOMS Symptoms can vary from a very subtle lameness, perhaps only evident now and again, to complete carrying of the affected leg and severe pain when the leg is touched or even approached. Confusingly, some conditions cause the dog to be lame on more than one leg, which can make diagnosis harder. Swelling on the leg may indicate the site of the pain due to inflammation, fractures, dislocations or the site of an open wound.

It is worth remembering that spinal or neck pain may appear as a lameness. This type of pain can be very severe, completely immobilising the dog which stands rigid and becomes afraid to move in any direction.

Remember that all dogs in pain may bite when handled if they are hurt or are afraid that they may be. If you have to move a dog in pain, applying a muzzle or tying a tape around the nose may be advisable so that you can help the dog more effectively and avoid being injured yourself.

Paralysed limbs tend to hang loosely or drag along on the ground. There is no pain or sensation and the dog may walk on the upper side of the paw without realising it.

DIAGNOSIS Diagnosis of lameness involves careful observation of the moving dog, examination of the limbs and body and X-rays when necessary.

TREATMENT This depends on the final diagnosis. Individual conditions are discussed below.

OUTLOOK Again, depends on the diagnosis and is discussed below.

Traumatic Injuries

FRACTURES

CAUSE In most cases, bone fractures are caused by trauma such as falling, being hit by a car or, in small dogs, getting stood upon. A rarer kind of fracture (called a pathological fracture) occurs because of underlying disease in weakened bone; this usually means severe bone infection or a tumour involving the bone. With this type of fracture, trauma is not necessary – the fracture can suddenly occur during normal movement. Avulsion fractures are detachments of small pieces of bone at the position where tendons attach. The free piece of bone is pulled away by the elastic recoil of the tendon after this type of injury.

In young dogs, a fracture may occur at the zone from which the bone is growing (the growth plate). Bone is weaker here and prone to separate from the rest of the bone. Growth plate fractures or injuries may result in the dog developing an abnormally shaped limb if not treated promptly.

Fractures are classified in different ways according to how much damage has been caused. Open fractures (i.e. fractures where the bone has been exposed to the environment) are at a high risk of developing bone infection (osteomyelitis – see page 172). This is a serious complication.

Comminuted fractures are when the bone shape has been completely fragmented. These are difficult fractures to repair. 'Greenstick' fractures can occur on the shaft of the bone of young animals. The term 'greenstick' is used because the soft young bone splinters in the way that a green stick or sapling would when bent.

SYMPTOMS Fractures cause pain which can be very severe, and swelling. Sometimes the swelling is difficult to appreciate if the fracture is near the top of the limb because the haircoat and muscle mass may mask it. The leg may adopt an abnormal shape or position and, with open fractures, wounds are present. Lameness occurs and most dogs with fractures are totally lame – the leg is completely carried.

The veterinary surgeon may detect 'crepitus' (grating) over the fracture site as the bone fragments move against each other.

Considerable haemorrhage may have occurred from the broken bone ends but with closed fractures this will not be noticeable except as swelling and, in thin coated dogs, severe bruising under the skin.

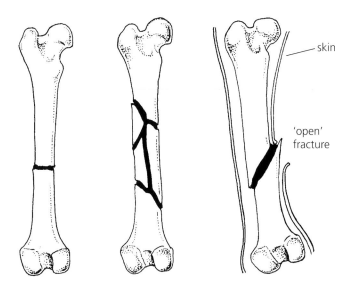

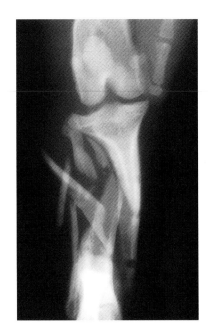

skin

'open' fracture

ABOVE Several ways in which a bone may fracture. RIGHT X-ray of a severe (comminuted) fracture of the tibia (shin bone) following a road traffic accident.

DIAGNOSIS Fractures can be detected by clinical examination in many cases, or else there may be a strong suspicion of them. Some dogs are in so much pain that anaesthesia is needed if any examination of the limb is to take place at all. To find out the type of fracture present, and therefore the best way of treating it, several X-rays are needed.

TREATMENT Initial treatment may be for shock or other immediately life-threatening injuries, rather than the fracture itself. Any injury severe enough to fracture a bone could also have caused internal injuries such as lung bleeding, diaphragmatic hernia or rupture of the bladder. These take priority over fracture repair and may well mean that fracture repair is delayed for several days.

Painkillers should be given before and after treatment for the fracture and dogs may be referred to specialist orthopaedic surgeons for repair of complex breaks. The precise treatment used depends on a number of factors including type and severity of the fracture, age and temperament of the patient and preference of the surgeon treating the dog. Some fractures are relatively straightforward; others require intensive treatment over many weeks or even months.

Commonly used techniques of repair are:

Bone plate. A metal plate is secured to the bone with screws to hold the fractured ends together while they heal.

Bone pin. A metal pin is driven down the marrow cavity of the bone to hold the fractured bone together. Loops of wire may also be added to secure loose fragments or prevent rotation.

Bone screws. These may be used on their own, as well as with plates.

External skeletal fixators. These metal frames appear on the outside of the leg and are connected to pins which secure the fractured bone in a position suitable for healing. They are often used for complicated fractures but are equally suitable for more routine injuries.

Casts. Casts made from synthetic materials (or plaster of Paris) may occasionally be used. They are used for fractures on the lower parts of limbs (below the elbow and stifle joints). Dogs with casts on need careful supervision as the technique is not without its problems and complications.

Cage rest. This may be used for fractures of the pelvis which, if not too displaced, will heal well due to the strong muscular support in the pelvic area acting as a splint. Dogs with unstable fractures which have been repaired may also be prescribed cage rest in order to give the fracture the best chance of healing without complications.

X-rays may be taken throughout the healing process of a fracture to monitor the bone as it gradually heals together.

Once a fracture has successfully healed (this takes weeks to months depending on the type of fracture and age of the dog) any implants used to repair the fracture may need to be removed – this entails a further set of X-rays and an operation. Sometimes, metallic implants are left in position in the dog if they show no signs of moving or causing problems. Many animals (and people) have implants within their bodies which cause no problems at all long term. Your veterinary surgeon's recommendations should be followed.

OUTLOOK Most fractures treated appropriately heal well. However it should always be remembered that orthopaedic surgery is a major procedure. Complications such as bone infection, loosening of implants before healing has occurred and poor healing or even re-fracture do occasionally occur and must be dealt with, usually by further surgery.

The most complex fractures are open fractures where bone has been exposed to the environment or where there has been extensive shattering of bone. Prolonged treatment may be necessary to get these fractures to heal. Also, fractures involving the radius and ulna (bones of the forearm) in toy breeds are associated with a higher incidence of delayed healing than other fractures.

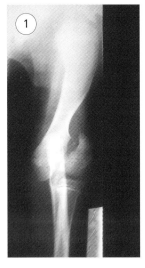
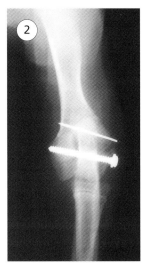
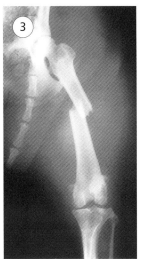
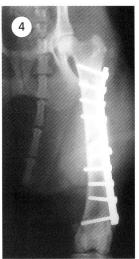
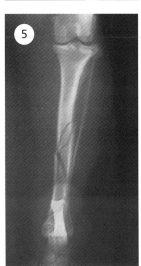
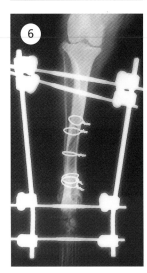

 ## How you can help: home nursing

- Follow your veterinary surgeon's instructions to the letter.

- Active small dogs may need to be kept in a cage or indoor kennel. Other dogs are best restricted to one room and kept calm. All dogs need to be taken out four times daily to empty their bladder and bowels. They should not be left unsupervised when out and, if necessary, they should be kept on the lead.

- *Controlled* exercise and use of the leg actually encourages the fracture to heal and helps prevent muscle stiffness and wastage. Your veterinary surgeon may give advice about physiotherapy, regulated exercise and possibly swimming appropriate for the treatment your dog has received.

- Report any changes or concerns to the veterinary surgeon promptly.

Danger signs after treatment for fractures

Things may not be going well if:

- The dog seems depressed, off colour and is reluctant to eat

- The limb or foot swells up

- Pain seems to be increasing rather than decreasing

- A discharge is noted from underneath any dressing or around the pins of an external fixator

- Surgical wounds are swollen, discharging or not healing

- There is no attempted use of the leg several weeks after surgery

X-rays of bones before and after fracture repair.
1 &2: Elbow fracture in a puppy treated with a screw and wire.
3 & 4: Femur fracture in a Labrador treated with a bone plate.
5 & 6: Tibia fracture in a Collie treated with an external fixator and wire loops.

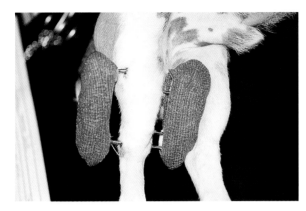

External fixator used to treat the severe tibia fracture shown on page 156.

Great care is needed when caring for an animal which has had a bone repaired. Instructions and all re-check appointments must be followed.

DISLOCATIONS

CAUSE Dislocation means disruption of a joint so that the normal position and relationship of bones is lost. Usually the soft tissues of the joint (joint capsule, ligaments and surrounding muscles) are also torn or stretched. Dislocations are caused by trauma such as motor accidents or getting the leg caught (e.g. on a fence while jumping). Jaw dislocations can also occur due to trauma.

Dislocations can occur on their own or be associated with fractures. Combined fracture-dislocation of a joint is a severe injury, with potential for complications even after surgical repair. Occasionally, congenital dislocations are encountered in newly born puppies.

SYMPTOMS Severe lameness and swelling around the area of the joint is the main symptom. With the hip joint, where the joint itself is buried deeply in muscle, lameness may be the major sign, together with a slight shortening and turning of the affected leg.

In the jaw (temporo-mandibular joint), a dislocation will cause irregularity in the meeting of the teeth and difficulty/pain in opening the jaw or in closing it completely.

DIAGNOSIS Manipulation of the joint will usually reveal a dislocation but X-rays are needed to assess how bad it is and whether there are any associated fractures.

TREATMENT Provided no fracture is present, some dislocations can be corrected by careful manipulation, carried out under anaesthesia. If this is successful a support dressing is usually applied to keep the joint in position while the surrounding tissues heal up and stabilise. Careful restriction on use of the joint is important during the healing phase. Surgery may be needed if it is impossible to replace the joint by manipulation or if it keeps re-dislocating. The aim of surgery is to correct the dislocation and take measures to stregthen or support the joint to keep the adjacent bones in place.

Chronic dislocations can be very difficult to correct and may necessitate removal of part of one of the bones of the joint to create a functional 'false joint'. This applies particularly to the hip or to the temporo-mandibular joint of the jaw, where the operation is called an excision arthroplasty. Elsewhere, the joint may need to be completely fused – a procedure known as arthrodesis. This major operation is not suitable for every joint, but when successful it can save the leg and result in adequate function.

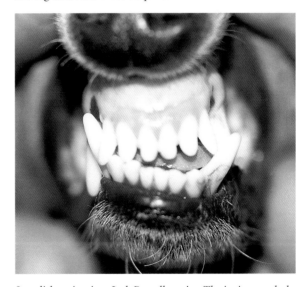

Jaw dislocation in a Jack Russell terrier. The incisor teeth do not meet perfectly, indicating that one side of the jaw has been displaced.

Are joint replacements performed in dogs?

The only joint that is currently replaced with an artificial one in dogs is the hip joint. Good success can be expected when a specialist performs this surgery. However the operation is very expensive, and not every case is suitable. Other alternatives such as excision arthroplasty or arthrodesis (see page 159) will often give good results in suitable cases if drug treatment is failing to control symptoms. As a last resort, amputation can be considered. Although this sounds drastic, it has to be remembered that most dogs cope extremely well after this operation, with a good quality of life.

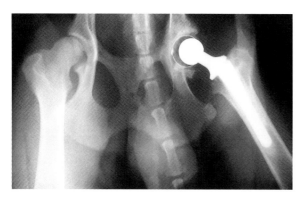

Total hip replacement using an artificial joint for chronic pain in a malformed hip joint. Following this surgery, most dogs show vast improvement in symptoms.

OUTLOOK A dislocation is a severe injury and a proportion of animals can be expected to develop arthritis in the joint afterwards, especially if a fracture was present in addition to the dislocation. In most cases, good return of function occurs – this applies even if an excision arthroplasty or arthrodesis had to be carried out.

RUPTURED CRUCIATE LIGAMENT

CAUSE The cruciate ligament is an important ligament in the stifle (knee) joint, rupture of which leads to instability and lameness. This is one of the commonest injuries causing lameness in the dog and is also a very frequent injury among human footballers!

The usual cause is trauma. Turning quickly whilst weight is being put on the leg or the leg entering a hole or depression whilst running fast are two of the usual mechanisms of injury. Progressive degeneration and weakening of the ligament occurs in some (especially overweight) dogs and can lead to rupture after even quite minor trauma. Some dogs with luxation of the patella (see page 165) also develop cruciate ligament rupture.

SYMPTOMS Initially there is pain and lameness on the affected limb. Dogs often stand with just their toe touching the ground. The onset of the lameness is sudden and may follow a period of exercise during which the dog abruptly pulled up lame.

DIAGNOSIS X-rays may be taken but diagnosis rests on the veterinary surgeon demonstrating instability in the joint, usually in the sedated or anaesthetised dog. When the ligament has ruptured, the two bones (femur and tibia) which are connected by the ligament slide over one another more readily – the so-called 'cranial drawer' sign of ligament rupture which provides the diagnosis.

TREATMENT A number of factors must be considered in treatment including the weight of the dog, its age, breed and also the severity and duration of symptoms. The usual treatment is an operation to replace the ligament using fibrous tissue taken from adjacent muscle. Surgical repair using this or related techniques is nearly always carried out in medium and large breed dogs, as this gives the best results long term. In smaller dogs, conservative treatment (strict rest) may be employed and if this seems to be working surgery may not be needed. In general, though, surgery is best for all patients. Recuperation after the operation takes 6–8 weeks during which time the dog's activity must be carefully controlled.

In a dog which is severely overweight, surgery is not without some risk because, during the postoperative period, the other leg will need to carry all the dog's weight. Occasionally, this can result in a second cruciate ligament rupture occurring on the opposite side, which may completely incapacitate the dog since now both hind limbs will be out of action. Note that this can also happen even when the affected leg is not operated on – overweight dogs with cruciate ligament rupture in one leg must therefore be looked after very carefully and a veterinary-supervised reducing diet is imperative. Such dogs may therefore not be good candidates for surgery until their weight is brought under control.

If surgery is not carried out for whatever reason, the dog normally starts to use the leg within a few weeks and makes a steady improvement over the next few months. Long term, however, arthritis in the joint is very likely and this can be severe.

OUTLOOK Surgical treatment has a very good outlook overall. If an operation is not performed, the dog will gradually regain use of the leg but arthritis is likely to develop in the joint a number of months later, and this may then well require intermittent or continuous treatment.

SPRAINS AND STRAINS

CAUSE A sprain is a joint injury caused by traction or incoordinated movement which stretches the joint capsule or ligaments and causes inflammation and pain. A strain is a similar injury affecting muscles or tendons. More serious injuries of these structures may result in rupture of tendons or ligaments or tearing of joint capsule and muscles. Such severe injuries are often found in association with fractures and dislocations.

SYMPTOMS Pain and inflammation are the commonest symptoms. These are worst when the affected structure is used, so the dog may adapt its posture or gait to protect the sore area. This usually results in lameness. If complete rupture has occurred then the function of the structure concerned will be lost. Tendons may be ruptured after severe trauma or wounds; ligaments may also be ruptured after similar trauma or joint dislocations.

DIAGNOSIS Clinical examination supported by X-rays is used in most cases. Sometimes the extent of tendon or muscle damage can only be evaluated properly during surgery since these structures do not show up well on X-ray.

TREATMENT Tendons may have to be surgically repaired, and the same applies to important ligaments which have been severed. The commonest important ligament damaged in the dog is the cruciate ligament of the stifle joint (see page 160). Severe sprains/strains are treated by strict rest, painkillers and support dressings as needed. Physiotherapy may be helpful to restore normal function.

 Homoeopathic first aid

Simple strains and sprains often respond well to Arnica. See Chapter 18. Cold compresses may also be helpful immediately after the injury and for a few days. The simplest technique is to apply a bag of frozen food (e.g. peas) to the area for 10–20 minutes at a time, 4–6 times daily.

OUTLOOK After adequate treatment and rest the outlook is usually very good for most of these problems.

Problems in Young Dogs

BONE DISEASES CAUSED BY INCORRECT DIET

Deficiencies or excesses in the diet can cause a number of bone diseases in dogs. These disorders, particularly important in young growing dogs, can be avoided by feeding a reputable dog food in quantities advised by the manufacturer or veterinary surgeon. Most of these diseases have become rare since commercial pet foods gained in popularity, however those caused by over-feeding or over-supplementing young dogs are still fairly common, and any dog fed a home-made diet may be at risk if the diet is not properly thought out and balanced. Otherwise, the deficiency diseases are only seen in badly neglected or starving dogs.

Obesity

This is the commonest problem. Many pet dogs are overweight for their size and breed and this can have severe consequences for *all* body systems, not just the bones and joints. If there is any bone, joint or spinal disease, however, symptoms can be made much worse if the dog is overweight as added strain is placed on these structures. It is very important that young dogs are not allowed to become overweight and older dogs prone to arthritis will be much harder to treat if they are too heavy.

 What's the correct weight?

You can find out the average weight for your breed of dog by consulting breed standards or enquiring at the veterinary surgery. However this information is not very useful for cross-breeds! Also, it must be borne in mind that individuals within a breed may be smaller or larger than the average, so published weights may not be entirely accurate for them.

A good general guide is:

- You should easily be able to feel and count the ribs individually without there being a pad of fat lying between them at the skin.

- The flank region should be slightly indented when you look at your dog standing.

Over-feeding or over-supplementing the diet

This is a particular problem in large breeds, especially growing dogs. Owners and breeders may feel tempted to supplement these dogs using, for example bone meal or calcium supplements, or else the dogs may be generally fed on too high a plane of nutrition using an excessively nutrient-rich diet. Owners may believe they are doing the right thing with these particularly large breeds, unaware that they are actually contributing to problems.

Over-feeding or supplementation of the diet of a growing dog can result in severe abnormalities since

Should I give my young dog diet supplements to help bone growth?

The answer is always *no!*, unless a deficiency has been detected by a veterinary surgeon and needs correcting. Whilst vitamin and general conditioning tablets are unlikely to do any harm, supplementation with minerals (calcium, phosphorous, bone meal, etc) can produce serious problems in growing dogs. The fact is that good quality dog foods will satisfy all of a dog's nutritional needs. Disorders are usually only seen in dogs fed homemade diets or in those which are supplemented unnecessarily.

natural bone growth is accelerated in rate. Although this may seem like a good idea because it makes the dog 'grow faster', it can in fact result in multiple problems and deformities affecting limbs and joints. Some of these deformities can be permanent.

Slow bone growth is natural and results in controlled and coordinated development of both the skeletal and muscular systems. It is therefore very important that large breed dogs are fed a balanced diet without extra supplementation. All reputable dog foods are correctly balanced with respect to minerals, nutrients, etc. and veterinary advice should be sought regarding the correct type of food and quantities to feed a growing large or giant breed dog so that a normal growth rate to maturity is achieved.

Hypertrophic osteodystrophy

This disease causes swellings at the lower ends of bones in the fore and hind limbs. Young dogs of the medium and large breeds are most commonly affected. The limbs can be painful and affected dogs may be miserable, reluctant to move and have a high temperature. Diarrhoea is often present. The cause is not fully understood, but over-feeding and over-supplementing with minerals may be involved. In some ways the disease resembles aspects of scurvy (vitamin C deficiency) and has been treated using this vitamin but recent research on the disease has tended to go against this theory. Painkillers may also be prescribed. Most cases clear up of their own accord after several weeks.

Rickets

Natural rickets is hardly ever seen in domestic dogs. It results from a deficiency of vitamin D in the diet and would only occur in badly neglected or starving dogs, or in those fed entirely on poor quality cereal food without sufficient fats added.

However symptoms can be seen in puppies that are given calcium supplements, since this interferes with the body's own complex control mechanisms and produces signs of the disease due to an imbalance rather than an actual shortage of vitamin D. This is another example of the hazards of supplementing the diet of a growing dog unnecessarily.

In rickets, swellings occur near the ends of the bone at the growth plates and poor growth and limb distortion is seen. The dog may be unable to stand or move properly and in severe cases fractures may occur. X-rays and possibly bone biopsies are used for diagnosis. The treatment is simply to correct the diet and feed a reputable prepared dog food, but any limb deformities arising may be permanent.

Diets based on meat only

All-meat diets are not natural for dogs. Wild carnivores will frequently eat the stomach contents of the prey animals they catch, obtaining vegetable matter this way. An all-meat diet has a calcium/phosphorus imbalance: meat contains high levels of phosphorus but low levels of calcium. When fed long term this can lead to a disorder called secondary nutritional hyperparathyroidism. In this condition, because calcium is deficient, the body attempts to make up the defect by absorbing calcium from the skeleton. This weakens the bones and may result in a pathological fracture (a fracture which occurs due to bone disease rather than trauma). This process can occur in both young and mature dogs, though it is commoner in younger animals.

This is one of the rare conditions when supplementing with calcium may be carried out (in addition to correcting the basic diet). This should always be performed following veterinary advice. Cage rest may be needed while this is taking effect in order to reduce the risk of fractures.

HIP DYSPLASIA

CAUSE The term hip dysplasia means abnormally shaped hip joints. The normal hip joint is a closely fitting ball-and-socket joint. When hip dysplasia is present the shape of the joint and the relationship between the bones is altered, resulting in instability and pain.

Hip dysplasia is a developmental disease, in other words the disease begins in young dogs and worsens to a varying degree as the individual dog grows older (see Symptoms below). Hip dysplasia is a common cause of hind limb lameness in dogs, especially in medium to large breeds or crosses. It is likely that a number of factors come together to cause hip dysplasia in an individual dog, and not all of these are fully understood, but at least part of the problem is inherited.

Other factors which may be involved include too fast a growth rate in puppies and young dogs caused by over-feeding and the administration of feed supplements, which owners may give in the mistaken belief that this will help bone structure. The result is that the growth of the skeleton out-paces the growth of the supporting soft tissue structures (muscles), and problems of hip dysplasia are produced in susceptible dogs (see also Diseases caused by over-feeding or over-supplementation, page 162).

Usually, both hip joints are affected, although this can be to differing degrees. The instability that is caused leads on to so-called secondary changes. These changes alter the shape of the head and neck portions of the femur and result in bone deposition around the joint.

SYMPTOMS Symptoms are variable depending on severity. Generally, symptoms occur in either young dogs in which the bones are still growing (age up to one year) or in older dogs, which have developed signs of arthritis in the hip joints. The older dogs have always had hip dysplasia but the condition has remained 'silent' until arthritis eventually begins to cause problems for them.

Lameness and hind limb stiffness are the commonest signs. Difficulty may be encountered in getting up after rest, in negotiating stairs and in jumping

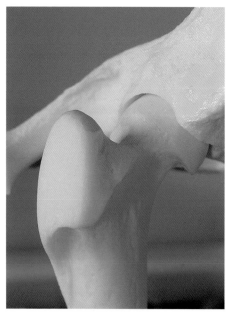

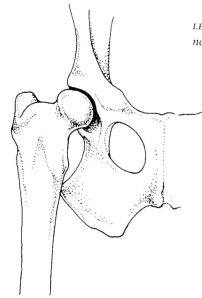

LEFT Model and diagram of a normal hip joint.

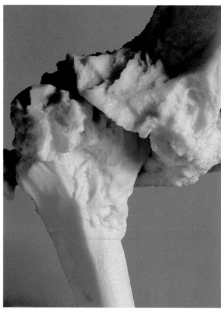

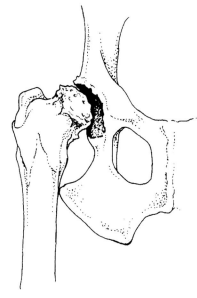

LEFT Model and diagram of an arthritic hip joint.

in or out of cars. Often the muscles of the hip area are noticed to be poorly developed or wasted in both young and older dogs. Young dogs typically show a sudden onset of signs. This can be the case in older dogs too (e.g. after strenuous exercise), or else there can be a more gradual onset of stiffness and lameness.

Some dogs develop a characteristic sitting posture with the legs pushed out to one side rather than folded underneath them or else the gait may be abnormal, e.g. a 'bunny-hopping' gait may be seen in the hind limbs when running. The veterinary surgeon may be able to detect crepitus (grating) over the affected hip when the leg is manipulated.

DIAGNOSIS The condition may be strongly suspected on the basis of the age, breed and medical history of the dog. Confirmation is obtained by X-rays, and these allow changes in and around the hip joint to be observed. X-rays are also necessary in young dogs having their hips 'scored' (assessed by a panel of experts) prior to possible breeding. Older dogs may show evidence of severe arthritis around the hip joint on X-ray.

TREATMENT Young dogs With rest, attention to the diet and weight control if necessary, many young dogs 'grow out' of the condition by 18 months of age. They become sound and symptom-free. In these dogs the soft tissues surrounding the hip joint have developed more fully and now provide additional support to the unstable joint. Painkillers may be given as needed, but these cannot replace adequate restriction of exercise, which must be diligently followed for a number of months in some cases. This is not always easy in active young dogs but without it, lameness is likely to continue.

The importance of good home care

Irrespective of what painkillers are prescribed in young dogs, adequate rest and restriction of exercise, sometimes for several months, is vital. Active young dogs made pain-free by strong painkillers may inadvertantly do more damage to their joints, storing up problems for later on.

It is likely that hip arthritis will occur in later life since the dysplasia has not disappeared, only become less troublesome.

Surgical operations are available in selected cases. A variety of techniques are employed and are almost always carried out by specialist surgeons who assess each patient individually and decide on the best course of action. Such surgery is expensive, but worth considering in severe cases.

TREATMENT Older dogs Older dogs are treated as for arthritis. Occasionally, an excision arthroplasty may be performed – part of the joint is removed to allow a 'false' joint to form, which may be less painful

---

Hip replacements

Hip replacements are increasingly performed in dogs with hip disease. Referral to specialist surgeons is required and not every case is suitable but for those that are, a good outcome can usually be expected. Other operations such as 'triple pelvic osteotomy' may also be able to used to help with severe symptoms of hip dysplasia. Again, specialist consultation and referral is required.

---

than the arthritic joint. This is unlikely to make a lame dog completely sound again, but it may alleviate symptoms in severe cases.

OUTLOOK Any problem which interferes with locomotion in larger breed dogs is potentially serious since if it becomes severe the dog may be unable to rise from a lying position. Most dogs which are treated by weight control and anti-inflammatory drugs as needed do quite well, and their mobility remains reasonable. Care must be taken not to over-exercise them.

Most young dogs with mild to moderate symptoms do well once they mature. Those severe enough to need surgery can often be considerably improved too, although may still suffer symptoms later on in life.

In very severe cases in old dogs, if there is a poor response to various treatments, euthanasia may be recommended rather than subject the dog to surgery that may anyway not prove very successful. Note that many old large dogs such as German Shepherds suffer from CDRM (see page 190) concurrently with hip dysplasia, so the treatment for hip dysplasia may improve overall symptoms but cannot be expected to cure these dogs entirely (there is no treatment for CDRM).

LUXATING (DISLOCATING) PATELLA

CAUSE Luxation of the patella (kneecap) is a common cause of hind limb lameness in dogs. The commonest form of patella luxation is a congenital disease, i.e. the dog is born with certain deformities which lead on to the problem after a few months or years. The initial problem is actually in the hip area but the effects are seen further down the leg, around the stifle joint and below.

The patella may also luxate after any injury which has damaged the supporting structures around the stifle joint. In these cases, the dislocated patella is the only abnormality found, whereas with the congenital form of the disease changes in the position and angulation of other bones may also have occurred.

The patella normally sits within a well-defined groove at the bottom of the femur or leg bone. If it comes out of this groove, a mechanical (pain-free) lameness results because normal function and extension of the stifle joint is interfered with.

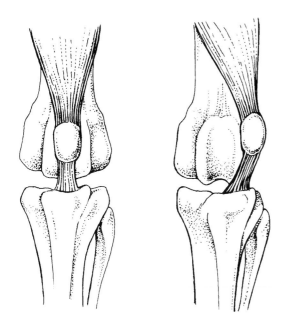

Diagram illustrating the problem of luxating (dislocating) patella or kneecap. The normal patella is shown on the left. The patella on the right has slipped out of its groove.

In the commonest type of luxation (medial luxation of the patella), the patella moves to the inside of the stifle joint. This is seen most in toy and small breeds, particularly Yorkshire Terriers, but a variety of other breeds may be affected including large dogs. Medium sized dogs generally do not get patellar luxation so frequently unless they have had an injury to

the joint, as described above. The patella can also slip to the outside of the stifle joint (lateral luxation of the patella). This is seen much less frequently.

SYMPTOMS The characteristic symptom is a 'skipping' hind limb gait caused by the patella slipping out of its groove and preventing the animal from bearing weight on the leg for a few steps. When the patella slips back in again the limb can be used as normal. Many toy and miniature breeds of dogs can be seen to have an occasional skipping gait of this type.

During dislocation, if the owner rubs the area of the stifle they can often shift the patella back into its normal position, particularly if the limb is straightened out while doing this (a click is felt as the patella slips back into place). The lameness will disappear but is liable to recur if there is underlying instability or deformation.

In severe cases the patella remains permanently out of its groove and this sets up a series of changes affecting the rest of the limb so that normal anatomy can be distorted. These animals have a very abnormal gait; they are usually bow legged and most of their weight is transferred onto the front limbs. Despite such severe changes, pain is not often a prominent symptom of this condition.

DIAGNOSIS This is usually a fairly easy disease to diagnose from the medical history and clinical examination. In order to discover how bad the problem is X-rays may be necessary to check on the alignment of the leg, and to look for complicating problems such as ligament rupture – a particular problem in large breed dogs when the important cruciate ligament (see page 160) may be damaged. A series of grades is allocated to describe the severity of the symptoms and abnormalities in the leg, with grade 1 being the mildest form and grade 4 the most severe.

TREATMENT Depending on the severity, a number of surgical operations are available to improve this condition. These range from simply tightening up the supporting tissues of the stifle joint in mild cases to more complex procedures involving deepening the patella's groove and re-aligning structures around the stifle joint. Which technique is chosen depends on a number of factors including age of dog, duration and severity of symptoms and changes within the joint.

Close attention should be paid to weight loss in overweight dogs. Generally, symptoms are not improved that much by painkillers or anti-inflammatories as pain is not a major feature of the condition in many cases, but it can still be quite disabling especially for larger dogs.

 First aid

Owners of affected dogs can often learn to replace a dislocated patella. The limb is straightened at the stifle (knee) joint (see page 152), and the patella slid or pushed back from its position on the inside of the joint. Sometimes, if the patella is particularly loose, simply rubbing the extended joint is all that is needed. In affected dogs the condition is, of course, liable to recur.

OUTLOOK Patellar luxation is a common condition and is usually non-painful. However in the most serious cases it can result in considerable deformity and interference with gait. If surgery is to be performed, it stands a much better chance of success if carried out in young dogs. While toy and small breeds cope easily with a poorly functional limb, larger dogs do not do so well and early treatment may therefore be recommended should this condition arise in a large dog.

OSTEOCHONDRITIS DISSECANS (OCD)

CAUSE This a problem found in many different species, including dogs, where abnormalities occur at the region from which bone grows (the growth plate) or at the joint surface within the cartilage layer. Like hip dysplasia, a number of factors is thought to bring OCD about, including inherited aspects and the influence of over-feeding in young dogs, resulting in too rapid growth.

The end result is a loose or detached flap of cartilage (sometimes called a 'joint mouse') within the joint or else a part of the bone near a growth plate

may remain unfused to the rest of the bone, causing problems of instability or abnormal growth. Larger breeds are affected most and male dogs seem more prone than females. Most dogs show symptoms before 18 months of age.

SYMPTOMS Affected dogs have a mild to moderate limp. The leg is rarely held completely off the ground (unlike a fracture or dislocation). Usually the affected joint is tender to manipulate and there may be some swelling. The commonest joints affected are the shoulder, elbow, stifle and hock joints.

DIAGNOSIS X-rays often show characteristic signs of problems with the cartilage in affected joints or failure of parts of the bone to fuse properly with the rest. Signs of arthritis may also be visible depending on the duration of symptoms.

TREATMENT As with hip dysplasia, restriction of exercise in young dogs is very important. They should be given short lead walks only. Any faults with the diet (over-feeding or the use of unnecessary supplements) should be corrected. Anti-inflammatory drugs may be given.

In cases where a flap of cartilage or section of bone is obviously causing problems, this may be removed by an operation. OCD has a number of different categories and the precise treatment depends on which joint is affected, how bad the changes are and the likely advantages of surgery over consevative (non-surgical) treatment.

OUTLOOK As with hip dysplasia, secondary arthritis can be a problem later in life. This tends to be worse when it affects the elbow and hock joints and many dogs with elbow and hock arthritis may have had OCD while younger. Treatment given is as for arthritis.

UNUNITED ANCONEAL PROCESS (UAP)

CAUSE This disorder is found mainly in young growing dogs of medium or large breeds. It is a developmental disorder of the elbow joint. The area known

167

as the anconeus on one of the bones of the elbow (the ulna) does not unite properly with the rest of the bone, as it should after 5 months of age. This causes inflammation and, eventually, arthritis within the joint. German Shepherds and Saint Bernards are prone to this condition.

SYMPTOMS These usually appear at about 7–10 months and consist of a limp on the affected leg as well as an alteration in gait pattern. Often, these dogs sit with the elbow rotated outwards and the toes spread. Pain may be produced on full extension of the elbow and joint swelling may be noticed on the outside of the joint.

DIAGNOSIS This depends on X-rays to show the section of bone which has not joined up with the rest of the ulna. Usually, both elbows are X-rayed since the condition may be present on both sides simultaneously.

TREATMENT The ununited section of bone can be removed or else attached to the ulna. Most often, removal is carried out as this is a more straightforward operation. This is undertaken soon after diagnosis in order to try to limit the degeneration and arthritis within the joint.

OUTLOOK Surgery performed early has the best chance of preventing arthritis developing.

PANOSTEITIS

CAUSE This is quite a common disease of young dogs of large breeds, with a particular tendency to affect German Shepherds. It is four times commoner in males compared to females. A large number of ideas exist as to the underlying cause of this disease but, as yet, none is proven.

SYMPTOMS Sudden lameness of one or more legs is the typical symptom. Different legs can be affected at different times and the lameness/pain can be severe. Some dogs have a high temperature during flare-ups. Recurrences are common but the disease eventually disappears completely. The dogs usually have no history of damage to the limb or over-exercise; the condition simply appears on its own.

DIAGNOSIS Characteristically, these dogs have painful areas on their bones without there being any fracture, dislocation or other problem such as OCD. The long bones of the limbs are affected and even gentle touching of sensitive areas can be very uncom-

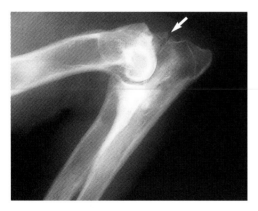
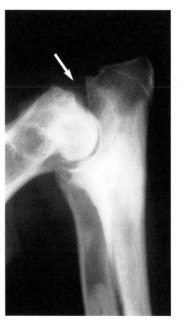

ABOVE Ununited anconeal process (arrow) as seen on the elbow X-ray of a young German Shepherd dog which had persistent lameness.
RIGHT A post-operative X-ray of the German Shepherd's elbow, showing where the fragment of bone has been removed (arrow). A steady improvement in symptoms is expected after this surgery.

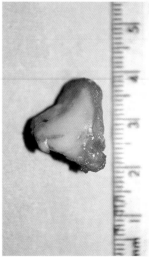

ABOVE The fragment of bone removed from the affected elbow joint.

fortable for the dog. Pain can usually be found in more than one area. This pattern of symptoms is very suggestive of the disease when it occurs in a young dog of large breed.

X-rays can show typical signs of this condition unless the pictures are taken very early on in the disease (in which case they may need to be repeated in order to detect the developing signs). X-rays are needed to rule out other problems as well as diagnose panosteitis itself.

TREATMENT Pain can be intense and painkillers are usually provided. In a few cases, hospitalisation may even be required for potent analgesic treatment. Treatment may need to be repeated during recurrences.

OUTLOOK Although symptoms can be dramatic at the time, and recurrences frustrating for owner and dog, the condition does eventually disappear, usually by about 2 years of age, and no lasting harm is caused to the dog.

LEGG-PERTHES DISEASE

CAUSE This disease of the hip joints in toy breeds and terriers is thought to be inherited or related to hormone imbalances. The result is that the neck of the femur undergoes destruction, causing inflammation and pain. It is usually seen under the age of 1 year.

SYMPTOMS Pain and irritability are the main symptoms together with progressive lameness. Muscle wastage can occur due to poor usage of the limb and in severe cases the limb may be totally carried.

DIAGNOSIS An X-ray allows the diagnosis to be made. Severe signs even extending to fracture of the head or neck of the femur may be seen in some dogs.

TREATMENT The femoral head and neck are removed in an operation known as excision arthroplasty. A 'false' joint then develops, which is usually much less painful for the dog. Most dogs regain a normal gait afterwards.

OUTLOOK The outlook is good after surgery. If no surgery was performed, arthritis would probably develop in the hip joint.

ACQUIRED LIMB DEFORMITY IN YOUNG DOGS

CAUSE Young dogs may develop limb deformity after an injury which damages the growth plate (the area of bone from which its length is increased). This injury need not be a fracture: any traumatic injury to the limb has the possibility of producing this problem. If damaged, the growth plate may 'close' (i.e. bone growth will stop). When this affects one of the paired bones of the radius and ulna in the foreleg, an angular limb deformity can result because the other bone keeps growing and eventually distorts the leg. This leads onto problems at the elbow and carpus joints. In severe cases it can be very disabling.

SYMPTOMS The injury may be forgotten or even unknown but some weeks after it, a deviation in the leg may be evident. Commonly, the foot turns outwards and the leg curves somewhat. This worsens progressively as the young dog continues to grow. The extent of deformity depends on the severity of the injury and the age at which it occurred.

> **Act early**
>
> Any deviation in the limbs of a young dog should prompt an early visit to a veterinary surgeon in case an angular limb deformity is developing.

DIAGNOSIS The condition is suspected in a young dog with deforming limbs and is confirmed by X-rays. A medical history of previous damage to the leg may be available and it can be assumed that this is what destroyed the growth plate and caused it to close.

TREATMENT Early surgical treatment is needed if permanent deformity and joint problems are to be avoided. Corrective surgery aims to straighten the leg,

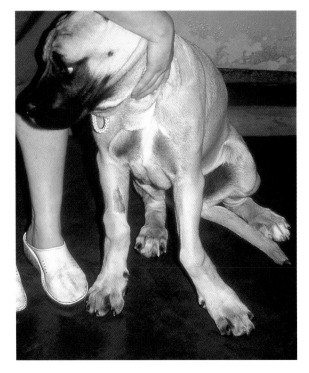

LEFT Angular limb deformity in a young dog due to premature growth plate closure.
LEFT BELOW The same dog following corrective surgery. The external fixator used will be removed after healing

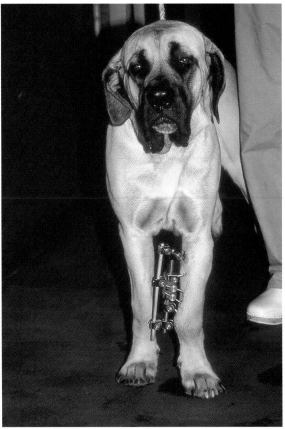

allow continued growth and prevent future joint problems. Degenerative joint disease can be expected if the problem is not treated.

OUTLOOK As long as the problem is treated early the outlook is fairly good.

Other Bone and Joint Problems

ARTHRITIS

CAUSE Arthritis, also known as osteoarthritis, is a degenerative condition which causes lameness due to joint pain in dogs. The term 'degenerative' refers to a progressive disorder which changes the composition of body tissues so that they no longer function as normal. In arthritis, the joint undergoes changes including swelling of surrounding and supporting tissues (especially the joint capsule), the formation of bony spurs and thickenings in and around the joint, inflammatory changes in the lubricating fluid in the joint (synovial fluid) and alterations in the cartilage cushions which cover the bone ends at the joint. All of these changes lead to reduced function and mobility and cause pain to varying degrees.

Any joint can be affected by arthritis and if the joint has been previously damaged (e.g. due to a fracture, dislocation or severe ligament injury) then arthritis is more likely to develop at some point in the future. Older dogs frequently have arthritis of the elbows, stifles or hips, and if they are overweight, symptoms can be severe. No injury need have been present to cause arthritis in older dogs.

Arthritis can also be caused by immune system disease, in which case it is likely to affect a number of joints simultaneously. A number of different immune-mediated types exist, some associated with certain breeds. Overall, this is a less common form of arthritis than the more usual degenerative joint disease.

normal joint

arthritic joint

cartilage

supporting ligaments of joint

fibrous joint capsule

menisci (cushions)

irregular bony deposits around the joint

pitted/ damaged cartilage

painful, swollen joint

damaged menisci

dense bone near joint

thickened joint capsule

Diagram illustrating the problem of arthritis in any joint. The structure of a normal joint is shown on the left.

SYMPTOMS Chronic lameness is the commonest symptom. The severity may vary from day to day and can be affected by changes in the weather, with symptoms being worst in cold, damp days. There may be a pattern evident within the day too. Some arthritic lamenesses are worst after rest, with the dog 'warming up' out of the lameness. On the other hand, if excess exercise is taken (e.g. a particularly long walk) in a dog with arthritis, the pain may be exacerbated on the following day such that lamenss is much worse than normal.

> ⓘ **Risk factors for arthritis**
>
> • Overweight dogs
>
> • Large breed dogs
>
> • Previous joint injury
>
> • Dogs with predisposing conditions, e.g. hip dysplasia, osteochondritis dissecans (OCD)

Any trauma such as a knock or sprain in a dog with arthritis can result in an exaggeration of the lameness, even to the extent of the limb being totally carried, as if fractured.

DIAGNOSIS Diagnosis is often strongly suggested by the dog's medical history, the pattern and type of lameness, the age and breed of the dog and if it is overweight. Examination of affected joints reveals stiffness, swelling, restricted movement and pain, and sometimes crepitus (grating) due to bony spurs or cartilage abnormalities.

TREATMENT The most important part of the treatment is weight control. Overweight dogs will often show a disappointing response to treatment no matter what type of drug is used, or else control of symptoms may require very high doses, which could be harmful long term. Conversely, dogs which lose weight will often show a great improvement in symptoms, perhaps to the extent that further treatment of the arthritis is not needed, is only needed

 171

intermittently or else can be achieved with very low drug doses.

Arthritis cannot be cured but symptoms can be eased by certain drugs, usually anti-inflammatories. The aim is to make the dog comfortable with the lowest dose that is possible, since it is likely that continuous or intermittent treatment may be required throughout the dog's life. In the initial stages after diagnosis, when pain may be severe, a high dosing regime may be adopted. This will then be tapered off as symptoms abate and as weight control (if necessary) begins to show positive results.

Arthritic dogs should still receive daily exercise. Several short walks are better than occasional long ones; the amount of exercise given should be constant from day to day. Swimming, if available, is a good form of exercise for arthritic dogs as it involves no weight-bearing on the diseased joints – but swimming should not involve excited jumping around on river banks or diving into the water!

Checklist for arthritic dogs

- Reduce weight if necessary (with veterinary advice). Note that weight loss must be achieved by modifying the diet and not by increasing the amount of exercise

- Give medication as prescribed but do not increase the dose without advice

- Ensure the dog's bedding is well padded

- Be prepared for symptoms to vary a little in intensity from day to day and week to week, even when on medication

- Keep daily exercise levels constant

- Swimming can be beneficial

In very severe cases, when other methods are failing, surgery may be indicated to relieve certain types of arthritis. In these circumstances operations to alter the shape of joints or to completely fuse a joint may be carried out if it is thought that this may help the symptoms. Most dogs, however, have arthritis in more

than one joint unless the problem is secondary to an injury affecting an isolated joint.

OUTLOOK Provided veterinary advice is followed, especially with regard to weight control, most dogs with arthritis can have their symptoms improved so that a good quality of life is possible as they grow older.

BONE INFECTION (OSTEOMYELITIS)

CAUSE This serious condition is caused when infectious organisms (especially bacteria) gain access to and multiply in bone. The usual cause is a puncture wound (e.g. bite or gun shot injury), a fracture or as a complication after surgery. Sometimes spread from infection elsewhere in the body may result in bone involvement. Any bone can be affected.

SYMPTOMS Bone infections are painful and affected animals are normally miserable with a high temperature in the early stages. The affected area may be swollen, discharging (if there is an open or surgical wound) and painful to touch or manipulate. If on a limb, severe lameness is usually present.

Chronic bone infections are less uncomfortable. Discharging wounds may be present with swellings and draining tracts around the area together with muscle wastage. Affected limbs are not used properly. Usually, dogs are relatively bright without the high temperature and lethargy seen in the acute stages.

DIAGNOSIS Examination, X-rays and blood tests are usually used. Often the medical history of the dog will suggest the condition, e.g. history of a deep wound or fracture, especially an open (compound) fracture.

TREATMENT Antibiotics are very important. Often, biopsies will be taken to ensure that the correct antibiotic is chosen to eliminate the bacteria causing the infection. Very long courses of antibiotics are needed and two months of treatment is not unusual. X-rays are taken to monitor progress.

Chronic bone infections can be extremely difficult

to clear up. If these are arising as a complication of fractures, then surgery is usually needed to establish drainage and stability at the fracture site. This may mean a second (or even third) operation if the first proved unsuccessful. Hospitalisation, continuous antibiotic treatment, frequent check X-rays and further minor or major operations to remove damaged tissue and create conditions for healthy healing may be required. In many cases, bone grafts are used to promote bone healing once the infection has been brought under control. Chronic bone infections occasionally recur many months after apparently successful treatment is stopped.

OUTLOOK Because chronic bone infection is such a problem, this condition is always taken seriously. Lengthy and expensive treatment may be involved. If associated with a fracture, once the fracture has healed and any implants removed, the infection may well subside. Problematical cases are often referred to specialists for treatment.

JOINT INFECTION (INFECTIVE ARTHRITIS)

CAUSE Joint infections are produced when bacteria enter the joint either from the bloodstream or via a penetrating wound. They can also occur as a complication of joint surgery.

Lyme disease, an infection which dogs may acquire from ticks (see page 26), can cause a severe arthritis of this type in affected dogs, as well as other more general symptoms. Always alert the veterinary surgeon if your dog has been exposed to ticks prior to developing lameness or joint problems.

SYMPTOMS Lameness will be present along with a swollen and tender joint. The pain can be severe and affected dogs may be miserable, reluctant to eat and have a high temperature.

DIAGNOSIS This is apparent from clinical examination and X-rays. Samples of joint fluid may be taken for analysis and to determine which is the best antibiotic to use.

TREATMENT Severe cases may require surgery to lavage (flush) the joint, obtain further samples and possibly insert drains or other treatments into the joint. Lengthy courses of antibiotics are used in addition.

OUTLOOK Joint infections are severe conditions, requiring intensive and prolonged treatment. Badly damaged joints may develop arthritis later on.

BONE CANCER

CAUSE Bone tumours are not particularly common in dogs but unfortunately when they do occur they are usually malignant. They can arise in the bone or else they may spread to the bone from primary growths elsewhere, e.g. from the mammary gland (females) or prostate (males).

Tumours arising directly from the bone are seen more frequently in large and giant breeds of dog (e.g. Great Dane) where they most frequently occur in the radius and ulna bones above the carpus (wrist) joint. Other usual sites include the humerus (arm bone) just below the shoulder, or in the femur (leg bone) or tibia (shin bone) in the hind limb. Bone tumours can arise or spread to other bones such as the skull or vertebral column.

SYMPTOMS Lameness is the commonest symptom of tumours affecting the limb bones. This can start off fairly mild but gradually worsens despite treatment. Alternatively, sudden lameness can result when fracture occurs after no or only a very slight injury. Bone tumours are considered in these cases since bones are strong structures and do not normally fracture easily unless seriously weakened by disease. Such fractures are termed 'pathological fractures', compared to the usual type of traumatic fracture after an accident.

A swelling may be felt on the limb if the tumour arises in an area that is not heavily muscled. Other signs include pain, poor appetite and lethargy and, possibly, signs of a growth elsewhere. In other areas (e.g. skull, ribs, spine) symptoms of a firm growth or of pain are usually present.

DIAGNOSIS X-rays of the affected area and of other areas of the body such as the thorax are normally carried out. Blood tests may also be performed and biopsies taken for specialist analysis in order to discover the type of the tumour and therefore, hopefully, plan treatment.

TREATMENT This does depends on the tumour type and its location. Where there is clear evidence of spread to other organs, the only treatment possible will be pain control to keep symptoms at bay and maintain quality of life. Euthanasia will be required once symptoms can no longer be tolerated.

Amputation may be carried out for limb tumours without obvious signs of spread elsewhere. If no tumour spread beyond the limb has occurred, this will cure the dog of its cancer and also remove the source of pain. Small and medium breed dogs cope extremely well with amputation; as do many larger dogs. A good quality of life is possible.

Because of the high risk of spread beyond the limb, a guarantee of a complete cure can never be given after amputation. In fact, in the majority of cases of the common bone tumours, spread will probably have occurred before diagnosis even if this cannot be readily picked up on X-rays. Amputation can however still be considered to prolong the dog's life and provide relief from pain. Some dogs are suitable for chemotherapy following amputation, and when successful this can lead to significant prolongation of life after bone cancer. In the future, chemotherapy may be used more and more for dogs with limb cancer.

Surgical techniques to preserve the limb affected by the cancer have been used in large or giant breed dogs where amputation is not desirable. These major operations involve removing the area of bone affected by cancer, inserting a bone graft and fusing nearby joints. It is highly specialised surgery and does carry a significant risk of complications, but can potentially give good results. As with amputation, the risk of spread having occurred elsewhere is still present. The surgery is expensive.

Bone tumours arising in areas like the skull or spine are much more difficult to treat as it is not possible to remove them easily. Re-growth of the tumour in its original location is likely after surgery.

How long will my dog live after treatment for bone cancer?

There are so many factors to consider that it is usually not easy to answer this question. The type of tumour, form of treatment used and possible complications vary a lot between patients.

In dogs with bone tumours present on the limb treated by amputation only (no chemotherapy) a survival of around 5 months can be expected. Some dogs may live significantly longer than this but, from the point of view of having a figure to think about, 5–6 months seems realistic.

When chemotherapy is included in the treatment, the survival time is likely to improve considerably.

OUTLOOK The outlook is always very cautious in cases of bone cancer. The disease cannot usually be cured. However treatment when successful can lead to prolongation of good quality life. Each case should be treated individually, taking into account age of dog, severity of symptoms, likely advantages and success rates of different treatments and wishes of the owner. Careful discussion of these points with your veterinary surgeon should result in the right treatment decisions being taken.

'LION JAW' DISEASE: CRANIO-MANDIBULAR OSTEOPATHY

CAUSE This is a fairly unusual condition affecting young West Highland White terriers and Scottish terriers. The exact cause is unknown but it is thought to be inherited. Young dogs of other terrier breeds and larger dogs are also occasionally affected.

SYMPTOMS There is pain when the jaws are opened and the dog may thus be reluctant to eat. A high temperature is often found as well as drooling, lethargy and pain when the jaws or head are touched.

DIAGNOSIS A characteristic appearance occurs on X-ray in which extra bone appears along the jaw line, somewhat resembling a lion's jaw (hence the name).

TREATMENT Severe cases may require hospitalisation and an intravenous drip. Most dogs however respond well to anti-inflammatory drugs and the condition usually resolves after several weeks.

Home nursing

Feed liquidised or slurried food to limit painful jaw movements if your dog is under treatment for this problem.

OUTLOOK Good in most cases; the condition eventually disappears though some changes to the jaw bone may persist and be visible on X-rays.

MUSCLE WASTAGE AND MUSCLE DISEASES

CAUSE Any painful condition which causes a dog to favour one leg is liable to cause muscle wastage in that leg. In order to maintain muscle mass, muscles must be used frequently; if they are not used sufficiently they shrink (atrophy). Muscle wastage does take a number of weeks to develop, so whenever it is discovered it indicates that pain or lameness arising from the bones or joints is chronic in nature.

Diseases of muscle itself are relatively rare but are occasionally encountered. Some of these are inherited with a tendency to occur in certain breeds, others are acquired and can affect any dog. The commoner muscle diseases are summarised in the box.

SYMPTOMS With muscle wastage, often the area of poor muscle development can be seen or felt. It is particularly noticeable when it occurs around the hip or shoulder areas.

Other muscle diseases produce problems with movement, posture or cramping. Swallowing may be affected in certain diseases. Problems with swallowing always carry the risk of aspiration pneumonia (when food accidentally enters the respiratory system due to incoordinated swallowing). This is a serious, potentially life-threatening, complication of any disease that interferes with the normal swallowing process.

Some of the commoner muscle diseases

Myositis – inflammation of the muscle. The commonest cause is a puncture wound or bite, resulting in an abscess that is treated by antibiotics or possibly surgery to allow drainage of infected fluid or material. Other causes of myositis may be related to problems in the immune system: the dog's immune system attacks its own muscle cells causing inflammation and pain. The best known example of this affects the jaw muscles (see below).

Myositis of jaw muscles (masticatory myositis) – this is one of the commonest muscle diseases in dogs. The jaw muscles are swollen and opening of the mouth is painful. Affected dogs are subdued, often with a high temperature. In chronic cases, severe wastage of the jaw muscles may occur. It is thought to occur due to an immune system malfunction which results in the dog's immune system attacking its own jaw muscles. In this condition, other muscles are not affected. The disorder is treated using corticosteroids, usually successfully. *Breeds with a high incidence:* German Shepherd.

Contracture – after an injury or inflammation, fibrosis may occur causing the muscle to seize in an abnormal position, causing pain or malfunction of a joint. The commonest muscles affected are the quadriceps muscle (hip area) and infraspinatus muscle (shoulder). Treatment is usually surgical but physiotherapy and swimming are also likely to be very beneficial.

Myasthenia gravis – this muscle disease can be congenital or acquired. Muscle weakness, easy tiring and problems with swallowing are seen; many dogs regurgitate food and can be prone to complications of pneumonia. The condition can often be controlled if complications have not developed.
Breeds with a high incidence: Jack Russell terrier (congenital form); larger breeds (acquired form).

box continued on page 176 ▶

Some of the commoner muscle diseases, (*continued from page 175*)

Toxoplasmosis – this is a parasitic condition caused by a minute organism called a protozoa. This is normally a parasite of the cat. In most instances, infection causes no symptoms in dogs but it may cause muscle disease in susceptible animals. Rigidly immobilised hind limbs may be seen in affected puppies or young dogs. Muscle biopsies are required for diagnosis. Treatment is possible but the response can be hard to predict.

Neospora infection – another parasite producing symptoms very similar to Toxoplasma. Treatment is the same.

Muscular dystrophy – this disease affects Golden Retriever male puppies. Abnormal gait, quick tiring and problems swallowing may be seen. The disease is thought to be similar to the human form of muscular dystrophy.

Labrador myopathy – young Labrador dogs are affected by this muscle disease. Signs include easy tiring, collapse, and a low head carriage. After a spell of rest the dogs recover from the weakness and are able to move again. Diagnosis is by muscle biopsy and other tests to rule out different conditions. Symptoms usually improve as the dog grows older but may never disappear entirely, however most pet dogs cope well.

DIAGNOSIS Muscle wastage itself is not a diagnosis. The veterinary surgeon aims to find what has been causing the muscles to atrophy in the first place. Usually, a cause of chronic lameness is found, e.g. hip dysplasia, chronic bone infection.

Muscle biopsies or other tests may be required to diagnose muscle problems that are not connected to bone or joint disease. A wide variety of such diseases exist; many are rare and/or restricted to certain breeds only. The box lists the commonest among them.

TREATMENT The underlying cause of the lameness or muscle problem should be treated whenever possible. When the problem is due to a bone or joint condition, swimming can be used to build up muscles without stressing the bones or joints themselves. Physiotherapy can be very helpful too.

Muscle disorders not related to the bones or joints may be able to be treated or improved using appropriate drugs.

OUTLOOK This depends on the condition that is eventually diagnosed, as some are not curable only controllable.

CHAPTER 10

The Nervous System

Common symptoms of nervous system disease
• Changes in behaviour • Incoordination/imbalance
• Tilting of the head • Fits or seizures
• Pain and inability to move • Paralysis or weakness
• Abnormal posture or gait

Structure and Function

The nervous system is the most complex part of the body. It is the 'central computer' which coordinates all aspects of life, but is far in advance of any computer yet invented by a human being. It is responsible for consciousness, individual personality, instinctive and learned behaviour and for the minute control of vital body functions such as blood pressure and breathing.

Because its function in the body is so all-embracing, the most important parts of the nervous system are very well protected. The brain lies within the bony covering of the skull which completely surrounds it, and the spinal cord is protected within the vertebral column. Even so, damage does occur and if severe and permanent it can have devastating consequences for the animal.

Central and peripheral nervous system

The nervous system as a whole is usually thought of as consisting of two parts:

1. The central nervous system, which consists of the brain and spinal cord.

2. The peripheral nervous system, which consists of all the individual nerves supplying the various organs and tissues of the body. The nerve cells which make up the peripheral nervous system are specialised, elongated structures which link the tissues and organs of the body to the central nervous system. In some ways, they are like the individual telephone lines leading to the central exchange.

Communication in the nervous system is by way of tiny changes in electrical current which pass along nerves and across the spaces between nerves, called synapses. The 'jump' across the synapse space is made by special chemical messenger compounds. These pass quickly across the tiny gap and then activate the next nerve cell they come to. In this way the nerve impulse is propelled towards the spinal cord or brain, where it may cause some change or other in body function, e.g. the heart rate speeds up, a foot is lifted quickly from the ground or a tail gives a wag!

The central nervous system constantly receives and processes information in the form of electrical impulses in its peripheral nerves. This huge data-processing task allows all of the normal functions of the body to operate smoothly and in a coordinated way.

Fortunately, no animal needs to think in order to keep its heart beating, to keep the breathing rate normal or to adjust the body temperature so that it is kept at just the right level. These and thousands of other adjustments are all made 'unconsciously' or automatically by the central nervous system. Different parts of the brain are responsible for each aspect of normal function and for keeping most of the processes in the body working within extremely tight controls.

However such is the ability of the nervous system

General anatomy of the nervous system

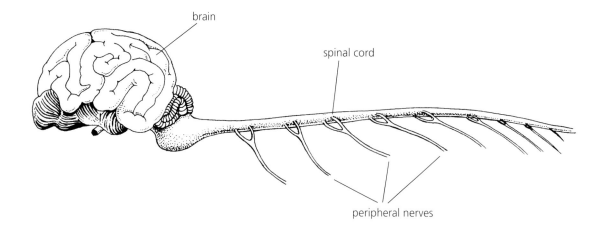

brain

spinal cord

peripheral nerves

that, with training, human beings can learn to adjust their own heart rate simply by thinking about it. This means that conscious effort is used to control something that is normally altered automatically. Usually, however, conscious control in the nervous system is reserved for other things such as movement and communication. The automatic functions which keep animals alive generally take care of themelves, unless disease is present.

Reflexes

Reflexes are important responses in the nervous system which happen automatically. Some of these have a protective function, e.g. the cough reflex prevents objects being inhaled into the respiratory system which could cause damage or suffocation. Other protective reflexes help to maintain posture so that when an animal becomes slightly imbalanced it doesn't always fall over. The pupillary light reflex in the eye (page 42) helps the eye adjust so that the animal can see in different lighting conditions. The simplest reflex is the patellar or 'knee jerk' reflex, which is used in dogs and people to check that part of the peripheral nervous system is working adequately.

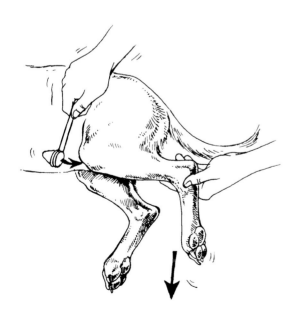

The patellar (or 'knee jerk') reflex tests one part of the nervous system.

Examination of the nervous system usually involves testing a number of reflexes which can be assessed easily. This can often give a good indication as to what, and where, a problem is.

Brain or spinal cord damage

One of the most severe injuries to the nervous system is damage to the brain itself, whether this be from trauma, infection or interruption of the blood supply. Brain damage, if it affects consciousness, produces some of the most obvious signs of nervous system damage, e.g. coma (loss of consciousness). More subtle damage to the brain may cause incoordination, imbalance or abnormalities in vision, hearing or any one of a number of body functions.

Damage to the spinal cord can be very serious, possibly resulting in partial or complete paralysis and interference with other organ function such as the bladder.

Paralysis

Paralysis results when a nerve supplying an organ or tissue becomes damaged. The result can be complete loss of function. For example, consider what happens when an important nerve in a limb gets damaged – perhaps the result of a road accident. Although the dog may send out signals from the brain which tell its limb to move, the message never gets through to the relevant muscles of the limb because the nerve has been severed or otherwise damaged somewhere along its path. The result is that no movement happens in the limb despite the dog intending it to.

Similarly, if the nerve which normally tells the brain that the bladder is full and requiring emptying gets damaged, the bladder can continue to swell with urine without the animal feeling any urge to urinate at all. The result can be permanent damage to the bladder and incontinence.

Veterinary Diagnosis and Treatment

Examination of the patient can usually indicate whereabouts the damage to the nervous system has occurred. However, it may not be possible to say, without further tests, what has caused this damage. The whole range of tests (X-rays, blood profiles, CT scans, etc) may be used in investigating disease of the nervous system.

Some causes of spinal disease, such as 'slipped' discs, may be able to be treated by rest or surgically. Other conditions are treated using drugs to try to limit further damage. Paralysis of a limb, if permanent, usually requires amputation.

Costs and prognosis in nervous system disease

Surgery inolving the nervous system is a very specialised form of treatment and is therefore expensive. Dogs requiring surgery of the spine are usually referred to specialist centres. The results can be excellent in many cases. A good insurance policy comes into its own if spinal surgery is needed.

Other conditions, such as epilepsy, have to be controlled rather than cured. This means on-going treatment, probably for the dog's life. Once initial diagnostic tests have been carried out, however, the treatment costs need not be that expensive as drugs for this problem are widely available.

Specialised techniques such as CT and NMR scans are becoming more widely available for pets. This makes diagnosis of nervous system diseases considerably easier. Currently, such scans are expensive but they are likely to become progressively cheaper as the technology becomes more commonplace.

Commonest Nervous System Diseases of Dogs

Brain Diseases

FITS, CONVULSIONS OR SEIZURES

CAUSE A fit or seizure occurs when brain cells malfunction and abnormal nerve signals spread throughout part of the brain in an uncontrolled way.

Commonest causes of fits/seizures/convulsions in dogs

- **Epilepsy:** This is the commonest cause. Epilepsy is inherited in certain breeds (inlcuding German Shepherds, Golden Retrievers and Dachshunds). The first fit or seizure normally occurs before age 3 years if true epilepsy is the cause.

- **Other diseases:** A variety of diseases such as liver disease, diabetes or other pancreatic disease, kidney failure and eclampsia (low blood calcium levels in lactacting bitches) can all be responsible. These problems cause symptoms because they produce disturbances in the chemistry of the body which interferes with normal brain cell function.

- **Young dogs:** Fits in young dogs may often be epilepsy, but can also be due to other congenital problems such as abnormalities in liver blood supply, hydrocephalus (page 185) or distemper.

- **Brain tumours:** Commoner in older dogs, these always have to be considered but are difficult to diagnose. Other symptoms like changes in behaviour may be present. Tumours may arise in the brain or spread there from elsewhere.

- **Poisons:** A wide variety of toxins and poisons can cause seizures. Usually, other symptoms are present too. Knowledge of possible access to toxins or poisons is important here.

- **Infections:** Distemper in unvaccinated dogs may cause symptoms as may other infectious diseases such as rabies in certain countries.

- **Traumatic injury:** Serious head trauma can result in seizures, often due to pressure build-up in the brain and/or lack of oxygen.

- **Hyperthermia:** Severe overheating caused by too hot an environment or diseases producing high fever can lead to fits/seizures as a serious complication.

The result is an abnormality in the behaviour of the dog which can range from minor trembling or twitching affecting a single area of the body such as a single limb (partial seizure), to loss of consciousness and generalised convulsions affecting the whole body (complete seziure).

SYMPTOMS A very limited focal seizure may be quite difficult to detect. The only sign may be a spasmodic twitching of a limb or other slight abnormality. A condition termed 'fly-catching' in Cavalier King Charles Spaniels is thought to be one type of partial seizure: the dogs behave as if trying to catch an invisible fly. Sometimes partial seizures may progress to become generalised ones.

A complete or generalised seziure is commoner in dogs. They have a fairly characteristic pattern which is often well recognised by owners of dogs with epilepsy (see box).

Typical epileptic fits have a predictable pattern as described in the box. They are undoubtedly very distressing for the owner the first time they are witnessed. However, the dog is not aware of what is going on and the fit promptly passes. They are only life-threatening if the fit persists for more than 10 minutes, i.e. the dog does not come out of the fit. This condition of continuous fits or 'status epilepticus' requires urgent veterinary treatment.

DIAGNOSIS Diagnosis usually involves careful consideration of the dog's age, breed and prior medical history. Access to any potential toxins or poisons may be enquired about. A precise description of the fit will be asked for, although veterinary surgeons realise that this can be difficult for owners who were extremely anxious the first time a fit was happening. It may therefore be difficult to recall all details that the veterinary surgeon needs to know, but a checklist can be provided for any future fits and the owner reassured that pain is not present, nor is death during the fit likely.

A clinical neurological examination may provide some clues as to possible causes. If the dog seems healthy, and it was only a single isolated fit, no further tests beyond perhaps some routine tests on a urine sample may be carried out at this stage, but the owner

---

Typical pattern of a generalised fit/seizure in a dog with epilepsy

Pre-fit phase

- Usually, a slight abnormality in behaviour is the first sign that a fit may be imminent. The dog may appear restless, anxious, and begin pacing about or seeking reassurance from the owner. Panting and whining may be noticed.

Fit or seizure

- This starts suddenly, with incoordination, loss of consciousness and falling over onto one side. The limbs are usually held rigidly extended and the neck is also tense. Breathing may appear to be interrupted. Some owners think their dog has died at this stage, but these symptoms usually only last 10 or 20 seconds. Death during a typical epileptic fit is very unusual.

- Paddling movements then start in the limbs, the dog may whine/bark, chomp its jaws and drool saliva. Urine and faeces may be passed at this stage. This activity can continue for up to 5 minutes.

Post-fit stage

- The symptoms subside and the dog gradually returns to consciousness.

- Complete return to awareness may take an hour or so. Some dogs may sleep or appear hungry (the muscular activity during the fit consumes a lot of energy).

---

may be asked to watch out for signs of future fits including any tell-tale signs that a fit has occurred when the dog was left alone in the house (e.g. urine or faeces on the carpet, disturbed bedding, etc.).

Alternatively, the veterinary surgeon may decide at this point to run blood tests to rule out such conditions as liver or kidney disease, diabetes or other pancreatic disease which interferes with the blood sugar levels, conditions causing low blood calcium, etc. Such blood tests can provide a wealth of useful information and can lead to a lot of conditions being considered and ruled in or out as causes of the fits or seizures.

How to cope with the fitting dog

1. Keep calm! The fit will end shortly in nearly all cases and the dog feels no pain.

2. Ensure the dog cannot damage itself by rolling into fires, obstructing its face, etc.

3. If necessary, gently extend the neck and pull the dog's tongue out – but take great care not to get bitten as the dog is not conscious of its actions and chomping/biting activities are frequently seen during fits. In fact, choking is not a common problem during most fits.

4. Switch off television/radio and keep the room quiet.

5. Dim or switch off bright lights.

6. Note the time on your watch.

7. If the fit is still going on 10 minutes later, telephone the veterinary surgery for advice.

Your veterinary surgeon should always be informed the first time a fit has occurred. Depending on the circumstances, tests may be done at that stage. If fits are very infrequent (e.g. one every few months), then treatment may not be given unless the frequency or severity increases.

Other possible tests include examination of the cerebrospinal fluid (the fluid that surrounds the brain and spinal cord), X-rays and scans. Hopefully, this information should lead to a provisional diagnosis.

TREATMENT Whenever possible, the aim is to treat or remove the cause of the fit. If this can be done successfully then no other treatment for the fit or seizure may be needed.

However, removal of the cause isn't possible in all cases – it is not known what causes epilepsy, for example, so treatment consists of preventing fits occurring by means of medication, which must usually be continued for life. Sometimes, if a dog has been on medication for a long time without any fits happening, a attempt to try without medication may be made. This should only be done under veterinary advice. A few

dogs may have no further fits and treatment can be discontinued at this stage.

In severe cases of epilepsy, it may not be possible to abolish fits completely, but usually their frequency can be substantially reduced.

OUTLOOK Most epileptic dogs can be controlled well with medication and, once settled on the correct dose, lead a good quality of life. Periodic blood tests may be needed to ensure the best dose is being used.

The outlook for other conditions is variable and depends on the severity and treatability of the underlying disease. In some cases treatment for both the fits/seizures and the underlying disease may be needed to adequately control symptoms.

GERIATRIC VESTIBULAR SYNDROME ('STROKE')

CAUSE 'Stroke' is not really the correct term for this problem since the condition is not quite the same as stroke in human beings, however it is often used as a useful shorthand by some veterinary surgeons and owners.

The cause is damage within the inner ear or the brain which leads to very characteristic symptoms, especially in older dogs. In most cases, the cause of the triggering damage remains unknown.

SYMPTOMS The usual symptoms are head tilt, incoordination, rapid eye movements and, quite often, vomiting. More severe cases can cause incessant circling or persistent falling over and rolling, which can be distressing for the unprepared owner. The circling and falling over are always towards the same direction, reflecting the side of the brain in which the damage has occurred.

These symptoms usually ease somewhat over 1–2 days.

DIAGNOSIS The symptoms are often characteristic in dogs over 10 years. The ears are usually checked to make sure there is no disease present and a general examination, possibly supplemented by blood and urine tests, will be carried out. Occasionally, a CT scan

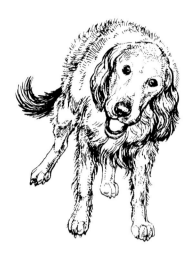
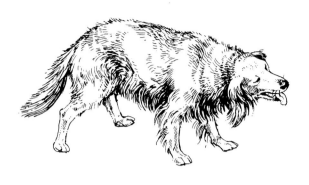

Head tilt and incoordination can indicate vestibular disease –
a problem which interferes with normal balancing and movement.

 Home nursing

Lots of patience is needed, especially in the first few days, as affected dogs will be staggery and incoordinated. It is best to restrict the dog to one room, or even an indoor kennel or cage if one is available and the dog will settle in it. Ensure that there are no obstacles around that could be stumbled into.

Hand feeding may be required and the dog may need to be supported, perhaps in a blanket sling, to be taken out to toilet 4 times daily. Fairly constant supervision is required in the more severely affected dogs.

Don't lose heart too soon. Despite the alarming signs, many dogs improve quite quickly. The condition is not painful but some dogs become agitated by feeling unbalanced and nauseous. Drugs from the veterinary surgeon may be able to help here.

may be suggested if facilities are available, to rule out other problems.

TREATMENT Sometimes drugs to ease vomiting and nausea are given. Other than this, no treatment seems particularly effective though various things have been tried. The condition usually improves on its own over a period of 2–4 weeks.

Severe cases with falling over and rolling may require hospitalisation in a padded kennel or very careful supervision at home to ensure that no damage is caused by the uncontrolled movement. Otherwise good general nursing care is required at home while the dog convalesces.

OUTLOOK Improvement can be expected in most cases. Occasionally, the head tilt may persist and may even be permanent in a few dogs, but most patients cope very well.

ENCEPHALITIS – BRAIN INFLAMMATION

CAUSE Canine distemper is the commonest infectious disease which can affect the brain and is possible in unvaccinated dogs. Distemper is discussed in detail on page 21.

In countries where rabies (see page 23) is seen, this disease can also affect the brain. Other infections are seen less frequently but can include various viruses, bacteria and protozoa. They all cause the brain to become inflamed and, in doing so, damage it, possibly permanently.

Granulomatous meningo-encephalitis (GME) is a fairly common cause of encephalitis in younger dogs, especially those of smaller breeds.

SYMPTOMS General signs of brain disease are seen, including head tilts, rapid eye movements, incoordination and seizures. Various other symptoms are possible depending on the specific areas of the brain that are affected.

DIAGNOSIS Diagnosis is not always easy and usually depends on an analysis of the fluid that bathes the brain and spinal cord (the cerebrospinal fluid), coupled with other tests to try to establish the exact cause.

TREATMENT Viral illnesses cannot be treated (only prevented by vaccination) therefore if brain disease results from a viral illness the extent of damage may not be apparent until after the infection has passed. Symptoms arising from this damage may be permanent. Sometimes the effects can be limited or controlled by drug treatments. In the initial stages, hospitalisation is likely in order to stabilise the patient and, hopefully, limit the damage to the brain.

OUTLOOK If permanent damage has occurred, and this is causing symptoms, the only hope is treatment to control or suppress these symptoms to give the dog a reasonable quality of life.

BRAIN INJURY

CAUSE The usual cause of head/brain injury in dogs is a road traffic accident which involves a severe blow to the skull, but any similar trauma (e.g. kick from horse) could act in the same way.

SYMPTOMS These can range from no immediate symptoms to unconsciousness, coma and rapid death. Symptoms depend on the nature of the injury and degree of brain swelling and bleeding that arise as a result of it.

Severe injuries lead to a progressive series of changes in the brain which worsen the original damage. This usually proves fatal.

DIAGNOSIS Diagnosis will be based on apparent or likely damage given the circumstances. Brain scans are

slowly becoming more available in large veterinary hospitals and it is likely that these will improve the chances of accurate diagnosis, and hence more specific treatment, in brain-injured patients.

TREATMENT Treatment is aimed at limiting brain swelling and preventing complications such as seizures or oxygen deprivation. This treatment can only be carried out effectively in a veterinary practice or hospital, so the injured dog must be transported there without delay.

OUTLOOK The outlook for severe brain injury is always poor. Early treatment may be successful in some cases. Fortunately, brain injury is encountered less often than might be expected in traumatised dogs due to the good protection afforded by the skull bone.

BRAIN TUMOUR

CAUSE Tumours may occur spontaneously in the brain as in other organs and tissues of the body. They are commoner in older dogs and may arise in the meninges (the covering layer of the brain), when they are known as meningiomas, or in the substance of the brain itself.

SYMPTOMS Fits/seizures are a frequent symptom. In young dogs, these are commonly associated with epilepsy but in older dogs a brain tumour does have to be considered as a possibility (as well as the other conditions mentioned under fits and seizures on page 180).

Other symptoms may include changes in behaviour/personality as well as incoordination and weakness. Changes in behaviour or personality are usually readily noticed by people who know the dog well. They can be quite subtle, but are nevertheless important.

Tumours which arise in the pituitary gland of the brain may produce more general symptoms of disease due to interference with hormone function. Cushing's disease, quite frequently encountered in dogs, is an example of this type of problem. These may be the only symptoms of this type of tumour and treatment is usually possible.

DIAGNOSIS Brain scans are gradually becoming more available to dogs and referral or university-based hospitals may be able to offer this technique. Such scans enable the tumour to be located and can often indicate the type of tumour present. Unfortunately, routine X-rays are not particularly helpful with brain tumours as the bony skull blocks out any image of the brain itself.

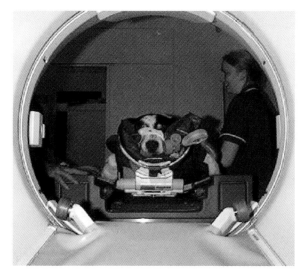

CT scans are now available for dogs and can give much more information than routine X-rays, especially for nervous system problems.

TREATMENT In line with the improving diagnosis of brain tumours in dogs, treatment techniques are also developing and some tumours are amenable to surgery or other forms of therapy, e.g. radiation treatment. Naturally, such treatment can be expensive and guarantees of cures cannot be given.

Medical treatment using 'steroid' drugs, which are relatively cheap and widely available, can often bring about an improvement in symptoms and extend the life in dogs with brain tumours. If fits are being caused, these may be able to be controlled using anti-convulsant drugs as for epilepsy.

Dogs whose symptoms are due to interference with the hormonal system (pituitary tumours) can usually be treated with specific drugs to counteract these effects.

OUTLOOK The long term prognosis is always very doubtful with a brain tumour, but this does not mean that a good quality of life cannot be attained in the interim. It all depends on the severity of symptoms and how treatable these are in an individual patient.

HYDROCEPHALUS

CAUSE This condition refers to a build-up of pressure within the brain caused by accumulation of cerebrospinal fluid – the fluid which surrounds the brain and spinal cord. Most cases of hydrocephalus are congenital and found in newly born puppies.

SYMPTOMS Affected puppies usually have prominent domed heads. Abnormal brain function may be present, including fits/seizures. Puppies may sleep excessively and be reluctant or unable to move as normal. Some puppies with this condition may die shortly after birth.

DIAGNOSIS This is usually suspected from the appearance of the puppy. The condition can be acquired in older dogs with brain disease, in which case analysis of the cerebrospinal fluid may be required in addition to other tests.

TREATMENT Treatment is difficult. In puppies, mild cases may not interfere with normal life too much and, provided the owner understands the condition, the dog may be able to have a good life as a pet. Severely affected puppies are more kindly put to sleep if they cannot interact normally with their environment.

In older dogs, treatment depends on the underlying problem and on the extent of brain damage caused.

OUTLOOK This is a serious problem in any age group. The best outlook is in mildly affected puppies who may manage to adapt to live a reasonably normal life.

NARCOLEPSY

CAUSE Narcolepsy is an unusual disease characterised by sudden attacks of sleep during normal wakening hours. The disease is inherited in dogs and certain breeds are especially affected, e.g. Beagle, Labrador, Dachshund, Doberman Pinscher.

SYMPTOMS Usually, excitement precedes the attacks, e.g. the owner returns home from work or the dog is fed. After a brief period of excitement the dog quickly falls asleep.

DIAGNOSIS The symptoms make diagnosis easy. Usually, the disease is first noticed in young dogs.

TREATMENT A cure is not possible but drug treatment can often help.

OUTLOOK Though inconvenient, this is not a dangerous disease and treatment may minimise the sleep attacks.

Spinal Diseases

PARALYSIS

CAUSE The cause of paralysis is nerve injury, which can be temporary or permanent. Several of the spinal conditions mentioned here can cause paralysis, so that paralysis is considered a *symptom* of a disease rather than a disease in itself: it is important to discover what is causing the paralysis in order to see if this can be cured.

Paralysis can be of a single limb (or the tail) or more than one limb, depending on exactly where the nerve damage has occurred. When the injury is in the spinal cord itself (rather than in a single nerve in a limb), the risk is that paralysis will affect more than one limb. Paraplegia refers to paralysis of the two hind limbs. Quadriplegia means paralysis of all four limbs.

Sometimes the word 'paresis' is used. This means weakness – in other words complete paralysis has not occurred but function is not normal.

SYMPTOMS Paralysis results in loss of voluntary function. The affected area cannot be moved, hangs loosely and may have no sensation. Partial or complete lack of sensation is dangerous because it means that the animal is not aware of injury, hence wounds can occur without the animal realising it.

Paralysis of the bladder, which can occur after pelvic injuries, means that the animal cannot feel its bladder filling up. No urge to urinate is produced and the bladder becomes over-full, which can cause permanent damage to it and possibly incontinence.

DIAGNOSIS Paralysis is diagnosed by examining the area and testing reflexes. X-rays may be used if the cause is thought to be in the spine or if a fracture is associated with the paralysis.

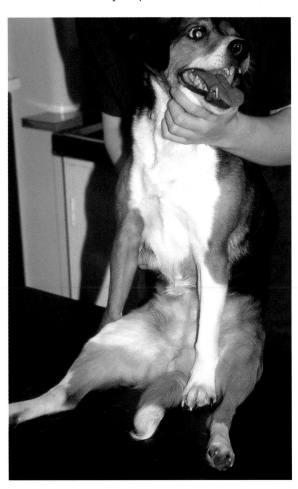

Dog with hindlimb paralysis following disc protrusion. The condition can usually be cured if treated early enough.

Nerves themselves cannot be seen on ordinary X-rays, so damage has to be implied from surrounding structures which are visible (such as bone). This does mean that it can be difficult to say exactly how severe the injury to a nerve is.

The spinal cord can be seen if a special X-ray called a myelogram is perfomed. In this technique, a contrast dye is injected into the space surrounding the spinal cord. This contrast dye outlines the spinal cord itself and shows up any areas of compression or damage.

TREATMENT Some causes of paralysis cannot be treated. If the nerve has been badly damaged then function may never return and the affected limb or tail may need to be amputated to prevent accidental injury.

Temporary paralysis caused by spinal problems can often be treated, but treatment or surgery must be carried out promptly in many cases for the best result.

OUTLOOK If some function remains in the nerve, the outlook may be encouraging. Sometimes however only time will tell how much function will return since it can be difficult to predict how severe the damage to the nerves is.

DISC PROBLEMS

CAUSE Spinal (inter-vertebral) discs are cushion-like structures which separate each spine bone and allow normal flexible mobility of the back. The disc consists of a soft centre and tough fibrous outer covering. As dogs grow older (or even in young dogs of certain breeds) the discs undergo changes which make them more likely to stretch or rupture, placing pressure on the nearby spinal cord and causing severe pain or paralysis.

Breeds especially prone to disc problems include Dachshunds, Beagles and Cocker Spaniels. These breeds can have problems at an early age due to premature degeneration of the discs. With other breeds, problems are generally seen later in life, after 5 years, as part of the normal ageing process.

SYMPTOMS The condition can be very painful indeed – dogs may scream when moved and stand rigid, with muscle spasms around the area of the spine that is affected. Pain is particularly severe when the spine in the region of the neck is compressed. There may be weakness of one or more limbs (paresis) or complete paralysis, when no pain is present.

Paralysis indicates a more severe injury and if more than one limb is affected such dogs will be unable to move voluntarily. Bladder problems are

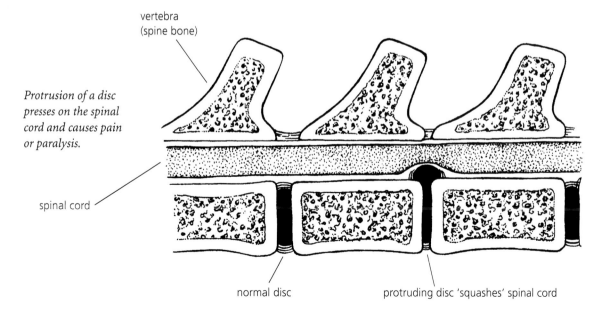

Protrusion of a disc presses on the spinal cord and causes pain or paralysis.

vertebra (spine bone)

spinal cord

normal disc

protruding disc 'squashes' spinal cord

frequently encountered in paralysed dogs. For this reason, any paralysed dog must be seen by a veterinary surgeon immediately in order to ensure that the bladder is protected and that treatment for the spine is started as soon as possible. This maximises the chances of success.

Less severe and more chronic symptoms include milder pain, inability to move properly and a reluctance to negotiate steps. The feet of the affected legs may 'scuff' the ground, causing abnormal wear of the nails or perhaps injuries on the skin surface. Such dogs may yelp out when their backs or hindquarters are touched in a certain way or when they move in an uncoordinated fashion themelves.

Dogs in severe spinal pain should be moved carefully. A muzzle should be applied or tape wound around the nose as they may bite accidentally.

DIAGNOSIS This requires a combination of neurological examination and X-rays. A myelogram (dye injected into the space surrounding the spinal cord) may also be performed if surgery is contemplated. The aim is to find the area of spinal cord compression and assess how bad the damage is. CT and NMR scans, as used in people, are becoming more widely available for dogs with spinal problems of this type and can greatly help the diagnosis.

TREATMENT For dogs with signs of pain but no abnormalities in their nervous system reflexes, careful confinement in a cage or indoor kennel may be tried. Any signs of worsening in condition may however require surgery.

More and more dogs with severe or recurring spinal problems are operated on since it has been found that if prompt treatment is received from a specialist surgeon, the recovery tends to be quicker with less likelihood of recurrences.

OUTLOOK The outlook is poor for dogs with the most severe form of damage – when reflexes have been lost entirely and there is no awareness of what veterinary surgeons call 'deep pain'.

The importance of the 'deep pain' response
The vital 'deep pain' response can still be present in

Essential requirements for cage confinement

- This is equivalent to strict bed rest in humans.

- A suitable size of cage or indoor kennel is required.

- The dog must remain in this *at all times* except when taken out (lifted if a small dog) to pass urine and faeces 4 times daily, at which times the dog must be carefully supervised and kept on a lead.

- The dog must be confined for the full duration of time as prescribed by the veterinary surgeon. Bringing the dog out sooner runs the risk of deterioration in condition, and possibly the need for immediate surgery.

- Effective cage confinement demands great perseverance by the owner and all members of the family. It may not be suitable for every dog as, temperamentally, some dogs may not settle well and rest as needed.

dogs which are completely paralysed. Checking for this reaction is the most important test the veterinary surgeon will do as the result affects the outlook considerably and can influence decisions about whether major spinal surgery is even attempted. The crucial thing is whether the dog is *consciously* aware of a painful stimulus. For conscious awareness to be present the dog must yelp or give another indication that messages about the pain are being received in the brain. Simple withdrawal of the foot without any signal of conscious awareness only demonstrates an automatic reflex and unfortunately cannot be taken as evidence that surgical or other treatment would give a good chance of recovery.

In severe cases which could be helped by surgery, an operation stands the best chance of success when performed by a specialist soon after the initial symptoms have appeared. Many dogs in this category are referred immediately for specialist treatment. If there is absolutely no deep pain response, euthanasia is usually considered the kindest option as no prospect for return to normal function exists.

Beagle with neck pain following protrusion of a disc. Note the unusual head position and hunched stance. This condition is very uncomfortable and affected dogs will often yelp when they move inadvertently.

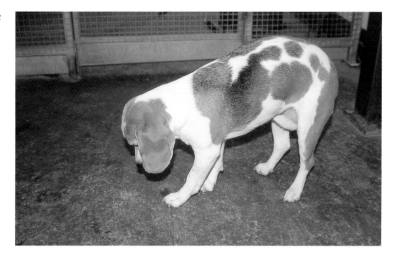

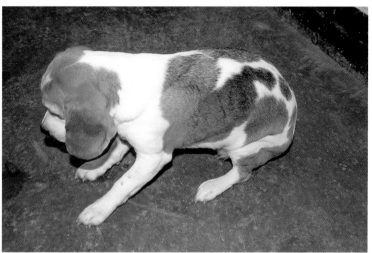

'WOBBLER' SYNDROME

CAUSE This is a disease of Dobermans, Great Danes and certain other large breeds caused by a number of abnormalities in the cervical (neck) area of the spine. Great Danes tend to show symptoms while they are young, whereas in Dobermans the condition is seen in mature animals. The term 'wobbler' comes from the unsteady gait that is produced in this disease – affected animals sway while walking.

SYMPTOMS The first sign is unsteadiness in the hind limbs together with an unusual 'choppy' stride pattern in the fore limbs. These symptoms worsen and the head may be held lower due to neck pain. Eventually, severe weakness may be present in all four limbs, even leading to quadriplegia (paralysis of all limbs). These symptoms are caused by progressive interference with nerve function caused by compression of the spinal cord by malformed or malaligned vertebrae.

DIAGNOSIS The condition is often suspected given the breed and the characteristic symptoms. It is confirmed using X-rays and usually a myelogram, when the exact problems in each individual dog can be picked up.

TREATMENT This can be a difficult disease to deal with. Some dogs respond well to anti-inflammatory drugs and improvement in symptoms can be achieved

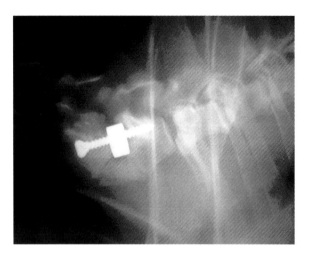

X-ray of a Doberman following spinal surgery for Wobbler syndrome. A screw and washer have been used to secure the unstable vertebrae and relieve symptoms.

for a considerable length of time. Usually, however, there is gradual deterioration in symptoms. A number of surgical treatments are possible – all of these are major operations. The aim is to stop the disease getting worse if possible. The outcome of the surgery can be difficult to predict in general, since dogs do vary in the severity of symptoms.

OUTLOOK Probably around three-quarters of dogs that are treated by specialist surgeons are improved, but the most severely affected dogs (those that are unable to walk at the time of treatment) carry a poorer outlook. Anti-inflammtory drugs can help but they will not cure the condition completely and gradual deterioration is to be expected.

CDRM

CAUSE The abbreviation of this disease stands for chronic degenerative radiculomyelopathy – a medical term describing the irreversible damage which occurs in the spinal cord of affected dogs. The condition is most commonly found in older German Shepherd dogs; the cause is unknown but the result is poor nerve function which slowly worsens over a period of months.

SYMPTOMS Initially, symptoms may be mild. The hind limbs are affected and coordination is poor. Abnormal wear of the nails occurs and the skin of the toes may be scuffed as the dog inadvertently drags these along. Worsening of symptoms results in more severe incoordination, a swaying gait and crossing of the hind legs while walking or turning. Severely affected dogs may knuckle over on their hind paws without feeling any discomfort. The disease is not painful at any stage but causes a progressive weakness, leading on to eventual paralysis and immobility.

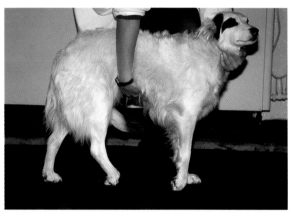

Loss of sensation in the foot shown by 'knuckling'. A normal dog would immediately correct the foot into its usual position but this dog stood like this indefinitely.

DIAGNOSIS Confirmation of the disease usually involves X-rays to rule out other problems. Many German Shepherds with CDRM may also be suffering from hip dysplasia and arthritis, which could be contributing to their problems.

TREATMENT There is no proven effective treatment for CDRM, however overall symptoms may be improved if other treatable problems are present. For example, if the dog also has arthritis, overall improvement in mobility may be possible if the arthritis is treated. The CDRM will still be present but its effects may be coped with better if the pain from the arthritis is managed.

OUTLOOK The eventual outlook with CDRM is poor because the disease is progressive. When the dog can no longer stand or move adequately, euthanasia is required on humane grounds.

ATLANTO-AXIAL SUBLUXATION

CAUSE This is a problem encountered in young toy breeds of dog such as Toy Poodles, Yorkshire Terriers, etc. It is a malformation of the first two bones of the spine: the atlas and the axis. A portion of bone is missing, with the result that these bones are more mobile than they should be. This can put pressure on the spinal cord and cause symptoms.

SYMPTOMS Neck pain is often seen, coupled with weakness, incoordination or sudden collapse. Dogs with this condition must be handled carefully and struggling, pulling on the lead etc. avoided at all costs.

DIAGNOSIS The age, breed and typical symptoms usually lead to suspicion of this condition, which is confirmed using X-rays.

TREATMENT The best results are obtained following surgery to stabilise the two bones, usually by fusing them together. Following this, symptoms normally disappear.

OUTLOOK This is usually good after specialist surgical treatment.

DISCOSPONDYLITIS

CAUSE This disease of the spinal disc occurs when bacteria gain access to it and set up infection. The infection often spreads to adjacent vertebral bodies on either side of the disc.

SYMPTOMS Most patients show spinal pain, a high temperature and poorly coordinated reflexes and movement. Affected dogs will be miserable and reluctant to move.

DIAGNOSIS X-rays are used to identify the infected discs and vertebrae.

TREATMENT Lengthy courses of antibiotics are prescribed. In severe cases, surgery may be needed to remove damaged tissue or pockets of infection.

OUTLOOK Most dogs respond to treatment and provided it is continued long enough a cure can be expected. Progress is checked by means of repeat X-rays.

SPINAL FRACTURES AND TRAUMA

CAUSE A fractured spine is normally caused by a road traffic accident, a fall or a kick from a large animal such as a horse.

SYMPTOMS A wide range of traumatic injuries are possible. Most animals with spinal trauma are in severe pain, cannot stand and may be paralysed.

DIAGNOSIS X-rays are important to assess the damage since, if the spinal cord has been severed or severely traumatised, there would be no prospect for recovery. It is important to differentiate damage to the bony vertebrae (which might be able to be repaired or heal by themselves) and damage to the spinal cord itself, which if severe cannot be treated.

Moving the spinal trauma patient

- In all cases it is safest to place a muzzle or tape around the dog's nose, as when in pain the patient may bite out of fear while you are trying to help.

- The best way to move spinally injured dogs is on a stiff board or stretcher, ideally with straps placed across the dog's body to limit movement or rolling as much as possible.

- In emergencies, a blanket held taut by two people makes a good stretcher.

- Try to reassure the dog so that it stays still while being moved.

- Go to the nearest veterinary practice or hospital.

Absence of a 'deep pain' response (see above) means that irreversible damage is very likely.

TREATMENT If the spinal cord is intact and functioning, spinal fractures can be treated. Unstable fractures are repaired in a manner similar to broken bones, using metallic implants and devices. If instability is less of a problem, the fracture may be treated with strict cage confinement or perhaps a body brace.

OUTLOOK This rests entirely on the state of the spinal cord. If it is intact and functioning then treatment carries a good chance of success. If not, euthanasia is the kindest option.

SPINAL TUMOURS

CAUSE Tumours may arise in the spinal cord itself or in the bony vertebrae which surround it.

SYMPTOMS Spinal pain is often caused and other neurological signs such as lameness, partial paralysis or weakness may be seen as the tumour enlarges.

DIAGNOSIS X-rays and, where available, CT scans or NMR scans are used in diagnosis. Biopsies may be taken to find out how dangerous the tumour is.

TREATMENT Some tumours of the spinal cord can be treated. Tumours of the bony vertebrae however tend to be malignant ones, and treatment other than pain relief is not possible.

OUTLOOK Overall, the outlook is poor for spinal tumours.

CHAPTER 11

Male Reproductive System

Common symptoms of reproductive disease in male dogs

• Straining to pass urine • Constipation • Blood in urine • Discharge from prepuce
• Testicular enlargement • Abdominal pain • Symmetrical non-itchy hair loss

Structure and Function

The reproductive system of the male dog consists of the testicles (two) in the scrotum, the prostate gland, penis and prepuce. Closely associated with each testicle and sitting on top of it is the epididymis. The male reproductive system as a whole produces and stores the male sex cells (spermatozoa or sperm) and, during mating, places these into the vagina of the bitch.

The epididymis stores mature spermatozoa that have been produced in the testicles. Production of spermatozoa occurs best at a temperature slightly *lower* than body temperature, which is why the testicles are present within the scrotum – the structure hangs outwith the body and is therefore a little cooler than the core body temperature. If a testicle was retained within the body (in the abdomen, for example – a common problem in dogs), sperm production would be slowed or stopped at the higher temperature, with consequent infertility. The 'retained' testicle would also be at an increased risk of disease such as cancer or torsion (see Retained testicles later).

The prostate gland, situated just behind the bladder, produces an important fluid which helps protect and nourish the spermatozoa. Spermatozoa together with its protective fluid (semen) is ejaculated into the vagina of the bitch at mating.

The penis consists largely of spongy tissue with a very good blood supply. The dog penis also has a small bone, called the os penis, within its tissue. During erection, spaces within the tissue of the penis become filled with blood, making the organ turgid. This allows effective sexual intercourse to take place. Further details of the breeding process itself are given in Chapter 15.

The prepuce is the skin which surrounds and protects the penis.

Veterinary Diagnosis and Treatment

Useful information is usually obtained from the general examination of the male dog. The testicles can be felt for growths (though some of these may be too small to feel easily) and, by conducting a rectal examination, the prostate can be checked. This is an

General anatomy of the male reproductive system

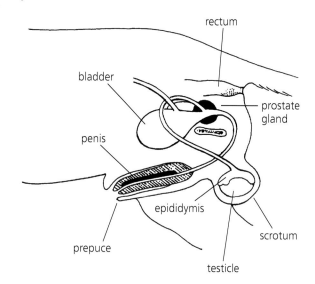

important part of the examination since problems here are so common in middle aged and older dogs.

X-rays and ultrasound scans are used a lot in investigating reproductive system diseases and usually provide very useful information.

Problems caused or worsened by excess male hormones are normally treated by castration of the dog. Although 'anti-male hormone' injections can be

---

What can go wrong with the male reproductive system?

Problems associated with infertility in male dogs are discussed in Chapter 15.

Commonly encountered problems in male pet dogs include retained testicles, testicular tumours and problems with the prostate gland in older male dogs which have not been neutered (castrated).

A number of conditions are associated with increased levels of male hormones, again mostly in older un-neutered dogs. In particular enlarged prostate, tail gland hypertrophy and anal growths (see page 97) and testicular tumours may occur, often together. Perineal hernias (see page 115) can also be associated with prostate problems.

Routine castration of male dogs is discussed on page 5.

given, these are a less satisfactory way of controlling most problems in the long term, except in very old dogs or dogs in which an anaesthetic would be especially risky. Such injections can be very useful initially however.

Older dogs often require blood tests, especially before an anaesthetic or any surgery is contemplated as they may have other 'hidden' diseases of the kidneys or liver which could increase the risk of these treatments.

Costs and prognosis in reproductive diseases in the male dog

Naturally, any problem which is associated with cancer has a poorer outlook than simple infections or inflammation. However cancer of the testicles carries a good outlook overall since these tumours do not often spread elsewhere.

In general, the problems caused by excess hormonal stimulation in the older male dog respond well to castration. Although there may be the expense of initial investigations and then surgery, this should in most cases put an end to the problem without the need for on-going treatment.

Severe infections and abscesses of the prostate can be expensive to treat if major surgery is needed in addition to castration.

Commonest Reproductive System Diseases in Male Dogs

Testes and Scrotum

RETAINED TESTICLES (CRYPTORCHIDISM)

CAUSE In this condition one or both testicles is missing from the scrotum. There are several reasons why this may occur (see box).

SYMPTOMS Male puppies should be checked frequently to ensure than both testicles are present. Any puppies which do not have both testicles at weaning

---

Possible reasons for missing testicles

• Puppy less than 12 weeks of age

The testicle or testicles are probably present but have not fully descended into the scrotum. They may be present in the inguinal area (inside the upper thigh near the abdomen) or else they could be retained within the abdomen, where they develop in the foetus. Note that most male puppies have descended testicles by 2 weeks of age.

Very occasionally, congenital absence of one testicle may be present (or, rarer still, absence of both). In the vast majority of cases, however, the testicle is within the abdomen, having failed to descend, or is found somewhere along the usual route of descent.

After 12 weeks, the dog is termed 'cryptorchid'. This medical term describes the situation of one or both testicles being absent from the scrotum.

• Dog over 12 weeks of age

In older dogs (6 months or more) that are newly acquired, the possibility of castration should be considered. Checking with previous owners or searching for a small surgical scar may provide the answer.

What causes cryptorchidism?
The likely cause is an inherited problem and affected animals should not be used for breeding. Neutering is also required for health reasons, as described below.

---

should be examined by the veterinary surgeon to confirm their absence.

Retained testicles are more likely to become cancerous and symptoms of testicular cancer may therefore be seen in older cryptorchid dogs which were not castrated when they were younger. In addition, the retained testicle will not produce sperm (since the temperature in the abdomen is higher than that in the scrotum) and in cases where both testicles are retained the dog will be infertile. A further potential problem in retained testicles is testicular torsion.

DIAGNOSIS Absence of one or both testicles should be confirmed by the veterinary surgeon after 12 weeks

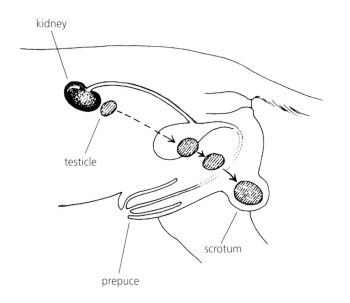

Path of descent of the testicle from the abdomen into the scrotum. The testicle may stop at any point – a condition known as cryptorchidism.

I don't know my dog's background. Is he cryptorchid or has he been castrated?

This can be a problem in rescue dogs or dogs acquired from other sources where their medical details are unknown.

The first step is a general medical examination. The veterinary surgeon may be able to detect a surgical scar if the hair is clipped off from the usual site. If one is present, castration can be assumed.

Otherwise, either an assumption of castration can be made or, in circumstances where confirmation is needed, response to a testosterone-stimulating injection could be measured. This should indicate whether or not retained testicles are present.

of age. (Some veterinary surgeons may elect to wait a little longer in the hope that the testicle may descend of its own accord however the chances are fairly low.)

TREATMENT The treatment for cryptorchidism is to remove both testicles. This is carried out even if only one is retained. The retained testicle, if present within the abdomen, may necessitate abdominal surgery as well as the more minor surgery normally used for testicles in the scrotum. A testicle which is partly descended may be accessible without major abdominal surgery.

OUTLOOK Provided castration is performed, the risk of testicular cancer or torsion is avoided.

INFLAMMATION (ORCHITIS; SCROTAL DERMATITIS)

CAUSE Inflammation or infection of the testicle is termed orchitis; that of the scrotum is called scrotal dermatitis.

Traumatic injury to the testicles may occur in road accidents or if a dog gets caught jumping over a fence.

Primary infection is rare but can be caused by *Brucella canis*, a bacterium which is found in some countries (not in the UK). Scrotal dermatitis is quite common as the skin on the scrotum is very sensitive. Clipper rash or irritant shampoos can cause a severe dermatitis; a few dogs may react to carpet cleaning products in this way. Dogs which are in kennels may develop a dermatitis in this area if they are sensitive to disinfectants or other products used to clean the kennels or runs.

SYMPTOMS Orchitis is extremely painful. Pain/lameness in the hind quarters may be seen and movement is likely to be stiff. A high temperature may be present and bruising or injury to the scrotum may also have occurred.

If it is only the scrotum itself that is affected, the skin can appear red and extremely sore. Any attempts to touch the sore area may be resisted. Affected dogs are usually miserable and irritable.

DIAGNOSIS These conditions are usually apparent on visual examination. Ultrasound is used occasionally for orchitis and if bacterial infection is suspected samples may be taken.

TREATMENT In most cases antibiotics and painkillers are used. Severe inflammation or abscess formation may necessitate castration of the dog. Scrotal dermatitis is often alleviated by topical creams or ointments containing anti-inflammatory compounds. Products that the dog may have been washed in or come into contact with should be avoided in the future.

First aid

Do not apply any antiseptic agents to inflamed or broken skin on the scrotum, as this may worsen inflammation that is already present. Bland creams (e.g. zinc and castor oil, or Calendula cream) can be used before a veterinary appointment. If the dog constantly licks the area, a 'buster' collar should be fitted to prevent worsening of the situation.

OUTLOOK The outlook is usually good but serious cases may require castration.

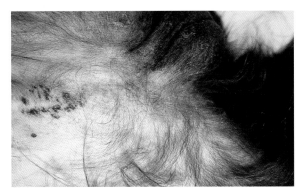

Dermatitis on the scrotum can be caused by allergy or by contact with irritants such as carpet cleaner, shampoos etc.

TESTICULAR TUMOURS

CAUSE These are common tumours in the male dog and a number of different types exist. They may cause enlargement of the affected testicle, but not all types do this. The tumours arise spontaneously and can affect any un-neutered dog.

Tumours are more likely to occur in retained testicles, i.e. testicles which have not descended into the scrotum and remain in the abdomen (see above). Any dog with retained testicles should be castrated at a young age to prevent this happening.

SYMPTOMS Testicular enlargement of one or both testicles can occur but this may not always be readily detected except by the veterinary surgeon. Some tumours cause 'feminising' syndromes because the tumours produce female-associated hormones. This can lead to female characteristics appearing in the male dog (see box).

DIAGNOSIS This rests on detecting typical signs of the tumour and/or feeling a tumour during routine examination of the male dog.

Feminising and other effects of certain testicular tumours

Dogs with testicular tumours may show some of these signs:

- Development of mammary glands
- Attractiveness to other male dogs
- Hair loss in the flank areas on both sides of the body
- Swelling of the prepuce area

TREATMENT Castration is required for testicular tumours. Both testicles are removed even if apparently only one is affected by the tumour.

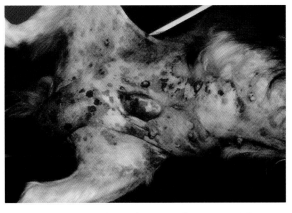

Skin symptoms in a dog with a testicular tumour. These symptoms usually disappear following castration.

OUTLOOK The outlook is usually good as these tumours do not spread quickly elsewhere in the body. Any hormonal effects caused by the tumour will gradually disappear following castration.

TORSION OF THE TESTICLE

CAUSE In this condition the testicle twists on its blood supply. The cause of this problem is unknown but the result is serious abnormalities in the testicle, with death of the tissue resulting from impaired blood supply. The condition is also extremely painful. Torsion is more likely to occur in cryptorchid dogs (see above).

SYMPTOMS Sudden onset of severe abdominal pain is seen. Vomiting and lethargy may occur.

DIAGNOSIS This is usually suggested by the dog's medical history of having an unremoved abdominal testicle, and also by X-rays and possibly ultrasound.

TREATMENT Surgery is necessary to remove the damaged testicle.

OUTLOOK The outlook is good after prompt treatment.

Prostate Gland

BENIGN ENLARGEMENT OF THE PROSTATE

CAUSE This is the commonest of a number of disorders which affect the prostate gland of the dog. It usually occurs in middle to old age and is a result of altered hormone levels in these dogs; occasionally, it may be seen in younger dogs.

RIGHT Diagram showing possible symptoms seen with enlargement of the prostate. Blood may be visible at the penis or during urination, the dog may strain to urinate and the enlarged prostate may press on the descending colon, causing constipation.

SYMPTOMS The enlarged prostate can press on the colon, causing constipation and straining, possibly leading on to a perineal hernia (see page 115). Other symptoms include straining to pass urine and passing blood in the urine.

DIAGNOSIS An internal examination performed by the veterinary surgeon will usually detect an enlarged prostate. This can be confirmed by X-rays or ultrasound. It cannot usually be said with absolute certainty that the enlargement is benign (i.e. not a tumour), but usually a good probability can be given especially if X-rays, ultrasound or biopsy techniques have been used. Urine samples are monitored for blood and/or protein in the urine and repeat examinations of the prostate are used to monitor its size as treatment takes effect.

Common indications of prostate disease

- Middle age or older dogs
- Straining to urinate
- Blood in urine or blood droplets at the penis
- Constipation
- Lethargy
- Abdominal pain

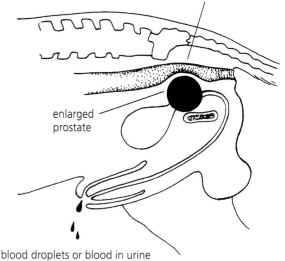

colon narrowed, causing constipation

enlarged prostate

blood droplets or blood in urine

TREATMENT The most effective treatment is castration. Sometimes, hormone injections are used – these may be tried prior to castration or used in very old or sick dogs where anaesthesia or surgery is not desirable. Hormone injections do however need to be repeated every few weeks, whereas castration provides a permanent cure.

OUTLOOK The outlook is good for benign enlargement.

ACUTE PROSTATIC INFECTIONS

CAUSE Bacteria may enter the prostate from the urinary system and set up a severe infection within the gland. This causes an enlarged and painful prostate. Dogs of any age may be affected.

SYMPTOMS This is a very painful condition and affected animals usually show signs of severe abdominal discomfort, vomiting and lethargy. There is usually a raised temperature and blood is present in the urine, which may be passed with difficulty.

DIAGNOSIS Symptoms of an 'acute abdomen' can arise from various diseases, but if the veterinary surgeon finds that the prostate is both enlarged and very painful, an infection in the gland can be assumed. As with benign enlargement, X-rays, ultrasound and biopsy techniques may be used and samples may be sent for culture of the bacteria causing the infection.

TREATMENT Antibiotics are important in treating this disease and some dogs will also need hospital admission for intravenous drip fluids and observation. A catheter may need to be passed if there is a risk of urinary obstruction.

OUTLOOK Most cases respond well but a few go on to develop chronic prostatitis/prostatic abscess, which will need further treatment.

CHRONIC PROSTATIC INFECTIONS AND ABSCESSES

CAUSE This condition can develop after an acute prostate infection. Chronic infection becomes established in the gland and causes recurrent bouts of illness. Chronic prostatic infections can be difficult and frustrating to manage.

SYMPTOMS The signs are usually less extreme than acute infections and may consist of discharge from the penis accompanied by straining to pass urine. The urine may be cloudy and/or contain blood. Some dogs have raised temperatures and may go off their food when experiencing symptoms.

If an abscess develops then pain can worsen considerably and vomiting and abdominal discomfort can occur as with acute infections.

DIAGNOSIS Palpation of the prostate combined with X-rays and ultrasound is used. In chronic infections, biopsies – which can be obtained from the prostate in several different ways – are often used to try to guage the severity of the condition and to help choose an effective antibiotic. Sometimes if an abscess is expected, exploratory surgery is carried out.

TREATMENT Very long courses of antibiotics are given for chronic infections; six weeks is not unusual. For abscesses, surgery may be required to deal with the severely diseased prostate. Usually, several days of hospitalisation are required as surgery on the prostate can be time-consuming and complex. An important part of the treatment of chronic and relapsing prostate conditions is castration.

OUTLOOK Chronic infections and abscesses are serious diseases that can be both time-consuming and expensive to treat. Complications and recurrences are both possible. Removal of the prostate is a very difficult operation that carries a high risk of incontinence; it is only rarely attempted.

PROSTATIC CYSTS

CAUSE These are another problem that may affect the canine prostate gland. Several types of cyst arise; the commonest type can become very large indeed.

SYMPTOMS The symptoms can be very much like an enlarged prostate, with constipation, problems passing urine and blood in the urine being common.

DIAGNOSIS Very large cysts may be felt through the abdominal wall, when they can be confused with the urinary bladder. X-rays and ultrasound help to make the diagnosis.

TREATMENT The most effective treatment is surgery to remove the cyst. Sometimes operations to promote drainage of the cyst may be carried out. Other forms of treatment are usually less effective.

OUTLOOK The outlook is usually good but recurrence is a possibility.

PROSTATIC TUMOURS

CAUSE Tumours can arise spontaneously in the prostate as in other organs and tissues of the body. Unfortunately, most tend to be malignant; however tumours are rarer than other diseases of the prostate.

SYMPTOMS Symptoms can resemble benign prostatic enlargement, with constipation, straining and blood in urine being present. Dogs may have a bloody discharge from the penis which occurs in between urinations. Pain in the hind limbs or back may be seen. Other general signs include weight loss and lack of energy. The tumour frequently spreads to the bones and produces signs of lameness/stiffness later in the disease.

DIAGNOSIS It is not always easy to separate benign enlargement, prostatic infections and prostatic tumours from each other. Usually a combination of diagnostic techniques are used including internal

examination, X-rays, ultrasound and biopsy. In this way, a reasonably secure diagnosis can be made.

TREATMENT Prostatic tumours are not very responsive to treatment, though symptoms may be controlled somewhat by castration or hormone therapy. Radiation therapy may extend the lifespan in dogs, but this technique is not widely available to pet owners. Generally, treatment aims to control the symptoms until quality of life is poor, when euthanasia should be carried out.

Removal of the prostate is rarely attempted in dogs as the operation is fraught with complications, especially incontinence.

OUTLOOK The long term outlook for dogs with prostatic tumours is poor.

Penis and Prepuce

DISCHARGE FROM PENIS/ PREPUCE

CAUSE Various abnormalities can cause discharge from the penis or prepuce including trauma, infection and tumours. Prostate disease (see above) can lead to bleeding from the prepuce.

SYMPTOMS A discharge which is yellowish or blood-stained may be present in addition to symptoms of irritation or excessive licking. An injury to the prepuce may be seen.

 Some preputial discharge is normal in male dogs

Most male dogs have some discharge from the prepuce area. This is quite normal and requires no treatment. The discharge is cloudy to yellow-greenish and usually starts in young male dogs around the time of sexual maturity. No blood is seen and the condition does not cause irritation or pain, nor any other symptoms.

DIAGNOSIS Usually the cause will be found once the lining of the prepuce and the penis is examined. Sometimes, however, the problem lies elsewhere, e.g. the prostate gland.

TREATMENT Any injuries or masses may need surgical treatment. Infections are often treated with mild antiseptic washes.

OUTLOOK The outlook is usually good.

PHIMOSIS

CAUSE In this problem the opening of the prepuce is very small. This may be a congenital problem or arise after trauma or inflammation.

SYMPTOMS Severe cases interfere with normal urination; less severe cases may not be noticed unless the dog is used for breeding, when the erect penis may not be able to be protruded, or else it may be protruded but be unable to be retracted back into the prepuce – see Paraphimosis below.

DIAGNOSIS Diagnosis is usually strightforward upon examining the prepuce.

TREATMENT A small operation is used to enlarge the opening of the prepuce.

OUTLOOK The outlook is good.

PARAPHIMOSIS

CAUSE In this condition, after erection or copulation, the erect penis becomes trapped outwith the prepuce. This can be a consequence of a smaller than normal preputial opening or other abnormalities in the prepuce involving its shape, muscle or nerve supply.

SYMPTOMS The erect penis is present outwith the prepuce. If a sufficiently long time has elapsed the tissue of the penis can become inflamed and damaged and the dog may lick or mutilate the penis.

DIAGNOSIS The problem is easy to diagnose and should be treated promptly.

TREATMENT Cold compresses, ice packs and lubricants may help to replace the penis, otherwise replacement under anaesthesia is required. If the cause is a small preputial opening, this can be enlarged surgically to prevent recurrences.

> **First aid**
>
> If this problem occurs, showering the penis/prepuce area with cold water for 10–15 minutes may allow its replacement. Otherwise, seek help from your veterinary surgeon promptly.

OUTLOOK The outlook is good provided the condition is treated early. If left too long, severe damage can occur to the penis.

TUMOURS OF THE PENIS

CAUSE Tumours of the penis are rare in the dog, but they can arise spontaneously here as elsewhere.

SYMPTOMS Usually bleeding from the prepuce is seen and the dog may lick excessively at the area.

DIAGNOSIS The tumour is usually evident once the prepuce is retracted.

TREATMENT Provided spread has not occurred, surgical removal may be possible. This would be likely to involve amputation of a substantial part of the penis.

OUTLOOK Good, provided spread has not occurred before surgery.

TRANSMISSIBLE VENEREAL TUMOUR

CAUSE This disease is thought to be caused by a virus and can affect either sex of dog. It is transmitted during copulation. It is very rare in the UK.

SYMPTOMS The symptoms in the male are of tumours arising on the penis. These bleed and ulcerate easily, causing a blood-stained discharge.

DIAGNOSIS A biopsy is usually required to diagnose this problem; however the symptoms are often suspicious.

TREATMENT Surgery may be possible. A large portion of the penis can be safely removed. If the tumours are too extensive then chemotherapy may be possible.

OUTLOOK This depends on the severity. The outlook is best for single tumours that are easily removeable.

'DOG POX'

CAUSE This disease, thought to be caused by a virus, can affect either sex of dog.

SYMPTOMS In the male, ulcers are seen on the penis, prepuce and possibly in the anal areas. In severe cases a large red ulcerated plaque may be present. Little pain is caused in most cases: the dog may be unaware of the condition. Some bleeding may however occur during mating.

In the female, ulcerated areas occur within and around the vulva.

DIAGNOSIS The characteristic appearance usually leads to the diagnosis being made.

TREATMENT Treatment is not always required but may involve mild antiseptic washes.

OUTLOOK Good.

PROLAPSE OF THE URETHRA

CAUSE In this problem either continued sexual excitement or else frequent straining to pass urine results in prolapse of the urethra at the tip of the penis.

SYMPTOMS A small area of red tissue is seen at the end of the penis. This tends to become swollen and may bleed.

DIAGNOSIS The veterinary surgeon makes the diagnosis after examining the penis.

TREATMENT The prolapsed portion of the urethra may be able to be replaced by a small operation; if the tissue is very damaged the tip of the penis may need to be amputated. Castration can help reduce recurrences.

OUTLOOK Good, especially if castration is performed.

CHAPTER 12

Female Reproductive System

Common symptoms of female reproductive system disease
• Irregular 'seasons' or oestrus • Vaginal discharge/bleeding
• Growths or thickenings in the mammary (breast) area • General illness
• Altered or unusual behaviour • Abdominal swelling or pain

Structure and Function

The female reproductive system consists of the ovaries, uterus, vagina and mammary glands. Overall, its function is to stimulate mating, conceive foetuses and retain these within the uterus until they are sufficiently developed to be born. After birth, the puppies are fed for a number of weeks on milk produced by the dam from the mammary glands (lactation). Following weaning they can be separated from their mother to live independently. The reproductive cycle is then complete and can be started again at the next oestrus or heat period. Further information on breeding and some associated problems is provided in Chapter 15. Neutering is discussed in Introduction, page 5.

Two ovaries are present in the abdomen, one lying on the right and left sides just behind the kidneys and surrounded by a fat-filled pouch or bursa. At the appropriate time during the reproductive cycle, the female sex cells (eggs) pass through the pouch-like ovarian bursa which surrounds the ovary and then on into the fallopian (uterine) tube. This slender tube connects each ovary to its uterine horn. Once in the uterus, the eggs are available for fertilisation by spermatozoa from the male dog. As well as storing eggs, the ovaries synthesise and release hormones into the bloodstream which influence reproductive cycling and pregnancy.

The uterus in the dog has a relatively short body and two long horns, giving the organ a Y-shape with long arms. The function of the uterus is to protect and nourish the developing puppies. It is capable of remarkable changes in size. During anoestrus, when the reproductive tract is inactive, the uterus is a fairly small organ, but towards the end of pregnancy, or if it becomes badly infected, it can occupy almost the whole of the abdomen.

Between the uterus and vagina is the muscular cervix. This structure acts as a barrier between the uterus and the outside world. It relaxes, however, during oestrus and at the time of whelping to allow spermatozoa to enter or puppies to leave the uterus.

The vagina, where the reproductive and urinary tracts open, leads into the vestibule. The vestibule lies immediately behind the lips of the vulva.

Dogs usually have five pairs of mammary glands running along the chest and abdomen. These glands are normally inconspicuous apart from the nipple areas, but following hormonal stimulation they can enlarge considerably and so provide milk for the offspring. Enlargement of the glands can also occur without pregnancy, in the relatively common condition of false pregnancy in the bitch (see page 207).

The oestrus cycle

Female dogs are generally considered mature at around 5–7 months, although there is considerable breed variation in this, with larger breeds maturing

General anatomy of the female reproductive system

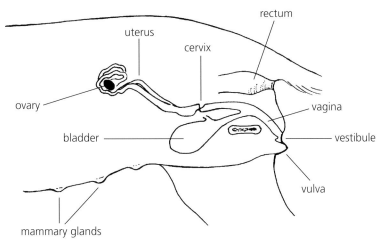

more slowly. The first oestrus or heat period may occur at any point after this time; in large or giant breeds, it may be considerably later than 6 months and can in fact be up to age 2 years. In addition, the first oestrus in many bitches goes unnoticed by the owner as few of the usual external signs may be seen and the overall duration may be shorter than normal.

Thereafter, entire bitches have approximately two oestrus cycles per year. Again, there is some variation. Few dogs have exactly 6 months between oestrus periods: in some it may be every 7–9 months. The oestrus cycle is divided into different phases for convenience and ease of understanding. These divisions are not absolutely clear-cut but they do represent important stages of the normal oestrus cycle.

Anoestrus is the longest phase and it takes up approximately 3–4 months of each 6 month cycle. During this time the reproductive tract is inactive and no indications of oestrus are shown by the bitch. Male dogs are not interested in them sexually.

Pro-oestrus marks the beginning of an oestrus or 'heat' period. It usually lasts around 10 days, but can vary somewhat. Signs of pro-oestrus include swelling of the vulva area with a clear or reddish-tinged discharge. Dogs may be interested in the bitch at this time, but the bitch will not allow mating.

Oestrus is the receptive stage of the cycle for bitches. It also lasts around 10 days. Red discharge continues from the vulva but it appears less watery. The most receptive time for a successful mating is around the time of ovulation, which occurs within the first few days of the oestrus period (this approximates to 12–14 days after the first signs of pro-oestrus were detected in most bitches).

Metoestrus occurs when a mating has not taken place. It lasts approximately 80–90 days and is associated with hormonal fluctuations which can lead to false pregnancy (see page 207) in some bitches.

Anoestrus follows on from metoestrus again.

The cycle operates *approximately* twice per year unless pregnancy has occurred. In dogs, pregnancy lasts approximately 63 days (see Chapter 15).

What can go wrong with the female reproductive system?

Apart from problems with pregnancy or whelping (discussed in Chapter 15) two fairly common but serious problems are infection of the uterus (pyometra) in unspayed bitches, and mammary or breast tumours. Other forms of cancer are infrequently seen in the reproductive system.

A number of problems such as irregular oestrus cycles, false pregnancy and juvenile vaginitis are fairly common but not on the whole serious diseases.

Veterinary Diagnosis and Treatment

Many diseases of the reproductive system are suspected on the basis of the bitch's medical history coupled with routine clinical examination. Further tests used frequently include X-rays, ultrasound examination

Stages of the oestrus cycle in the bitch.

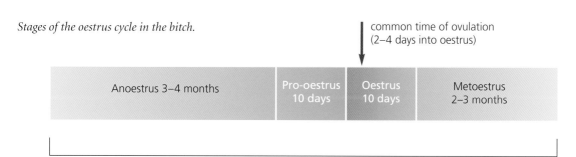

common time of ovulation
(2–4 days into oestrus)

| Anoestrus 3–4 months | Pro-oestrus 10 days | Oestrus 10 days | Metoestrus 2–3 months |

6 months average (but varies between dogs)

and endoscopic examinations (especially of the vagina area). Ultrasound is particularly useful in reproductive diseases.

With middle-aged or older dogs, blood tests may be recommended in order to check out function of important organs such as the liver and kidneys prior to an anaesthetic or lengthy operation. Additionally, in certain of the less common diseases, blood hormone levels may need to be measured to help with diagnosis.

Costs and prognosis in reproductive system disease

Several reproductive disorders require surgery for effective treatment; this, together with the necessary tests beforehand, can make them expensive to treat. However, a complete cure may well be achieved following a successful operation.

A few reproductive disorders require measurement of hormone levels or other blood tests to unravel the condition. Breeding bitches and problems they may encounter are a special case and are dealt with in Chapter 15.

Commonest Reproductive System Diseases in the Bitch

General Problems

IRREGULAR OESTRUS (HEAT PERIODS OR SEASONS)

CAUSE It should always be remembered that there is some variation between dogs in the interval between oestrus periods and in the length of the oestrus cycle itself. Although 'every 6 months' is often quoted, in fact many bitches do not conform so exactly. The length of each oestrus period is also variable, and some dogs show very obvious signs of oestrus whereas in others the external or behavioural signs are unobtrusive.

A number of possibilities exist for deviations from normal. These are outlined in the box.

Abnormalities with the oestrus cycle

• Delayed onset of puberty

This is when a bitch does not have her first oestrus period at the expected time. However the 'expected time' includes a very wide range of ages. First oestrus can occur from 6–22 months of age, with smaller breeds entering oestrus sooner than larger or giant breeds. If no oestrus has been observed by 2 years of age, then this is abnormal. It may be that oestrus is occurring but very 'quietly'. Hormone measurements can help here. Other health problems must be ruled out, such as low thyroid hormones.

• Too long a time between cycles

Again, some bitches show few signs of oestrus and these may be missed by the owner leading to an incorrect impression that too long a time is elapsing. Hormone measurements can reveal this. It is known that some bitches may only enter oestrus once per year (a feature of the Basenji breed). Other factors such as certain drug treatments, ovarian cysts and general illness may need to be considered and investigated as oestrus may be subdued by these things.

• 'Split oestrus'

This condition results in a bitch returning to oestrus several weeks after previously having an incomplete cycle. Mating would only be successful at the second, full, oestrus cycle as the first one did not progress beyond the initial pro-oestrus phase. 'Split oestrus' can occasionally cause confusing signs especially for those intending to breed from their bitch.

• Prolonged or persistent oestrus

Ovarian cysts or tumours may cause this problem, however they are rare. Many dogs in this category simply have longer oestrus cycles than the average. If signs extend beyond 4 weeks, however, veterinary advice should be sought since persistent high levels of oestrogen hormone in the body can cause anaemia.

SYMPTOMS These are as outlined in the box. It is important to separate out 'true' problems from variations, albeit it quite extreme ones, from the average.

Any other symptoms of general ill health should be reported to the veterinary surgeon as these may be relevant to the abnormal oestrus cycles.

DIAGNOSIS In cases where a true abnormality is thought to exist, diagnosis is likely to involve hormone measurements, tests for general health problems and ultrasound scans if applicable.

TREATMENT Treatment, when required, depends on the underlying reason for the problem. Several problems do not require specific treatment.

SIGNS OF OESTRUS IN SPAYED BITCHES

CAUSE The cause is a small fragment or fragments of ovary left behind after the ovariohysterectomy (spay) operation. If this small piece of tissue establishes a blood supply, it can produce and release the hormones which bring about signs of oestrus. This is a fairly uncommon condition.

SYMPTOMS A spayed bitch shows signs of oestrus.

DIAGNOSIS Since other problems can cause vaginal discharge, they may also need to be considered. However the characteristic twice-yearly pattern of oestrus is seen in these dogs and the bleeding stops after several weeks in correspondence with the normal oestrus cycle.

TREATMENT The condition is not life-threatening but may be perceived as a nuisance as the bitch will be attractive to male dogs. Treatment if followed consists of another operation to locate and remove the fragment of ovary. This will normally be carried out when the bitch is showing signs of oestrus as the tissue will be easier to find then.

OUTLOOK The outlook is good. Once the tissue is removed the signs will stop.

FALSE PREGNANCY

CAUSE This condition is a result of the hormonal changes which occur following oestrus in bitches. In many respects, it is considered a normal phenomenon but there is no doubt that some bitches show particularly marked signs, which can cause worry in owners.

SYMPTOMS Symptoms begin several weeks after oestrus and may continue for several months. Basically, symptoms mimick some of the behaviours which a pregnant bitch would be expected to show:

• Nest building

• Possessiveness: often a small furry toy will be 'adopted'

• Development of the mammary glands and lactation (production of milk)

Other symptoms can include:

• Poor appetite

• Restlessness or lethargy

• Uncharacteristic aggressiveness

In a few cases, even symptoms suggestive of whelping may appear, though this is very unusual.

DIAGNOSIS This is usually suggested by the symptoms and the fact that certain bitches seem prone to developing exaggerated signs after each oestrus when pregnancy has not occurred. Note that occasionally it may be possible that pregnancy *has* occurred without the owner having realised the dog was mated!

TREATMENT Mild cases require no special treatment, but more severe false pregnancies may be treated with hormones or other drugs. Ovariohysterectomy (spay) will prevent this condition but it cannot be carried out during a false pregnancy as this can lead to persistence of the signs after the operation.

OUTLOOK The condition is harmless. Dogs especially prone to it can be treated or spayed.

Vaginal Problems

VAGINAL DISCHARGE

CAUSE This is a symptom of reproductive disease rather than a condition in itself. As a symptom, it is fairly common and can be caused by a number of different problems arising throughout the reproductive tract (see box). Most of the conditions mentioned are considered in detail below or in Chapter 15.

Sometimes the cause of vaginal discharge is disease in the urinary system, such as severe cystitis (see page 146).

Some possible causes of vaginal discharge

General

- Normal oestrus cycling in unspayed bitches
- Oestrus cycling in spayed bitches in which a fragment of ovary remains in the abdomen and produces hormones

Vaginal problems

- Juvenile vaginitis in young bitches
- Vaginal tumours or cysts
- Injury from mating
- Vaginal prolapse
- Infantile vulva

Uterine problems

- Endometritis
- Uterine infection (pyometra) in unspayed bitches (usually middle-aged or older)
- 'Stump' pyometra in spayed bitches
- Abortion in pregnant bitches (see Chapter 15)
- Parturition (birth of puppies) in pregnant bitches (see Chapter 15)
- Cancer of uterus (rare)

Ovarian problems

- Ovarian cysts (rare)
- Ovarian cancer (rare)

SYMPTOMS A discharge is present at the vulva. The quantity, colour and type of discharge varies according to the underlying cause and is discussed under each separate condition below.

DIAGNOSIS The veterinary surgeon makes the diagnosis based on questioning the owner, examining the bitch and performing appropriate tests.

TREATMENT Medical or surgical treatment may be neccesary or (in some cases) no treatment is required.

OUTLOOK See individual conditions.

 Help your vet

If you are concerned about a vaginal discharge, let your vet know:

- If and when your dog was spayed (if this was not carried out at your usual practice)
- When your dog was last in season, if applicable
- When she was mated, if applicable
- The duration of the discharge
- The type of discharge: blood, red-tinged, cloudy, clear
- Whether the dog is well in herself, or has other signs of general illness such as increased thirst, vomiting or weight loss

---

JUVENILE VAGINITIS

CAUSE This problem is seen in young sexually immature bitches before their first oestrus. The cause is a usually low-grade inflammation within the vagina.

SYMPTOMS A clear to cloudy discharge is seen to come from the vulva. This, together with the inflammation of the vagina, may cause the dog some irritation and lead to 'scooting' in a similar way to anal gland irritation (see page 95). Otherwise, affected dogs are in good health with normal appetite, water intake and activity levels.

DIAGNOSIS The age, sexual immaturity and characteristic symptoms often lead to the diagnosis without any investigations beyond routine examination.

TREATMENT In many cases treatment is not necessary as the problem vanishes as the bitch matures. In severe cases, antibiotics may be given.

OUTLOOK The outlook is excellent for this condition.

VAGINAL TUMOURS AND CYSTS

CAUSE Tumours can arise spontaneously in the vagina as in any other organ of the body. Vaginal tumours are more common than uterine or ovarian ones. Fortunately, most vaginal tumours are benign growths. Cysts are also occasionally found within the vagina.

SYMPTOMS The vulval or vaginal area may seem enlarged or distorted in shape. Sometimes the first sign of a tumour is when it appears between the vulval lips. A clear to cloudy discharge is often present, sometimes blood-stained. If the growth or cyst is very large, difficulty passing urine may be noticed or else the mass may provoke straining or irritation in the dog.

DIAGNOSIS This is normally by physical examination, aided with the use of a small scope. X-rays using liquid contrast agents may be used. Biopsies can be taken to classify the growth.

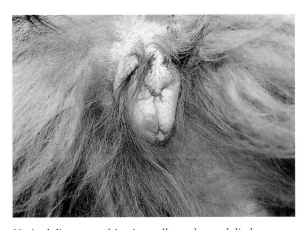

Vaginal disease resulting in swollen vulva and discharge.

TREATMENT Whenever possible the growth or cyst is removed surgically. Growths can be simple polyps or more serious tumours.

OUTLOOK Many vaginal tumours can be dealt with successfully and most tend to be benign. Occasionally, even benign growths may have reached a very large size before surgery, complicating their removal. Cysts can normally be effectively treated by surgery.

VAGINAL INJURY CAUSED BY MATING

CAUSE This problem occasionally occurs when the lining of the vagina is injured during mating with the male dog.

SYMPTOMS Sudden yelping during mating could indicate that the vaginal wall has become damaged. Bleeding in excess of that seen during oestrus may be observed after the injury has occurred.

DIAGNOSIS This requires examination of the vagina with the aid of a scope, and possible X-rays using liquid contrast material.

TREATMENT If severe, surgery is required since a ruptured vaginal wall allows communication with the abdomen, and the possibility of peritonitis.

OUTLOOK Though a fairly rare injury, this should always be checked and treated promptly to avoid possible complications.

VAGINAL PROLAPSE

CAUSE The lining of the vagina may thicken excessively and prolapse (protrude from between the lips of the vulva) during oestrus. This is fairly unusual but is encountered more frequently in Boxers and Bulldogs. The problem does seem to run in certain family lines of these (and other) breeds; it is not advised to breed from affected animals.

SYMPTOMS Pink tissue protrudes from the vulva area and may be accompanied by vaginal discharge caused by infection of the exposed tissue. The prolapsed vaginal mucosa can become traumatised if care is not taken. Excessive licking by the bitch can cause self-inflicted injury.

DIAGNOSIS The condition is evident on examination. Occasionally, a large vaginal tumour or prolapsed polyp can look similar to this.

TREATMENT Minor vaginal prolapses regress after oestrus. The tissue needs to be kept clean and lubricated during this time to prevent excessive damage. More severe prolapses may require surgical removal of the excessive swollen tissue.

 First aid

Fit a 'buster'collar if the dog tends to lick excessively at any prolapsed tissue and seek veterinary advice promptly.

OUTLOOK The condition does tend to recur during future oestrus periods. Ovariohysterectomy (spaying) may be advised.

INFANTILE VULVA

CAUSE The cause of this problem is not fully established. There may be an association with early (pre-puberty) spaying, making this a possible disadvantage of early spaying in contrast to the advantages gained with respect to prevention of mammary tumours (see page 214). However by no means every bitch that is spayed early develops this condition.

SYMPTOMS The vulva appears recessed and in this position the surrounding skin is prone to dermatitis. This is worsened considerably if the bitch is overweight. Frequent licking and pain at the vulva area is the main sign and the surrounding hair may be darkly stained from saliva.

DIAGNOSIS The small recessed vulva and dermatitis are characteristic.

TREATMENT The problem is often helped substantially by surgery to remove any excessive skin folds in the area.

 First aid

Bathing the area with warm saline solution or with antiseptic washes obtained from the veterinary surgeon can help keep the problem under control, though is unlikely to bring about a complete cure. A 'buster' collar can be used to prevent excessive licking.

OUTLOOK Surgery carries the best chance of eliminating problems in cases where there are significant skin folds causing dermatitis. (See Skin fold problems in Chapter 5, page 87). Weight loss in overweight dogs may result in significant improvement also.

Uterine Problems

ENDOMETRITIS (METRITIS)

CAUSE Endometritis means inflammation of the lining of the uterus. This condition normally occurs either after oestrus or whelping, since the cervix relaxes at this time and there is the possibility of bacteria entering the uterus and setting up an infection.

SYMPTOMS A yellowish or red-tinged discharge is noticed several weeks after the end of oestrus or after whelping. Most dogs are slightly off colour.

DIAGNOSIS The symptoms are fairly typical but are also similar to the serious condition of pyometra (see overleaf), which tends to affect older dogs. If symptoms are seen in a younger dog that has recently had puppies, endometritis is more likely. Ultrasound may be used in the diagnosis.

TREATMENT Antibiotics are given and a careful watch is kept on the dog for any deterioration, which might require ovariohysterectomy (spaying) to be carried out.

OUTLOOK The outlook is normally good. If the bitch is not being used for breeding purposes, spaying should be considered.

PYOMETRA

CAUSE This term means 'pus in the uterus'. Pyometra is a common – and serious – disease of unspayed bitches and usually affects older dogs. It occurs shortly (several weeks) after an oestrus cycle, though occasionally this oestrus cycle is not noticed by the owner.

SYMPTOMS Symptoms develop over a few days to a week and consist of lethargy, poor appetite and increased thirst and urination, progressing to vomiting, abdominal swelling and collapse. Some dogs seem unsteady on their hind legs and have pain when touched in the abdomen area. There may be a vaginal discharge, in which case it can be yellowish or red/brown. Some dogs with pyometra have no vaginal discharge. These cases of 'closed pyometra' (the cervix is closed, allowing no drainage of pus to the exterior) are particularly serious as toxins are absorbed into the bloodstream to a greater extent and the uterus is at an increased risk of rupture, causing massive and life-threatening peritonitis.

Warning signs of pyometra

- Older unspayed dog

- Recent oestrus

- 'Off colour' symptoms: poor appetite, lethargic, occasional vomiting

- Drinking and urinating to excess

- Possibly a vaginal discharge

- Abdominal swelling

DIAGNOSIS Typical symptoms often point to this diagnosis but blood tests and X-rays/ultrasound are also usually required. Blood tests are important to assess the functioning of the kidneys and liver, and also to calculate how dehydrated the patient is. Both of these aspects have an important bearing on the necessary anaesthetic risk. As many patients will be older dogs, they may be suffering from undiagnosed kidney and liver disorders as well as pyometra. Knowing this beforehand allows the veterinary surgeon to take action to try to limit such complicating problems.

Several other disorders can produce symptoms quite like those of pyometra, e.g. chronic kidney or liver disease, diabetes.

TREATMENT Most bitches with pyometra require hospitalisation for cage rest and treatment. Initial treatment usually consists of starting on antibiotics by injection. In addition, an intravenous drip will nearly always be given to correct dehydration and the effects of absorbed toxins. Once these treatments have improved the dog's circulation and overall condition, an ovariohysterectomy (spay) operation is performed. Continued drip fluids and antibiotics are normally required, possibly necessitating hospitalisation for 24–48 hours after surgery. Careful recuperation at home follows, provided the dog's appetite has returned and overall symptoms are gradually improving.

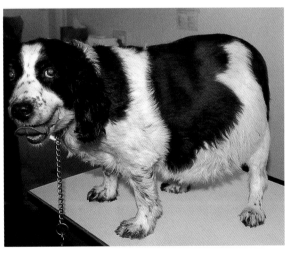

Pyometra is a serious condition of older, unneutered bitches. It nearly always requires surgery.

OUTLOOK Many bitches recover extremely well from this serious disease. There are, however, risks – especially that of toxaemia, kidney and liver complications and peritonitis. Most veterinary surgeons will give a cautious prognosis until the dog has cleared the first 48 hours after surgery. Thereafter most dogs do very well.

'STUMP' PYOMETRA

CAUSE In this condition, a 'mini' pyometra develops in the residues of the uterus of a spayed bitch.

SYMPTOMS Yellowish or yellow-red persistent vaginal discharge is the commonest finding. There may also be symptoms of general illness: increased thirst and urination, poor appetite, lethargy and possibly vomiting.

DIAGNOSIS X-rays and/or ultrasound are used, and blood tests can indicate that there is a source of infection in the body.

TREATMENT The diseased area of uterus (the stump) is removed by surgery; antibiotics are normally prescribed.

OUTLOOK The outlook is good. Symptoms usually disappear quickly.

CANCER OF UTERUS

CAUSE Tumours may arise spontaneously in the uterus, as in all other organs. However this is a rare condition in the dog.

SYMPTOMS Vaginal bleeding may be seen. Sometimes there is an accompanying pyometra.

DIAGNOSIS X-rays and ultrasound can help, but the diagnosis is usually made at surgery.

TREATMENT Ovariohysterectomy would normally be performed as long as there was no sign of spread to other organs within the abdomen or elsewhere.

OUTLOOK The outlook is good for a benign tumour completely removed but poor for malignant ones.

Ovarian Problems

OVARIAN CYSTS

CAUSE A number of cysts of different types can arise on the ovary. Frequently, the ovary of a normal dog undergoing routine overiohysterectomy (spay) is found to contain a cyst or cysts. This is not considered abnormal. Other dogs may have multiple cysts present which may interfere with reproductive cycling.

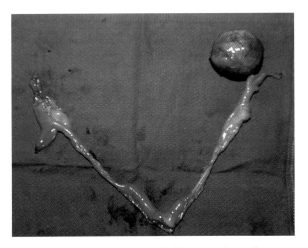

Ovarian cyst treated by removal of both ovaries and uterus in a middle-aged bitch.

SYMPTOMS Persistent signs of oestrus can be a sign of an ovarian cyst. Other possible symptoms include abdominal pain, drinking excessively and vomiting. Persistent oestrus signs can be dangerous if they last for several weeks as prolonged exposure to the hormone oestrogen can result in anaemia.

DIAGNOSIS This is based on examination of the dog, an understanding of its reproductive history and tests such as ultrasound. Exploratory surgery may be advised to rule out other problems such as ovarian cancer.

TREATMENT Hormonal treatment may be suitable. In many cases, ovariohysterectomy is the best treatment for pet dogs.

OUTLOOK The outlook is usually good.

OVARIAN TUMOURS

CAUSE Ovarian tumours arise infrequently in dogs.

SYMPTOMS Some ovarian tumours secrete hormones, resulting in a prolonged or permanent state of oestrus. Alternatively, if other hormones are produced, pyometra can result. General symptoms

include weight loss, increased thirst and urination and poor coat.

Tumours which do not produce hormones may cause symptoms by pressing on other organs in the abdomen or even, if very large, changing the shape of the abdomen.

DIAGNOSIS This usually involves X-rays and ultrasound but often a clear diagnosis depends on exploratory surgery.

TREATMENT Ovariohysterectomy (spay) is the treatment performed.

OUTLOOK As long as spread of the tumour has not occurred the outlook is good.

Mammary Gland (Breast) Problems

MASTITIS

CAUSE Mastitis results when the mammary glands (breasts) develop a bacterial infection or are injured. Infection may enter through the teat (nipple), through small skin wounds or from the blood supply to the glands.

SYMPTOMS One or several glands may be affected. The affected areas are swollen, tender and warm. The bitch's temperature is often raised and, if nursing puppies, she may be reluctant to let them suckle. Her appetite may be reduced. If milk is expressible from the affected gland it may be blood-flecked or a brownish colour.

DIAGNOSIS This is usually straightforward but very occasionally, mammary cancer can be mistaken for severe mastitis and vice versa.

TREATMENT This consists of antibiotics and drugs to bring down the temperature and ease the pain of the condition. Very severe cases may require that the dog is hospitalised for an intravenous drip.

First aid

Warm compresses applied to the mammary area can often help. If possible, hand-feeding or early weaning of puppies should be considered (hand feeding may anyway be necessary if the bitch refuses to let the puppies suckle). Gentle exercise may promote the reduction of the painful swelling.

OUTLOOK The outlook is good in most cases. In very severe cases, where the gland undergoes necrosis (death of tissue), an open wound may occur or else surgical removal of damaged tissue may be required at a later date.

MAMMARY (BREAST) TUMOURS

CAUSE Mammary tumours are common in the bitch. Most of these occur in the middle or caudal (back) glands. Both benign and malignant tumours are encountered with a frequency of about 60:40 for benign versus malignant, i.e. slightly more are benign compared to malignant.

The cause of these tumours is not certain but most of them are dependent on hormonal stimulation. Most tumours occur in middle-aged or older dogs; mammary cancer is rare below the age of 6 years.

SYMPTOMS A growth is felt or seen in the mammary area. The entire mammary area runs from the axilla (inside of the elbow) to the groin on both sides. The growth can range in size from a small pea-shaped mass to a large tumour the size of an orange in chronic cases. Sometimes, discharge from the nipple of the affected gland is seen.Most of the time the mass is fairly mobile under the skin and can be moved around between the skin and the underlying muscle of the body wall.

In severe cases, there is marked ulceration of the skin and it is difficult to detect where the tumour starts or stops. These 'inflammatory' tumours are the most malignant and are well connected to surrounding tissues. They cause considerable pain.

On occasion, other skin tumours may be mistaken for mammary lumps. Skin tumours are discussed in general on pages 88–89.

Spaying at a young age is protective

It is known that bitches spayed when they are very young are less likely to suffer from mammary tumours when they are older. This is related to the fact that mammary tumours are in part responsive to hormone levels. Spayed dogs do not experience the hormonal fluctuations seen in entire bitches, so this could explain why the incidence of this form of cancer is reduced. However the protective effect of spaying only occurs when the bitch is spayed at a young age (before 1 year old).

- If a bitch is spayed before her first oestrus (i.e. at age 4–6 months for most dogs), the likelihood of mammary tumours occurring is negligible.

- A low risk is encountered if the bitch is spayed after the first season and before the second one.

- Beyond this, the protective effect of spaying is less noticeable.

The advantages and disadvantages of spaying bitches are discussed on page 6.

DIAGNOSIS The presence of an unidentified lump is checked out by careful examination for any additional lumps and enlargement of lymph glands, as tumours may spread along lymphatic drainage vessels as well as via the bloodstream. Biopsies may be taken. In most cases, though, any suspicious lump is completely removed surgically and then analysed afterwards. The exception may be in very elderly dogs, or in dogs suffering from another disease which makes anaesthesia less desirable. In these cases, it may be possible to take a small 'fine needle' biopsy without incurring any risk of anaesthesia or even sedation. This can sometimes help with decision-making when various aspects of treatment have to be weighed against each other.

X-rays of the chest are often taken when investigating mammary tumours. This is to check for possible

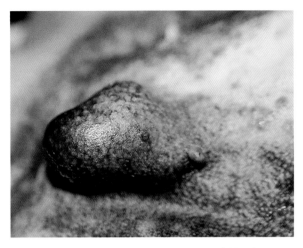

A mammary (breast) tumour in an 8-year-old bitch.

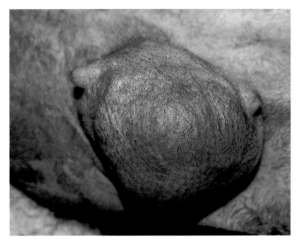

Mammary tumour in a 10-year-old Collie.

spread to the lungs, which can occur with malignant tumours. If signs of such spread were present, surgery would not be performed but palliative treatment (pain control, etc.) could be provided instead.

 The danger of tumour spread

X-rays are often taken to see if malignant tumours (which make up about 40% of the tumours seen) have spread to the lungs. If the lungs look clear, then surgical removal of the tumour is usually carried out. Very occasionally, lung X-rays *look* normal but tumour seeds are in fact present. They are simply too small to see on the original X-ray. In most cases, though, normal-looking X-rays are a good sign that the condition is indeed potentially curable.

Signs of a malignant tumour

- Does not have distinct edges

- Is fixed to underlying tissues

- Grows rapidly

- Ulcerates and reddens the skin

- Causes severe pain

- The dog has a cough, lameness or other symptoms (spread to lungs or elsewhere may have occurred)

TREATMENT Complete excision of the lump or lumps is the usual treatment, except in cases of malignant inflammatory tumours or other tumours that have shown signs of spread within the body. In these situations, surgery would be pointless and would be unlikely to extend the life of the dog.

In very old dogs, or dogs ill with another condition, careful monitoring of the lump may be carried out and if it seems slow growing or harmless, no action may be taken. In other words, a balanced judgement as to the risks of removal versus non-removal will be taken.

When surgery is decided on, it is normal to remove a large area surrounding a mammary tumour in order to try to ensure that all the abnormal cells have been taken away. Thus surgical wounds after this operation can be large – in some cases extending from the elbow area to the groin. Although such a large wound can look alarming, it often heals uneventfully. If complications occur they are usually caused by wound tension or perhaps fluid accumulation beneath the stitches. Such problems do resolve given time although if large areas of wound breakdown occur some resuturing may be required. Small areas of breakdown are often left to heal as open wounds and medication to encourage rapid healing may be prescribed to put on the surface of these wounds.

First aid

If wound seepage occurs after a mastectomy operation, a 'buster' collar may need to be used to prevent excessive licking at the stitches by the dog. Fitting an old tee-shirt over the dog's chest and abdomen can help prevent mess from fluid dripping onto carpets, chairs, etc. Exercise should be restricted to prevent tension on the stitches and veterinary advice should always be obtained if the wound looks reddened, angry or moist. A small degree of wound leakage is often seen after these operations and usually settles within a day or two.

OUTLOOK The outlook is good for benign tumours and for malignant tumours which have not spread from the mammary gland by the time of treatment. Sometimes dogs develop tumours in other glands after treatment. This may be related to the original tumour, or can sometimes be a new tumour arising at a different site. It is investigated and treated in the same way as already discussed.

If the tumour is sent off for analysis, detailed information on its malignancy and future prognosis will usually be available.

CHAPTER 13

Hormonal Diseases

Common symptoms of hormonal diseases
• Increased thirst and increased urination
• Changes in coat quality
• Lower energy levels • Changes in weight
• Vague or unusual symptoms
not responsive to other treatments

Introduction

A variety of hormonal (or endocrine) diseases occur in dogs and can cause a wide range of symptoms, affecting many of the body's organs and tissues. Hormones are chemical compounds produced by glands in the body. They can be thought of as 'messenger' compounds which control other organs and tissues and maintain normal health and body function. Disease can be caused when either too much or too little of a hormone is produced, so that many of these diseases are caused by either underactive or overactive glands. Many people are familiar with the term 'underactive thyroid gland', which is used to describe the disease of hypothyroidism which affects people. As can be seen from the table below, dogs also suffer from this condition.

The commonest glands affected by disease in the dog are shown in the table. These diseases are then considered separately. Diagnosis usually involves specialised blood tests. In most cases, the underlying disease cannot be cured but treatment to control the symptoms may be very successful.

Several of these diseases can produce a baffling array of symptoms. Addison's disease is often called 'the great mimicker' because of the varied nature of the symptoms produced. Quite often, dogs with confusing symptoms that seem unresponsive to routine treatments turn out to have one of these diseases.

Thirst and urination in hormonal diseases

Many hormonal diseases cause disturbances in thirst and urination. Usually, both of these are increased, often to a very marked extent. Normally well house-trained dogs may be unable to retain urine overnight and will pass urine in the house. These dogs should never have their water intake restricted until a diagnosis is made because, in most instances, they are unable to regulate their body water properly and restriction of intake could lead to dehydration and even kidney failure.

An assessment of daily water intake can help in diagnosis. Guidelines on how to measure the water intake accurately are given on page 142.

Hormonal diseases in the dog

Gland affected	Name of disease	Reason for disease	Frequency
Pancreas	Diabetes mellitus ('sugar diabetes')	Insulin deficiency	Commoner
Pancreas	Insulinoma	Tumour in pancreas	Rarer
Adrenal gland	Cushing's disease	Benign brain tumour	Commoner
Adrenal gland	Addison's disease	Gland destroyed	Rarer
Thyroid gland	Hypothyroidism	Underactive gland	Commoner
Pituitary gland (in brain)	Diabetes insipidus	Underactive gland or failure to respond to hormone	Rarer

Commonest Hormonal Diseases in Dogs

DIABETES MELLITUS

CAUSE Diabetes mellitus (or 'sugar diabetes') is usually seen in middle-aged dogs, and more often in females than males. The cause is a deficiency of insulin, which is normally produced by specialised cells in the pancreas. Why this should happen is not entirely clear in most cases. Some forms of diabetes ('secondary diabetes') are caused by factors such as obesity, drug therapy and other hormone imbalances, but 'primary diabetes', caused by a real deficiency of insulin, is commoner.

Another type of diabetes, diabetes insipidus, is also found in dogs and is discussed on page 225. It is much less common.

SYMPTOMS Diabetes has a number of common symptoms, but these are not very specific and various other diseases can appear in a similar way. Most dogs show excess thirst, increased urination, increased appetite and weight loss. Other symptoms associated with diabetes include urinary infections, cataract, and muscle wastage.

Diabetes symptoms usually develop over a number of weeks but, if left untreated, severe cases can show vomiting, poor appetite, depression, coma and death from dehydration and kidney failure.

DIAGNOSIS Routine urine tests may give the first indication that diabetes is present since glucose (sugar) will be found in the urine sample; it is usually absent. Blood tests are then performed and these reveal high levels of glucose and also fats in the blood. Conditions which can occur at the same time as diabetes are liver and pancreatic disease (see Chapter 6), and also disease of the adrenal glands (Cushing's disease, discussed on page 223).

TREATMENT Human beings suffer from different types of diabetes and some patients can be treated using tablets. The form of diabetes which affects dogs, however, requires insulin to be given since diabetic dogs do not make enough of their own.

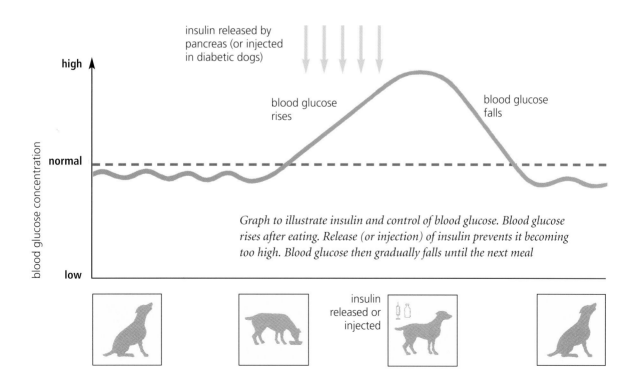

Graph to illustrate insulin and control of blood glucose. Blood glucose rises after eating. Release (or injection) of insulin prevents it becoming too high. Blood glucose then gradually falls until the next meal

Diabetes: some extra facts

- Diabetes often occurs in female dogs. If they have not already been spayed (neutered) then this operation should be carried out as soon as possible since it greatly helps in keeping the dog on a level plane. The hormone changes associated with the dog's oestrus cycle can otherwise make diabetes very difficult to control at these times. In a few cases, the diabetes does not require further treatment after the dog has been spayed.

- Various different types of insulin are available. Most dogs receive one daily injection but some require two. As each patient varies slightly, the dosage and treatment pattern will be tailored to whatever works best at controlling glucose levels in an individual dog. There is no standard dose of insulin.

- Accurate records of the daily amount of insulin given, the amount of water drunk, food eaten and dog's weight should be kept. Additional information such as blood and urine test results can also be noted here. These details, kept by the owner, are invaluable in assessing the day-to-day and week-to-week progress of the diabetic dog. They also help greatly in unravel-

ling any problems that may occur. Most insulin manufacturers produce charts which contain boxes for all the relevant details to be added to, but many owners make out their own notebooks for this purpose and adapt the charts accordingly.

- Insulin should be kept in the fridge and inverted (but not shaken) before administration. Shaking the bottle can destroy the insulin molecules.

- Children should never be allowed near insulin or needles/syringes as if accidentally injected it could be extremely dangerous.

- Veterinary practices often supply literature on diabetes and videos explaining about the disease and how it is treated are also available. These demonstrate the techniques involved in caring for the diabetic dog.

- Although it can seem daunting at first, once a daily routine is established the tasks can usually be timed to fit in with most people's lives. Many veterinary practices may agree to board their diabetic patients while owners are on holiday, since boarding kennels may not have the facilities or expertise to cope with the demands of diabetic residents.

Unfortunately, insulin cannot be given as tablets because it is digested in the stomach and small intestine and therefore cannot do its job of lowering blood glucose by encouraging the transfer of glucose into the body's cells. Insulin therefore has to be administered by injection each day.

Dogs which are very ill with diabetes require hospitalisation and stabilisation using intravenous drips, and also treatment of any complicating disorders.

More routine cases can usually be started on treatment as out-patients, but may have to attend the clinic daily for the first few weeks until the diabetes is gradually brought under control. This also gives owners the chance to learn the techniques of how to look after their dog under expert supervision.

OUTLOOK The outlook depends on how successfully the dog can be stabilised. Diabetes does shorten dogs' lives and makes high demands on owners. A very careful management routine has to be followed every day,

with attention to diet, water intake, and administration of injections. Exercise should also be regulated. The dogs that do best are those that receive a regular schedule and similar amounts of exercise every day – the less the daily routine is changed, the better. It is better, too, if one person looks after the dog and performs the necessary tests and treatments.

While there is no doubt that a diagnosis of diabetes is a daunting prospect for any dog owner, most people cope very well. There is an initial learning curve and owners should receive lots of support and encouragement from the veterinary practice regarding necessary techniques to be learned. Many owners are wary of giving injections, and are then pleasantly suprised at how easy this is using the very fine needles that are on insulin syringes. They soon become confident and there is no doubt that it is a rewarding experience to see a diabetic dog return to better health and to play an active part in that process.

Most dogs have periods of instability, which may

need to be investigated by blood tests, etc, and of course syringes, insulin, urine testing materials (if used) and special diets all constitute additional expense. Regular general health checks are also impor-tant. Despite these considerations, most dog owners would say that treatment of their pet (rather than euthanasia) was worthwhile and rewarding and good quality of life can result.

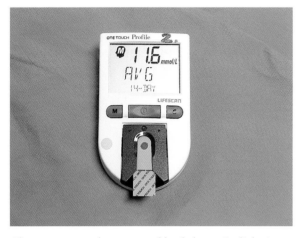

Glucose meter used to measure blood glucose in diabetic dogs.

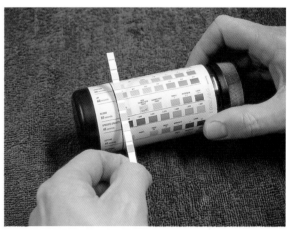

Testing a urine sample for glucose and other substances using a diagnostic strip test.

Date	Breakfast @ 8.30 am	Insulin @ 9 am	Tea @ 5.30 pm	Water drunk	Notes
1st Oct	3/4 tin	10 units	1 1/4 tin	820ml	Urine 2%
2nd Oct	3/4 tin	10 units	1 1/4 tin	900ml	Could not get a urine sample!
3rd Oct *Vet. Appoint. 3pm	3/4 tin	10 units	1 1/4 tin	790ml	Weighed at vets– 13.4 kg. Blood test taken. Insulin to be 11 units from tom.
4th Oct	3/4 tin	11 units	1 1/4 tin	Spilt all water	Urine 1%

Typical record chart kept by owner of a diabetic dog.

Diabetes problems and first aid: action to take

Always contact the veterinary practice if you suspect a problem is ocurring in caring for your diabetic dog. Several commoner problems can occur in the diabetic dog on treatment, as discussed below.

Problem 1: Too much insulin is accidentally given

Result: Blood glucose will become lower than normal.

This can happen quite easily if more than one person is involved in the care of the dog. The dose could be accidentally repeated, or perhaps the wrong dose was drawn up in the first place. A form of overdosage can also occur when the usual dose has been given but the dog, for some reason, does not eat its meal (this is why the insulin injection is normally given *after* the dog has eaten in the morning).

A serious insulin overdose means that blood sugar will be reduced to dangerously low levels, a condition called hypoglycaemia. Symptoms include disorientation/incoordination, apparent blindness, muscle tremors leading on to fits, depression, stupor and coma. Eventually death occurs.

Action: These dangerous symptoms are easily reversed by supplying glucose. A concentrated solution can be made up and smeared around the gums and tongue. If no powdered glucose is to hand, any sugar-containing product can be used, e.g. orange juice, confectionery, etc. The symptoms normally resolve quickly, but the veterinary practice in charge of the dog should be called for further advice.

Note: It is a good idea to keep powdered glucose (available from chemists) to hand in case of an emergency of this type.

Problem 2: Too little insulin is given

Result: Blood glucose will become higher than normal.

This is less serious than insulin overdosage in most patients, who have often lived with the disease for some time before diagnosis.

A common cause of this problem is in the early stages of treatment, before owners have become proficient at giving injections: the owner may miss and end up losing some of the injection onto the dog's coat.

Action: If the dog received no insulin, it is safe to draw up another dose and give this. If you are unsure how much, if any, the dog received, it is best not to give any more until the next injection is due. Missing one injection will slightly destabilise the dog but should not cause any lasting harm since it takes some time for serious consequences of high blood sugar to develop. Simply observe your dog carefully until the next injection is due.

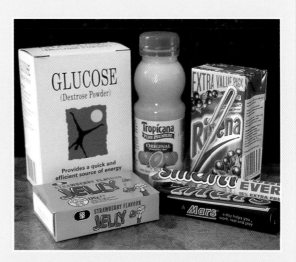

Common everyday sources of glucose which can be used in emergency situations to treat insulin overdose or hypoglycaemia.

Problem 3: Dog is found disorientated or having seizures

Result: It is unknown whether under or overdosage may be the problem.

The safest course of action here is to quickly supply glucose as described under Problem 1 above. If this has no effect, then the veterinary practice should be called and the dog transported to the clinic immediately as an emergency case.

INSULINOMA

CAUSE Tumours of the pancreas are fairly uncommon in dogs but of those that occur, this one is the commonest. It is known as a 'functional' tumour because the tumour growth produces the hormone insulin, which is secreted by the normal pancreas. In insulinoma, however, far too much insulin is produced. Insulinoma is therefore the 'opposite' of natural diabetes. The symptoms are similar to the effect of giving too much insulin to a diabetic dog. Symptoms are usually seen in middle to old aged dogs.

SYMPTOMS Affected dogs tire easily and may even collapse after moderate exercise. Incoordination with altered behaviour may be seen and apparent blindness can occur. Many dogs show fits or seizures, similar to epilepsy. Symptoms are improved after feeding.

DIAGNOSIS Blood tests to measure glucose concentrations (which are low) are used and insulin levels are also assessed. As a number of other diseases can produce rather similar signs, additional testing may be required to rule these out.

TREATMENT Surgical removal of the tumour is normally carried out. Unfortunately, in most cases, spread of the tumour has already occurred, however surgery does alleviate the symptoms for many months and a good quality of life can be obtained.

Drug treatments can also be used to control the symptoms and attention to the diet will also offset some of the signs of this disease.

 First aid

An incoordinated or collapsed dog which is already known to have an insulinoma should receive glucose/sugar by mouth, as in the case of insulin overdosage mentioned on page 222.

OUTLOOK Long term, the outlook is not good due to progression and spread of the tumour but most dogs gain a year of good quality life after successful treatment and some live longer than this.

CUSHING'S DISEASE

CAUSE This is quite a common hormonal disease of middle and old aged dogs. Most dogs with this disorder have benign hormone-secreting tumours in the pituitary region of the brain. An excess of hormone is produced. These brain tumours do not usually cause other symptoms apart from the over-supply of hormone. Smaller breeds, especially terriers, seem prone to this type of Cushing's disease.

A less common cause of Cushing's disease is adrenal gland tumours, and these can be either benign or malignant. The benign tumours do not spread but the malignant ones usually do. About 15–20% of naturally occurring Cushing's disease is caused by adrenal tumours and these seem commoner in larger breeds of dog and in females.

Finally, Cushing's disease can be caused by drug treatment with steroid drugs used for other diseases. When steroids need to be used long term, a dosing schedule is usually chosen which aims to limit the possibility of Cushing's disease. If Cushing's disease-type symptoms occur, they can usually be removed by gradually reducing the dose of the steroids, but this can mean that the problem for which the steroids were originally prescribed returns.

SYMPTOMS A wide variety of symptoms is possible. The commonest ones include drinking to excess and passing increased volumes of urine, increased appetite, abdominal distension giving a 'pot-bellied' appearance and skin disease with hair loss. Many animals show loss of muscle mass, overall thinning of the skin and general weakness. Infertility is possible in breeding dogs. There is no single symptom that is diagnostic of Cushing's disease, and this can mean that diagnosis is occasionally delayed, but a general matching of several different symptoms usually leads to suspicion of the condition. The disease often starts fairly slowly and many owners may put down some of the symptoms to 'age' at first.

DIAGNOSIS This requires general blood profiles and specialised blood tests. A number of abnormalities are usually found. If the dog is currently receiving treatment with steroid drugs, this may need to be reviewed as it could be causing the symptoms. Otherwise, the aim is to find out which type of Cushing's disease is present. Most dogs will have the pituitary (brain) type. X-rays can also be useful in diagnosing Cushing's disease as the liver is often enlarged.

TREATMENT Most patients require drug treatment using powerful drugs and this is often started off in a hospital environment to assess response. Once stabilised they are sent home on an appropriate dosage.

Surgery may be performed for Cushing's disease. Although it is theoretically possible to remove the tumour from the pituitary gland in the brain, in practice surgery is only used for the adrenal gland form of the disease, when an abdominal operation is required. Even so, this is a specialised procedure.

OUTLOOK Most dogs respond well to treatment but do require drugs for life and careful monitoring of their condition. In those minority of cases where a malignant adrenal tumour is the cause, the outlook is poor as tumour spread occurs frequently. Benign adrenal tumours removed by surgery have a favourable outlook once the immediate operation and recovery phase is over.

ADDISON'S DISEASE

CAUSE This disease is the 'opposite' of Cushing's disease, discussed above, and is much less common. It results in a deficiency of hormones normally produced by the adrenal gland, whereas Cushing's disease results in an excess.

The cause of Addison's disease is often a faulty immune system response which leads to the gland being destroyed by antibodies directed against it, i.e. the dog's own immune system destroys the gland. As a result, hormone production is reduced. Addison's disease is commoner in young to middle aged female dogs.

SYMPTOMS As with Cushing's disease, a large variety of symptoms can be found. Addison's disease is a characteristically vague illness but most dogs show lack of energy, occasional vomiting and poor appetite, occasional diarrhoea and, possibly, drinking and urinating to excess. Sometimes, a 'crisis' in the disease develops and affected animals collapse when stressed. Most often, typically vague symptoms have been present for some time prior to the diagnosis being made. It is a 'waxing and waning' illness, i.e. symptoms often seem to improve, possibly after some sort of treatment, only to come back again later. This will continue until a definite diagnosis is made.

DIAGNOSIS Because of the vagueness of the symptoms, a number of diagnostic tests are usually required. Blood tests are certainly necessary and are usually combined with X-rays and an ECG. Specialised blood tests are needed to confirm the diagnosis.

TREATMENT Collapsed animals require emergency resuscitation and treatment with intravenous drips. Hormone replacement treatment is then started which must be kept up for the rest of the dog's life.

 First aid

Dogs suffering from Addison's disease may not cope well with stress. Often, additional medication may be supplied for use during potentially stressful situations to compensate for the dog's deficiencies of steroid hormones. Advice and recommendations from the veterinary surgeon as to when and how to use this medication need to be followed.

OUTLOOK Provided treatment is kept up, the outlook is good.

HYPOTHYROIDISM

CAUSE This is a common hormonal disease of dogs and affects middle aged dogs. Dobermans are among several breeds that seem prone to this disease. Also, dogs which have been neutered (spayed or castrated)

Breeds with a higher incidence of hypothyroidism

Doberman	Dachshund
Golden Retriever	Poodle
Airedale	Boxer
Irish Setter	Miniature Schnauzer

are slightly more likely to suffer from hypothyroidism. In most cases, the dog's immune system attacks the thyroid gland, destroying the tissue and resulting in a deficiency of thyroid hormone.

SYMPTOMS Like other hormonal diseases, this can be a vague and confusing illness with a variety of symptoms involving many different organs. Many dogs become lethargic and dull and seek to lie in warm places. Weight gain may be noticed and coat quality deteriorates with poor hair growth. If hair is clipped off for any reason, it may take many months to re-grow.

Often dogs have symmetrical patches of hair loss on their flanks and a denuded tail. The skin often thickens and becomes darkly pigmented. Around the face, this may result in an increase in skin folds giving the so-called 'tragic expression of hypothyroidism'. Infertility is a common finding in entire dogs. Heart

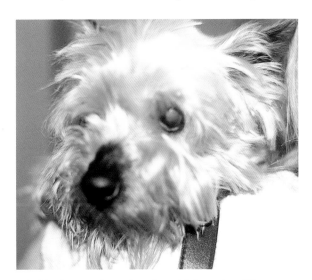

A bald, pigmented nose in a dog with hypothyroidism.

rates are often slower than normal and the periphery of the dog (ears, paws, etc.) seem cool. The skin of the underside of the abdomen may feel cool and clammy. Weakness and partial paralysis may be seen.

DIAGNOSIS With such a large variety of possible symptoms, diagnosis may not be straightforward. Some dogs show many symptoms; others may only display one or two. Blood tests can provide vital clues to the disease and specialised tests to assess thyroid function can then be performed. A confusing factor is that dogs which are ill for other reasons often commonly show depressed levels of thyroid hormone, leading to a possible mistaken diagnosis of hypothyroidism. However further tests can be used to distinguish between 'true' and 'false' hypothyroidism.

TREATMENT Thyroid replacement hormones are given in tablet form and this is required for the rest of the dog's life. Response to treatment is quite slow and improvement in the condition of the skin can take several months.

OUTLOOK The outlook is good but permanent treatment is required.

DIABETES INSIPIDUS

CAUSE This disease should not be confused with the much commoner diabetes mellitus (sugar diabetes) described earlier. The cause of most cases of diabetes insipidus is unknown, but for some reason the pituitary gland in the brain fails to release an important hormone which controls the concentration of urine. The result is that large quantities of very dilute urine are passed, and thus the dog requires to drink much more to replace the lost fluids.

Occasionally, the disease results from a problem in the kidney. In these cases normal amounts of hormone are produced by the pituitary gland in the brain but the kidney does not react to them (by concentrating the urine) as it should.

SYMPTOMS Dogs with diabetes insipidus pass copious amounts of urine, often in the house. To compensate for the fluid loss, excess thirst is present; the thirst can seem unquenchable.

DIAGNOSIS Urine tests reveal very dilute urine. The disease is confirmed by a carefully conducted test in which water is withheld and urine concentration measured. Many other diseases can cause disturbances in water intake and urine output. These will normally need to be ruled out by other tests.

> **Caution**
>
> Water should never be witheld at home in an attempt to control excess urination as serious illness could result.

TREATMENT Hormone replacement, required for life, is used to control the symptoms. Usually, the hormone is given via drops placed in the eye which are then absorbed into the body.

OUTLOOK Most occurrences of diabetes insipidus have a good outlook with appropriate treatment.

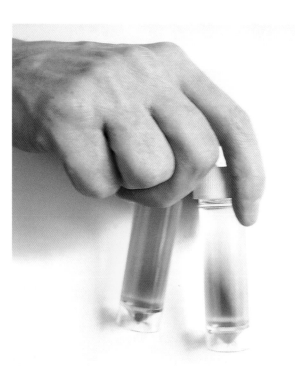

Normal and very dilute urine samples. The dilute sample is pale and watery and came from a dog that had diabetes insipidus.

Diseases of the Blood System

Common symptoms of blood system diseases
• Poor energy levels • Pale gums • Easy bleeding
• Irregular breathing • Collapse
• Enlarged lymph glands • Vague symptoms of illness

Structure and Function

Blood is the vital fluid of life and is made up of a collection of different cells suspended in liquid (plasma). Every part of the body requires an adequate supply of blood in order to stay alive and to function normally. It is the job of the heart and circulatory system to ensure that enough blood reaches each organ to provide oxygen and nutrients and to remove carbon dioxide and waste products. Failure of the circulation soon produces death of individual cells due to oxygen deprivation and accumulation of poisonous waste products. If this situation persists, more and more cells and eventually whole organs and even the animal itself may die.

Red blood cells give blood its colour. The redness comes from a substance called haemoglobin, a chemical present within the cells which has the unique ability to trap and transport oxygen. Oxygen is picked up in the lungs from the air that is inhaled by the animal. It binds to the haemoglobin and is then transported in blood and distributed to all the tissues of the body. In the tissues, the haemoglobin releases its oxygen and picks up the waste gas carbon dioxide, which is taken back to the lungs where it is removed from the body in exhaled breath. This constant system of transport and exchange of gases is a fundamental part of life; without it, no cell could exist.

Blood also contains white blood cells which are important in fighting infection and in protecting the body from the host of potentially harmful organisms it constantly encounters. Finally, very small cells called platelets have a vital role in producing blood clots after injury. If blood did not clot, constant bleeding would soon lower the blood pressure and lead to oxygen deprivation and death.

As well as these vital functions, blood also acts as a transport system for all other substances used by the body. Hormones travel in blood to their target organs; the products of digestion are moved around the body in blood, and so on. Blood itself is filtered and maintained by the liver, kidneys and spleen – dangerous toxic substances, bacteria or waste products are removed and the immune system monitors the blood for any signs of infection.

Production of blood

In young dogs blood is produced in the bone marrow of all bones but in older animals it is mainly flat bones such as the ribs, pelvis and vertebrae which produce blood cells. If there is a severe shortage of blood, the liver and spleen can also produce blood cells.

Commonest Blood Diseases of Dogs

ANAEMIA

Cause Anaemia occurs when there are fewer red blood cells than normal. This can occur because of external or internal bleeding. For example, a major wound may damage a large artery or vein leading to severe blood loss. Internal bleeding can also occur after injury, and certain tumours can bleed internally, leading to chronic blood loss over a long period

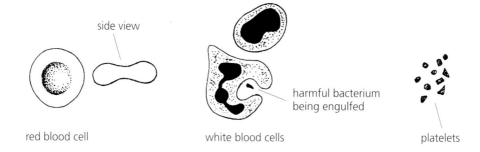

side view

red blood cell

white blood cells

harmful bacterium being engulfed

platelets

Red blood cells, white blood cells and platelets.

of time or sudden severe blood loss if the tumour ruptures.

Anaemia can also occur when red blood cells are destroyed within the body. Some immune system diseases produce this problem; also, poisonings and toxicities can lead to anaemia through destruction of red blood cells or interference with normal blood clotting.

Certain infections can also damage blood cells and in diseases such as kidney failure (see page 145) anaemia can be a complicating feature. An unusual cause of anaemia in dogs is onion toxicity – chemicals present within onions may damage and destroy red blood cells.

SYMPTOMS Anaemia has to be quite severe before symptoms are seen. It can be detected by examining the dog's mucous membranes, e.g. the gums or the lining of the eye. These membranes are normally a salmon pink colour but in anaemia they become pale, even white – a condition known as pallor.

Other symptoms can include increased breathing rate, as the dog works harder to deliver oxygen to its tissues, poor ability to take exercise and even complete collapse.

DIAGNOSIS Anaemia itself is quite easily diagnosed. It is usually suspected from examining the animal and then confirmed by taking a blood sample and counting the number of red blood cells present. Diagnosis of anaemia has to take account of the large range of possible causes. Tests on blood samples, X-rays, ultrasound and other techniques are all used to try to find out the reason.

TREATMENT Emergency treatment may consist of a blood transfusion or intravenous drip fluids. The animal may be placed in an oxygen tent or cage and be kept quiet and rested. This is used to save the animal's life and buy time while the underlying cause is identified. Once this has been discovered, appropriate treatment can be given.

OUTLOOK This does depend on the cause and can only be predicted once a diagnosis has been made. Certain problems, such as tumours bleeding inter-

 First aid

Any anaemic animal must be kept quiet, warm and stress-free. The appetite should be tempted and exercise strictly limited to short lead walks for toilet purposes only.

nally, may carry a poor outlook, but others can be completely cured or, at least, controlled to prevent future attacks of anaemia.

BLEEDING

CAUSE Bleeding is a natural reaction to injury. Blood flowing from a wound helps to flush contamination away from the wound and so protect against infection. Bleeding is only a problem when the injury is so severe that a major blood vessel has been damaged, resulting in loss of large volumes of blood and a fall in blood pressure, or when the blood flow does not stop as expected, i.e. there are problems with blood clotting.

Blood clotting is a very complex series of reactions which, in normal animals, take place in a coordinated way so that a few minutes after injury, blood flow slows and then eventually stops. If this does not occur, blood loss from even minor wounds can be severe and the animal's life may be threatened.

SYMPTOMS Bleeding from an injury can take two forms:

Arterial bleeding: This form of bleeding comes in strong jet-like bursts in time with the heart beat. The blood is bright red.

Venous bleeding: Here, the blood flow is more constant and the blood is dark red in colour. This is the usual type of bleeding after injury.

Both arterial and venous bleeding can threaten life if a large enough vessel is damaged. Bleeding can also occur internally, in which case there may be no outward symptoms at all apart from anaemia if the bleeding is severe. Bleeding under the skin may show as a large swelling or bruise (a haematoma). Haematomas can also occur in the ear flap (see page 66) – in this case the volume of blood is low and there is no risk of severe loss; the condition is however uncomfortable.

Bleeding into the chest or abdomen is a serious concern after any traumatic injury such as a road accident, and treatment for this must be carried out before other injuries such a broken bones are dealt with. Another quite common cause of bleeding into the abdomen is a splenic tumour (see below).

DIAGNOSIS The diagnosis of a bleeding wound is usually obvious. Internal bleeding can be harder to pick up. It may be suspected after trauma or surgery if certain subtle signs are shown by the animal (including pale gums, increased breathing rate or abdominal swelling), in which case tests such as X-rays may be used for confirmation.

Blood clotting problems require specialised diagnosis in order to find out what aspect of the clotting process is defective. Certain poisons (e.g. warfarin) interfere with normal blood clotting so any possible exposure to these substances is important to know about. Some forms of defective blood clotting show up as small red dots on the gums or inside the lips. These may be single or grouped together. They occur when blood leaks from minute blood vessels.

TREATMENT Minor injuries are treated by bandaging or possibly sutures. More severe bleeding may require emergency surgery and resuscitation techniques such as intravenous drips or even blood transfusions. Blood clotting problems may be treated initially by transfusion and then by medication designed to improve the blood clotting ability.

 First aid

First aid for bleeding wounds is described in Chapter 18.

OUTLOOK Severe bleeding is a major threat to life and must be stopped promptly. This is an area where intelligent basic first aid can make the difference between life and death. Chronic lower-grade bleeding usually reflects the presence of an underlying disease which must be diagnosed and, if possible, treated to ensure the blood loss stops.

SPLEEN DISEASES

CAUSE The spleen is positioned near the stomach. It is an elongated organ which stores blood and filters it for signs of infection. Although these are important functions, the spleen is not necessary for life – other organs can take over its job should removal of the spleen be necessary.

The main problems with the spleen are injury caused from trauma (such as a road accident) and tumours. Occasionally the spleen may undergo torsion (this can be associated with gastric dilation, see page 109). Splenic tumours are commoner in medium to large dogs, and German Shepherds seem prone to them.

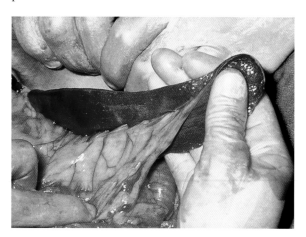

The normal spleen as visualised during abdominal surgery.

SYMPTOMS With tumours, symptoms may be vague including weakness and lethargy, poorish appetite and, possibly, swelling of the abdomen. Many dogs with splenic tumours have paler than normal mucous membranes (gums, lining of the eye) and altered breathing patterns. If the tumour starts to bleed, extreme weakness and collapse may occur, even leading to sudden death.

Traumatic injury to the spleen, causing bleeding, produces similar signs when the bleeding is severe; minor injuries probably cause no signs and bleeding stops quite quickly. Torsion of the spleen can produce severe symptoms such as pain, dehydration, fever and jaundice. Breathing and heart rate are likely to be irregular with weak pulses and collapse.

DIAGNOSIS Diagnosis usually relies on X-rays or ultrasound. Often, a sample of fluid from within the abdomen may be withdrawn to check for any bleeding as there should be no blood in normal abdominal fluid. Blood tests can be used to see whether anaemia is occurring, and to check the function of other organs such as the liver and kidneys.

TREATMENT Initial treatment may involve correction of dehydration using intravenous drips and treatment of anaemia by a blood transfusion. Once the animal is stabilised, surgery is often needed to treat the spleen.

OUTLOOK Tumours which have not spread within the abdomen can be treated by removal of the spleen. Sometimes, spread has occurred but is not obvious at the time of surgery, in which case surgery will prolong the dog's life but the underlying cancer is likely to return in the future and affect organs such as the liver.

Badly damaged spleens are usually removed (partially or completely) and, provided the circulation has not failed, such dogs usually make a good recovery.

LYMPHOMA (LYMPHOSARCOMA)

CAUSE Lymphoma is a form of cancer which affects the lymphatic tissue. The lymphatic tissue (or system) comprises a network of vessels and nodes spread throughout the body. 'Lymph', a milky fluid, flows through these vessels and is filtered in the nodes, where any signs of infection are detected by the immune system. Lymphoctyes, a type of white blood cell that is important in fighting infection, are contained within the lymph.

Most affected dogs are middle aged, although this disease can affect younger animals too. Some breeds, such as Boxers and Scottish Terriers, are thought to be at increased risk from lymphatic cancers.

SYMPTOMS Several different types of lymphoma exist and symptoms can vary somewhat. Enlargement of the lymph glands (e.g. in the throat, shoulder and hind limb areas) can be a frequent finding. These glands are usually non-painful even though they may be enormously swollen and firm. The dog may show no other symptoms apart from enlarged glands.

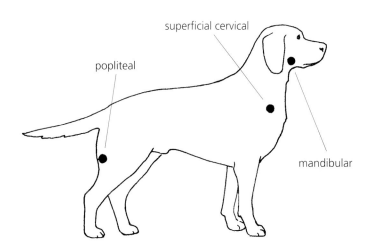

Location of the major lymph glands that can be felt easily in the dog.

superficial cervical

popliteal

mandibular

A 'non-specific' illness

Signs of lymphoma are often non-specific. In other words, owners feel that affected dogs are 'just not quite right', although it can often be difficult to pin-point exactly why. Obviously, a great many other diseases can produce just such a picture – it does not necessarily mean that lymphoma is present. But, when many diagnsotic tests have been carried out with unconvincing results, the veterinary surgeon may begin to suspect a disease like lymphoma.

Lymphoma can affect the organs within the chest or abdomen, in which case signs associated with these areas may be seen, e.g. coughing/breathing problems, vomiting, diarrhoea and weight loss. Forms of lymphoma may also affect the skin and disease can occur in the eye too, often part of a more general presence of the disease. Sometimes, the disease is first picked up in a less usual site such as the eye.

DIAGNOSIS A number of tests are likely. Blood tests and X-rays will usually be performed to try to localise the disease or discover any spread of the cancer. Biopsies of the lymph glands or of other body areas (e.g. the bowel) are important in confirming the diagnosis.

TREATMENT Lymphoma can quite often be treated reasonably successfully using chemotherapy and some forms are also treated by surgical removal of the tumour, followed by chemotherapy to deter recurrences. The form of treatment depends on the type of disease present and how advanced it is at the time of diagnosis.

OUTLOOK Chemotherapy may be able to extend life for some time by putting the disease into remission. Some dogs live for many months or even several years; others, with more serious disease, do not respond so well. Chemotherapy can be expensive, and regular general blood tests may also be required, however most pet insurance policies should cover initial treatments.

LEUKAEMIA

CAUSE Leukaemia is a form of cancer which originates within the bone marrow. Cells within the bone marrow multiply in an uncontrolled way and are found within the blood. The abnormal cells grow to outnumber the normal ones and symptoms are produced. Two forms of leukaemia are seen: acute and chronic, and carry different outlooks (opposite).

SYMPTOMS Symptoms are usually vague and can include features such as weight loss, lack of energy, vomiting, diarrhoea and high temperatures. Many dogs drink to excess and pass more urine than normal and have paler than normal mucous membranes.

DIAGNOSIS Examination of the blood to detect abnormal cells is required. X-rays may be used to check other organs and bone marrow is examined to establish which cells are being affected by the cancer.

TREATMENT Chemotherapy can be possible, depending on the type and severity of the leukaemia.

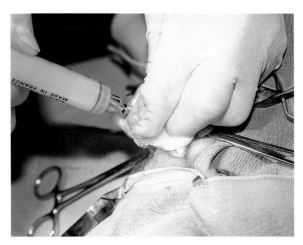

Aspiration of bone marrow may be required for diagnostic purposes and requires a small operation.

OUTLOOK For acute leukaemia, which is commoner, the outlook is not good as the disease is not very sensitive to chemotherapy and tends to progress; also, problems relating to the very strong treatment that is used can also develop (side-effects).

Chronic leukaemia carries a better outlook and some dogs can live for many months. Chemotherapy and frequent monitoring is used to keep the disease in remission for as long as possible.

Breeding and Whelping

Breeding

Successful breeding and whelping requires a normal male and female reproductive system as well as an inclination to copulate by both the male and female dog. An understanding of the female oestrus cycle is important in order to appreciate the time interval during which mating is likely to take place. This information is briefly summarised in the box. The normal oestrus cycle is discussed in Chapter 12.

Receptivity and pregnancy in the bitch: average figures

- *On average,* the bitch will pass through an oestrus cycle twice every 12 months.

- The first oestrus will occur at age 6–22 months, with larger dogs taking longer to become sexually mature than smaller dogs.

- For the first 7–10 days of the oestrus cycle, although a male dog may be interested in the bitch, the bitch will not allow mating. The vulva area is swollen at this time and there is a clear or reddish discharge (unless the bitch fastidiously cleans herself of this).

- The optimum time for mating is usually 10–14 days *after the first signs* of the bitch being in oestrus (or 'heat') were observed. At this point the discharge is smaller in volume and somewhat thicker.

- Normal pregnancy is 63 days.

- A certain amount of variation in all of these timings is possible between bitches. In this sense there are no hard and fast rules.

Both physical disease and behavioural factors can prevent normal mating behaviour. Physical disease can usually be ruled out by veterinary examination and tests. Behavioural influences are more difficult to predict and some bitches or dogs may simply not show interest in sexual behaviour with specific dogs, or at all. In most cases, however, mating will occur provided the correct times are chosen.

The normal mating process

Assuming the bitch is in the correct phase of the oestrus cycle, her acceptance of the dog is indicated by a reluctance to move as the dog approaches her hind quarters. The tail is usually held elevated and to one side and the bitch shows no objection as the dog sniffs her perineal area.

The dog will then usually mount the bitch. The shape of the dog's penis is such that once inserted into the bitch's vagina, further swelling results in the two animals becoming locked together – this is referred to as 'the tie'. The dogs cannot be separated at this stage.

The male then alters position such that both dogs are 'tied' tail-to-tail. This position is retained for 30 minutes or so while the enlarged penis remains within the vagina. Once the penis reduces in size, the dogs can separate.

Signs that the bitch is ready to accept a dog

- The bitch stands still when the dog approaches

- The tail is raised and held slightly to one side

Signs that the bitch is not ready or willing to mate

- The bitch does not allow the dog to approach her hind quarters or else she continually turns to face the dog

- There may be aggression or desire to escape

Problems with mating

Some of the commonest problems are as follows.

Owner/breeder does not choose the correct time for mating. This is very common and can arise because of problems in identifying the start of the pro-oestrus phase of the cycle (see page 235), or because some dogs simply do not conform to the 'average' time intervals quoted.

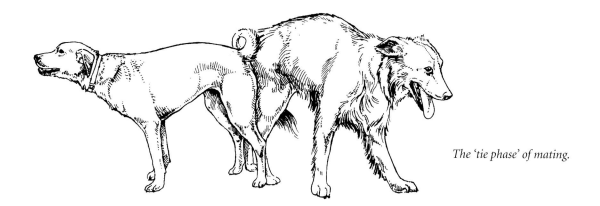

The 'tie phase' of mating.

Is a 'tie' necessary for a successful mating?

Most dog breeders prefer to see a 'tie' occurring. The process is considered a natural event which ensures that sufficient spermatozoa reach the uterus after ejaculation by the male dog. However a 'tie' does not invariably need to occur for fertilisation to take place. For this reason, one cannot assume that because the bitch and dog have *not* 'tied', no puppies will be born in cases of mis-mating!

SOLUTION: Best results are obtained when the bitch and dog are allowed unrestricted access to each other for several hours each day from the middle of the pro-oestrus phase, i.e. about a week after first signs of vulval swelling and bleeding have been noticed. Mating will usually take place at the appropriate time and if several matings occur it is likely that the optimum period of fertility of the bitch will be utilised.

Anxiety. Anxiety and inexperience on the part of the bitch or dog can occur and can prevent normal mating.

SOLUTION: For a first mating it is better if one of the dogs is more experienced. Alternatively, keeping the dogs together most of the time may result in eventual success. Too many human beings involved in the process may adversely affect some dogs. If the dogs are left quietly together and observed from a distance they may mate naturally.

Incompatibility. There is no doubt that some dog partners do not 'get on' for whatever reason and mating may not take place. Other factors should be ruled out too, but even in experienced dogs this incompatibility is known to occur.

SOLUTION: Either another mate should be tried or else artificial insemination carried out if breeding these specific dogs is very important.

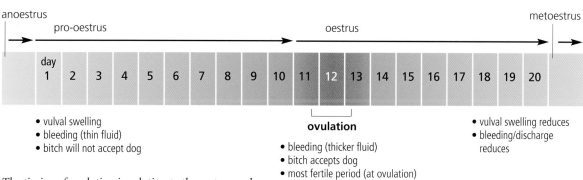

The timing of ovulation in relation to the oestrus cycle.

Human-oriented pets. Pet dogs who have bonded extremely strongly with their owners may be reluctant to mate while the owner is present.

SOLUTION: If the owner withdraws, successful mating may occur.

Medical conditions. Pain may prevent mating. For example, hip or back pain may affect either male or female dog adversely such that the process of mating is uncomfortable and will be resented. Male dogs may suffer from a narrow preputial orifice (the conditions of phimosis or paraphimosis, see page 201) which could render copulation painful or impossible. The female dog may have vaginal injuries. Young dogs of either sex may have congenital problems with the sexual organs which result in painful or impossible mating, yet cause no symptoms at other times.

SOLUTION: Prior to mating, both male and female dogs should be checked over by a veterinary surgeon.

Misalliance (unplanned mating) has occurred. Even with great vigiliance on the part of owners mating can occur between dogs. Normally obedient bitches may stray when their hormones and instincts indicate that time for mating has come; male dogs can be extremely persistent – and resourceful – in gaining access to receptive females.

SOLUTION: One solution for pet dogs which are not intended to be bred from is, of course, overiohysterectomy (spay). This operation is carried out *between* oestrus periods and is discussed, along with its advantages and disadvantages, on page 5. If a mis-mating has occurred, the pregnancy can be terminated at an early stage by an injection from the veterinary surgeon – but this must be received several days after mating. The veterinary practice should be contacted on the day the mating occurred and an appointment will be arranged for the misalliance injection, usually given on the 3rd day after the unintended mating.

Infertility

Infertility can have a large number of causes and may affect either the dog or bitch.

Males

In the dog, infertility can be caused by failure to produce sperm, by the production of abnormal sperm or by the lack of an ability or desire to mate. Dogs may be born infertile or they may acquire the condition in later life.

Lack of ability or desire to mate

Possible causes are as follows:

• Some of the medical conditions affecting the male reproductive organs (Chapter 11) when these may cause inflammation, pain or malfunction of the sexual organs, can result in a physical inability to mate or a reduced desire to do so if this causes pain. In this case, examination and treatment of the dog may cure the infertility if the underlying problem is responsive to treatment.

• Medical conditions affecting other body systems which have an effect on the reproductive system can also result in infertility. Hormonal diseases (e.g. underactive thyroid gland, Cushing's disease), infections and psychological or disease-associated stress can all be responsible. Review of the dog's medical history, reproductive examination and diagnostic tests may uncover the reason and allow treament.

• Congenital problems may be present which remain unnoticed until mating is attempted. Possibilties include malformed penis, phimosis, poorly formed testes or epididymis and various other anatomical or functional abnormalities. Examination of the dog should reveal these conditions. Some of these conditions are not however treatable.

Abnormalities in semen

If the ejaculate which the dog produces is abnormal, then infertility is likely. Microscopic or laboratory examination of the ejaculate may reveal the problem. Possibilities are as follows.

The dog does not produce sperm. This may be a temporary problem arising from disease in the reproductive system or general disease. Treatment of the underlying condition may result in sperm production resuming in 2–3 months. Some congenital problems may result in non-production of sperm, in which case there is no treatment.

Insufficient sperm are produced. This can occur in dogs which are over-bred, i.e. there are too many matings in too short a period of time. Sexual rest is required. Otherwise, a search must be made for diseases which could be affecting the production of sperm.

Abnormal sperm are produced. If more than a third of the sperm are abnormal in shape, infertility is likely. Similarly, if the sperm show poor mobility then it is unlikely that a fertilisation will be possible.

Females

As with the male, infertility can be caused by lack of a desire or ability to mate or by diseases which interfere with normal reproductive and hormonal function. Possible causes of infertility in the female are outlined below. Other common causes are described on pages 234–236, and some of the reproductive system diseases mentioned in Chapter 12 could also lead to failure to mate or conceive. In investigating a case of infertility, all of these possibilities would need to be taken into account.

There is no oestrus cycle. Be aware of the large variation in appearance of the first oestrus cycle, especially in large breed dogs. This may not occur until they are almost 2 years of age and a 'normal' twice per 12 months pattern may take some time to establish. Some dogs cycle at longer or irregular intervals, i.e. it is not always 6 months between cycles.

POSSIBLE REASONS AND TREATMENT: Treatment may simply be waiting for the oestrus to appear if the bitch is young. Usually, small and medium dogs have had their first oestrus by 12–14 months and larger dogs by 22 months. After this time, investigation may be required if it is intended to breed from the bitch. Sometimes, simply keeping the bitch with another bitch in oestrus for a few days will initiate events.

Oestrus cycles are present but there is a long time between them. There is a degree of variation in the interval between oestrus cycles and this must be accepted as normal. Certain breeds, notably the Basenji, only cycle once every 12 months, but most bitches cycle *approximately* twice every 12 months.

Basenjis are unusual in that the females only enter oestrus on average once per 12 months.

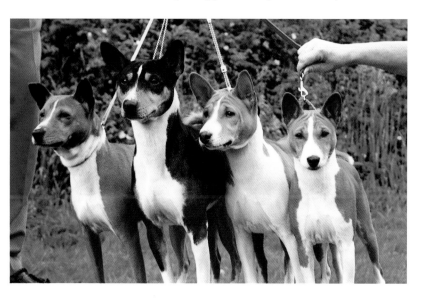

Note this does not necessarily mean twice per calendar year!

POSSIBLE REASONS AND TREATMENT: Hormone problems may be to blame in some cases. Underactive thyroid glands can be checked and, if necessary, hormone replacements given. Other possible causes are drugs being given for co-existing medical problems. Certain types of ovarian cyst can also have an effect. If these causes are ruled out then it may be possible to induce oestrus in breeding bitches if mating at a specific oestrus is important.

Oestrus occurs but very few signs of it are displayed. Greyhounds typically have 'silent' oestrus of this type. Fertility is however normal. Other bitches may clean themselves excessively and apparently show few external signs of oestrus. Again, fertility is normal. No treatment is required.

Split oestrus. The bitch shows initial signs of coming into oestrus, but events do not proceed. Then, some weeks later, a complete oestrus cycle is seen. The symptoms of this pattern are similar to ovulation failure (see below).

TREATMENT: With split oestrus, fertility is normal when the complete oestrus cycle takes place. Mating should be successful at this time. No specific treatment is required.

Ovulation does not occur. Ovulation – the movement of an egg from the ovary into the uterine (fallopian) tube and uterus – is required for fertilisation to occur. Conception is impossible if this process fails.

TREATMENT: Failure of ovulation can be diagnosed by measuring progesterone concentrations in the blood. If failure of ovulation is occurring in a bitch, induction of ovulation may be attempted by hormonal injections. Bitches which fail to ovulate tend to return to oestrus sooner than normal – the next oestrus would occur at approximately 4 months rather than approximately 6 months after the previous one.

Implantation does not occur. Implantation is the process by which the fertilised egg takes up position in the uterus and pregnancy begins. Implantation may not occur if the uterus is diseased or malformed. Similarly, if damage to the uterus occurs during pregnancy implantation can fail and abortion occur (see below). The commonest reason is however a simpler one: the timing of the mating has not corresponded with the most fertile period of the bitch's oestrus.

TREATMENT: Investigation for problems in the uterus (infection, malformation) or hormonal irregularities may be necessary if implantation failure is suspected. Giving the male dog repeated access to the female over the course of several days is the best way of ensuring that optimum timing of mating is achieved.

Pregnancy and Whelping

Normal pregnancy

63 days is the average length of pregnancy in the dog but several days variation on either side of this is also considered normal. Bitches vary a lot in the changes they show while pregnant and much of this is due to the huge variety of dog sizes and shapes that exist. Some bitches show very few signs until pregnancy is well advanced; in others changes will be seen at a much earlier stage.

The chart opposite can be used as a guide to follow the progress of pregnancy in the bitch but, as with all aspects of reproduction, bear in mind that individual dogs can vary considerably in the signs they show at different times. The information presented represents the 'average' dog.

Health checks for the pregnant bitch

- Bitches should be checked over prior to mating to ensure they are fit to enter pregnancy

- Vaccination and worming schedules should be checked at this time and advice will be given on worming throughout pregnancy

- Based on the size of the dog, conformation and weight, advice on feeding during pregnancy can also be given at this time

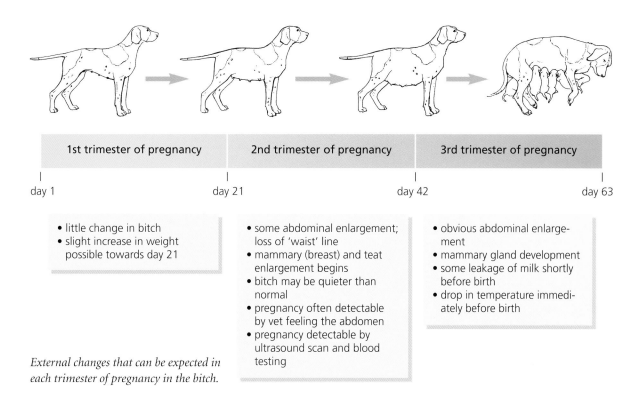

1st trimester of pregnancy	2nd trimester of pregnancy	3rd trimester of pregnancy

day 1   day 21   day 42   day 63

- little change in bitch
- slight increase in weight possible towards day 21

- some abdominal enlargement; loss of 'waist' line
- mammary (breast) and teat enlargement begins
- bitch may be quieter than normal
- pregnancy often detectable by vet feeling the abdomen
- pregnancy detectable by ultrasound scan and blood testing

- obvious abdominal enlargement
- mammary gland development
- some leakage of milk shortly before birth
- drop in temperature immediately before birth

External changes that can be expected in each trimester of pregnancy in the bitch.

Preparations for whelping

It is very important that preparations for whelping are made beforehand. The main consideration is in providing a whelping area that is quiet, warm but not overheated and easily observed. Breeding kennels often have special whelping areas with facilities to hand. Pet dogs kept in a house may choose to have their puppies in certain places, e.g. in a cupboard or in the corner of a bedroom. If you prepare a place like this and introduce the bitch to it about a week before the puppies are due to be born, it is quite likely that she will choose to go to this place when she starts to give birth. Otherwise, it is a simple matter to move blankets etc. to the place she has chosen.

Important features of the whelping area or box are:

- It should be able to be cleaned easily. Lining with newspapers or incontinence pads is best.

- It should be secure and safe. Wire mesh, irregular corners and projections can be dangerous for puppies as they may become stuck. If the bitch goes into a cupboard, placing some sort of barrier across the door opening is required to stop the puppies rolling or moving out.

- It should be draught-free. The best temperature is a comfortable room temperature for humans. If it is too hot, the bitch may be reluctant to stay in the box; if it is too cold, hypothermia may develop in the puppies (puppies cannot regulate their own body temperatures when newly born). A heat lamp can be used if there are concerns that the temperature is too low, but overheating of the bitch must be avoided.

- It should be possible to observe the bitch and puppies easily.

- The whelping area or box should be well away from busy parts of the house or noisy children.

- Ample bedding should be provided.

- Near the whelping box or area water and food bowls should be provided for the bitch.

Normal whelping

The birth of puppies is referred to as whelping, parturition or labour and is divided up into several different stages. It is important to be able to recognise these so that, if problems occur, appropriate action can be taken. Most bitches whelp uneventfully if not unduly disturbed. Common sense and a calm approach are necessary from the owner.

The normal stages of labour

STAGE 1

The initial stage of labour is usually marked by restlessness and slight anxiety in the bitch. It is at this point that she desires to find and make a nest. She should be gently encouraged to investigate the area chosen for her beforehand.

There is usually a fair amount of digging and scrabbling around as her instincts instruct her to make a suitable bed. She may whine somewhat and pant, settle a little and then become restless again.

This stage lasts several hours in most bitches, occasionally extending even longer than this. It is important to recognise that this is normal and not a sign of severe pain or distress at this time.

Eclampsia (milk fever)

Very occasionally, eclampsia (milk fever – see p.242) can occur before the puppies are born. Initial symptoms of this serious problem can resemble first stage labour. If you suspect eclampsia, veterinary advice should be sought as soon as possible. Developing eclampsia would be indicated by severe muscle tremors, incoordination and collapse of the bitch.

STAGE 2

During this stage uterine contractions begin in preparation to deliver the puppies. At this point the bitch should be settled in the whelping box and will probably be lying down most of the time. Some anxiety may still be present. She may get up and turn around, investigate her rear end and whine or pant. Try to gently encourage her to remain in the whelping box. Ensure there are not too many distractions in the form of noise, excited children or other animals. She can be left alone, perhaps in the dark, and checked on every 15 minutes or so.

The uterine contractions gradually increase in frequency and strength as stage 2 progresses. The contractions are often visible through the abdomen.

Second stage labour usually results in the delivery of a puppy within 30 minutes, but this can take well over an hour and still be normal. Over 2 hours of strong unproductive straining is usually abnormal and telephone advice should be sought from the veterinary surgeon at this point if no puppies have been born.

When a puppy is born, it appears at the vulva in the amniotic sac ('water bag'). This sac may rupture as the puppy is being born; alternatively the bitch may rupture it herself by licking before delivery is complete or just after delivery. All of these are normal.

At this stage the bitch normally shows interest in the puppy and will commence licking it vigorously. This stimulation helps to establish normal breathing patterns in the puppy. The afterbirth (placenta) may be still attached to the puppy, in which case the bitch may eat it while cleaning the puppy. Alternatively, the afterbirth may be passed separately a short time later.

This process of stage 2 labour is repeated for each puppy that is born. Note that puppies are not always born immediately after each other. There is usually a delay, even a delay of over an hour or so. The bitch will rest during these times and possibly direct her attention to the puppies that have already been born. Onset of uterine contractions again means that another puppy is on its way.

STAGE 3

This stage is the passage of the afterbirth or placentas. This can often happen as part of stage 2 above, or else the afterbirths may appear separately a short while later. It is quite normal for the bitch to eat these.

The end of whelping

Litter size varies considerably in dogs but usually the end of whelping is marked by the bitch settling down and showing increased interest in the puppies she has produced. She may get up out of the whelping box or area for a short time and can be let outside briefly or given a small amount to eat. However she should not

What if the bitch ignores the puppy in its bag?

- Gently tear and remove the membrane surrounding the puppy. Fluid will escape. Gently pick up the puppy and hold it head downwards. Rub the puppy with a towel and open its mouth to wipe away any fluid or mucus and encourage breathing. If the afterbirth (placenta) is still attached to the puppy, tie thread tightly around the umbilical cord and then cut the cord between the knot and the placenta.

- Take care not to pull hard on the cord as this can cause a hernia in the puppy's abdomen at the umbilicus. Give the puppy to the bitch or place it near a teat.

- Often bitches will not give puppies their full attention until the whole litter is born.

- Do not take the puppy away from the bitch at this point except to resuscitate it. Handle it as little as possible.

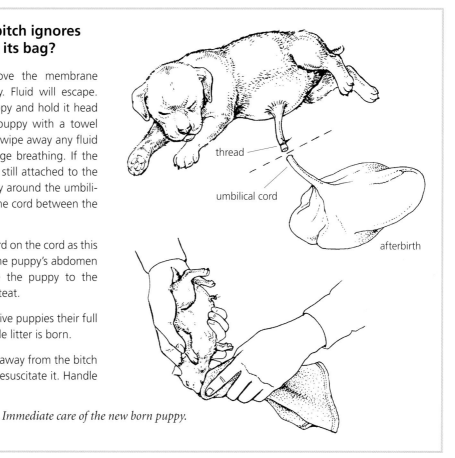

Immediate care of the new born puppy.

I have not seen all the afterbirths. Are some retained?

- It is quite possible that the bitch has eaten an afterbirth when you have not noticed.

- The afterbirth may yet be passed by the bitch. This can take up to 30 minutes after the birth of the puppy.

- The afterbirth of one puppy may be passed with the next puppy to be born.

- An afterbirth may indeed be retained in the uterus. If this happens, it gradually dissolves there, possibly causing a slight vaginal discharge for several days or a low grade infection. If necessary an injection can be given to aid in the expulsion of the retained afterbirth from the uterus.

be separated from the puppies for more than a few minutes at this stage, and the puppies should not be handled excessively. Most bitches settle best with their puppies if left alone at this time. This ensures good maternal bonding takes place.

What can go wrong?

Difficulties with giving birth are termed dystokia and can arise for a number of reasons. The commonest problems encountered in dogs are as follows.

1. Owner misunderstanding
Quite often, there is no problem but the owner thinks there is! This can arise when there seems to be lengthy delays between stages of labour or between puppies.

2. No uterine contractions
In this situation the second stage of labour does not

> ### ! Remember...
>
> - Stage 1 labour can on occasions last for 12–24 hours. The bitch will appear unsettled, anxious and may whine or growl. She may scratch or dig in attempts to make a nest.
>
> - Problems are only likely to have occurred if strong, unproductive straining has persisted for 2 hours or more without a puppy being produced.
>
> - There can be lengthy delays between puppies.
>
> - The afterbirths (placentas) are not always passed immediately.

seem to start. Many cases are simply due to a lengthy delay between stage 1 and stage 2 labour, but if 24 hours have elapsed the bitch should be checked.

The problem may be uterine inertia (inactivity in the uterine muscle). If the birth canal is open and clear, a uterine stimulating injection may be given. Otherwise Caeserian section may be recommended.

3. Uterine contractions start but then stop without a pup being born after 2 hours

This may be because a pup has become lodged, perhaps because it is oversized, malformed or approaching the birth canal in an incorrect position. Sometimes vaginal examination reveals a pup that is partly delivered but stuck in the birth canal or else two pups may be present and causing a blockage as they cannot be delivered simultaneously.

Simple cases of obstruction can be corrected by experienced owners or breeders, but generally such cases should be checked by the veterinary surgeon. Vaginal delivery may be possible, or else a Caeserian section may need to be peformed.

Puppies are normally presented for birth:

- Head and front legs first

- Tail and back legs first

A breech presentation is when the tail and hindquarters (but not the legs) are presented, and usually results in obstruction. A similar situation can result if the forelegs do not come with the head – this shape, like a breech, is not streamlined enough to pass easily through the birth canal. These presentations are normally easily corrected without recourse to Caeserian section. The legs are hooked forwards to allow normal delivery.

4. Exhaustion of the mother

If significant straining has occurred to deliver one puppy, exhaustion may prevent the delivery of the rest of the litter. Sometimes uterine stimulants and calcium injections, perhaps aided by an intravenous drip, can result in birth without the need for a Caeserian section.

Other conditions requiring Caeserian section

Several other situations means that a Caeserian is required:

- Bitches with pelvic deformities may be unable to produce any pups naturally. This usually arises after road traffic accidents which have caused pelvic fracture. When the fracture heals it results in narrowing of the birth canal. It is unwise to attempt breeding in the first place in these patients.

- The cervix does not dilate. This will appear like an obstruction and will be apparent on gynaecological examination. A Caeserian is performed.

- If only one puppy is present, or if only one horn of the uterus contains puppies, normal processes may not operate and the cervix may not dilate. Also, a single very large puppy may not be able to be passed naturally. Again, Caeserian is required.

- Uterine rupture or torsion, both quite rare, require emergency Caeserian section (and usually hysterectomy).

Problems of Pregnancy and the Post-natal Period

ECLAMPSIA (MILK FEVER)

CAUSE This serious disease is caused by a deficiency of calcium and may occur in late pregnancy or (more

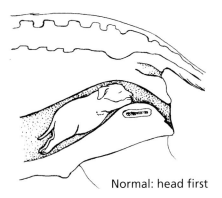

Normal: head first

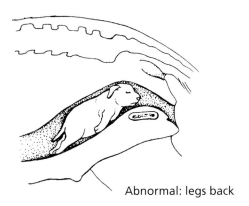

Abnormal: legs back

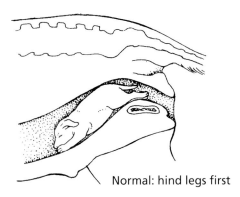

Normal: hind legs first

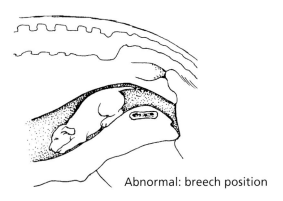

Abnormal: breech position

Diagrams showing normal (ABOVE) and abnormal (RIGHT) presentation of puppies at birth.

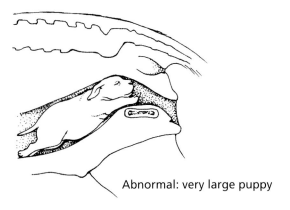

Abnormal: very large puppy

usually) after the puppies are born. It is associated with the loss of calcium that can occur into the milk supply of the dam and is commoner in smaller breeds, especially if litter size is large.

SYMPTOMS Initial symptoms are restlessness and panting. These can progress to nervous twitches, shivering and incoordination leading to rigidity and collapse with muscular spasms as the low blood levels of calcium affect the central nervous system.

Note that initial symptoms can appear similar to first stage labour. However muscle twitches, shivering and incoordination are not seen in first stage labour. It is commoner for eclampsia to occur after the puppies have been born, when milk production (and hence calcium loss) is at its peak. Nevertheless, if you suspect this condition in a bitch which has yet to give birth you should contact the veterinary surgeon for advice.

Important key symptoms of eclampsia

- Trembling/shivering or muscular spasms
- Incoordination or fits
- Collapse

DIAGNOSIS The symptoms are characteristic of the disease.

TREATMENT Emergency treatment is required. A calcium solution is injected intravenously by the veterinary surgeon. The effect is a dramatic improvement in symptoms but must be carried out quickly.

OUTLOOK Good with prompt treatment. Following an attack, the puppies should be weaned or fed artificially to avoid depleting the dam's calcium reserves further. Occasionally, calcium supplements may be given in late pregnancy in small dogs expected to have large litters; this is continued throughout lactation and then stopped when the puppies are weaned.

VAGINAL DISCHARGE OR BLEEDING AFTER WHELPING

CAUSE Whilst a small degree of vaginal discharge is to be expected, any profuse discharge, especially if associated with other signs of ill-health in the bitch, must be taken seriously as it may indicate metritis (infection of the uterus).

Normal bitches do have a slight vaginal discharge of brownish material for 5–10 days after whelping but do not show any other symptoms and continue to eat normally and feed their litter.

SYMPTOMS Serious cases have a profuse foul-smelling vaginal discharge, as well as symptoms of lethargy, poor appetite and milk production, and high temperature.

DIAGNOSIS Metritis usually takes several days to develop following whelping, and if this timing fits with the symptoms the condition may be assumed.

TREATMENT Antibiotics are prescribed together with drugs which help speed involution (reduction in size) of the uterus. Severe cases may require hospitalisation for intravenous drips and even hysterectomy. During this time, the puppies must be hand raised (see page 246).

OUTLOOK The outlook is usually fair to good with effective treatment.

FAILURE OF MILK PRODUCTION (AGALACTIA)

CAUSE This is fairly uncommon but may occur at the first litter or if a Caeserian section was carried out. Undernourished or ill bitches may also have a poor milk supply.

SYMPTOMS The mammary glands are poorly developed, milk is not expressible from them and puppies cry constantly from hunger.

DIAGNOSIS The condition is easily diagnosed from the symptoms and examination of the mammary glands.

TREATMENT Some cases may be helped by an injection of oxytocin, to promote release of milk, but supplemental feeding of the puppies using an approved milk replacement product will also be required.

OUTLOOK Hand-rearing puppies (see page 246) requires a lot of patience and effort but is usually successful if advice is followed.

MASTITIS

CAUSE Mastitis means inflammation in the mammary gland. It is usually caused by an infection that has entered via the teat, a skin wound (e.g. caused by a puppy) or via the bloodstream.

SYMPTOMS The affected gland tends to be warm, swollen and tender with either no milk production or a brownish coloured milk. The bitch is unlikely to let the puppies suckle from this gland, and if the mastitis is severe may not allow suckling at all. Severe mastitis is a painful, unpleasant condition.

DIAGNOSIS This is usually straightforward. In severe cases, the bitch may have a high temperature and also be off food, requiring an intravenous drip.

Treatment Antibiotics are used and the puppies must be hand-fed or weaned (see page 246). Drugs to lower the temperature and relieve pain may be given.

First aid
Warm compresses and gentle exercise can help relieve the discomfort of mastitis.

Outlook The condition usually resolves in a few days. Occasional severe cases result in necrosis (death of tissue) in the mammary gland that may necessitate surgery or wound management.

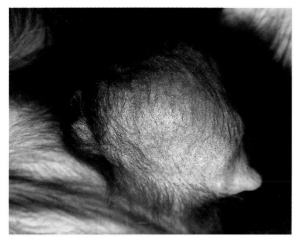

Mastitis is painful inflammation of one or more mammary glands.

FOETAL DEATH/ABORTION

Cause The causes of loss of a foetus or entire pregnancy can be many and varied. Most likely are infections, trauma, birth defects or abnormalities in the maternal reproductive system such that pregnancy cannot be supported or maintained. Death of one foetus may occur without the whole pregnancy being jeopardised.

Symptoms The only symptom may simply be that pregnancy does not occur after an apparently successful and correctly-timed mating. Obviously, problems of infertility (male or female) need also to be considered in this case.

If pregnancy has become established and is then lost, a vaginal discharge may be noted during the time the abortion is occurring and for a period afterwards. Usually the bitch will also appear unwell and, if infection is the cause, other symptoms are likely depending on the specific disease that is involved.

Some infectious causes of abortion in dogs
- *Brucella canis* bacteria (not in UK)
- Canine distemper
- Canine herpes virus
- *Toxoplasma* infection
- Other bacteria or viruses

Diagnosis Ultrasound and X-rays may be helpful in confirming that foetal death or abortion has occurred. Tests on the dam or aborted material may allow a diagnosis of the exact cause of the abortion to be made. This is not always possible however.

Treatment Hospitalisation may be required in bitches that are significantly ill, e.g. dehydrated and with high temperatures. Otherwise antibiotics and drugs to help expel residues from the uterus may be given. Ovariohysterectomy is usually required for severe metritis and toxaemia.

Outlook If the cause was a one-off infection then, provided this was cleared up adequately, there is no reason why a future pregnancy should not be successful. If the cause was a physical or hormonal problem with the reproductive system, then the outlook depends on trying to establish a precise diagnosis and seeing if the problem could be corrected for future pregnancies.

POOR MOTHERING BY THE BITCH

CAUSE Most bitches' maternal instincts take over when puppies are born but problems can be encountered with inexperienced bitches and their first litter, especially if a Caeserian section was required. Similarly, sensitive bitches which were excessively disturbed during labour (e.g. noisy room, excited children) may have problems bonding with their puppies.

SYMPTOMS The bitch shows no interest in the puppies, may even appear frightened of them and refuses to stay in the whelping area.

DIAGNOSIS It is usually readily apparent that the bitch does not wish to be with the puppies.

TREATMENT Sometimes, with patience and reassurance, the bitch will accept the puppies and allow them to suckle. Oxytocin injected by the veterinary surgeon may help promote milk let-down and hopefully instinctive responses should take over.

Mild sedation may be beneficial in the short term, but if these attempts seem fruitless, hand-rearing of the puppies will be required.

OUTLOOK It is worth persisting for several days (during which time the puppies will need to be hand-reared using an approved milk replacer, see below) before abandoning all attempts to have the bitch rear the puppies.

OVER PROTECTION OF THE PUPPIES

CAUSE A few bitches become very protective of their puppies and may growl at or even bite other animals or human beings they know well.

SYMPTOMS Usually warning growls are given by the bitch as the nest area is approached.

TREATMENT If the bitch will accept one person, then this individual should be responsible for looking after her and the puppies. Often, as time passes, the bitch becomes less protective. However, for safety reasons, a muzzle may need to be used to allow examination of the puppies or cleaning of the nest area. Strangers should not be allowed near the bitch or her puppies. The bitch and puppies should be moved to a quiet area of the house.

OUTLOOK The bitch's behaviour usually returns to normal after a few days.

Checklist for Puppies

Basic checks

- Newborn puppies should be checked to ensure there is no infection or hernia at the umbilicus, that they are suckling effectively and receiving milk and that the bitch is interested and caring for them.

- During the first 12–48 hours the milk produced by the bitch is called colostrum. It is important that each puppy receives this as it contains antibodies to common diseases. By drinking colostrum, the puppies will receive immunity which should last approximately until the time of their first vaccination.

- Each puppy should be checked over for obvious congenital abnormalities. Signs of milk refluxing down the nose could indicate a cleft palate, for example. A veterinary examination should be arranged if this problem is suspected.

- Other common birth abnormalities include under or overshot jaw, hare lip and atresia ani (absence of an anal opening – this can be treated by surgery if not too severe).

Hand-reared puppies

- Hand-reared puppies require feeding and assisted elimination every 2 hours initially. The frequency is gradually reduced as the puppies grow older and consume larger amounts of milk at a time. Only an approved puppy milk replacement powder should be used, and manufacturers' dilutions and feeding frequencies should be followed according to the age of the puppies. Puppy feeding bottles make hand feeding easier.

- Puppies pass faeces and urine in response to the bitch licking their perineal areas. If the puppies are being hand-reared, this process must be mimicked by gentle rubbing with a warm, damp towel or cloth after every feeding.

- If at all possible, hand-reared puppies should receive colostrum within the first 12–24 hours of life. It may be possible to withdraw some colostrum from the bitch even if she refuses to feed the puppies herself. This can then be given to the puppies via the feeding bottle. Veterinary advice should be sought.

- If the bitch is not present in the nest area a heat lamp should be used. A constant temperature of 75°F should be maintained. Puppies cannot control their own body temperature when newly born and are thus prone to hypothermia.

- Make sure the nest/box area is safe, with no projections, recesses or holes where puppies could get trapped. A thick layer of newspaper underneath a synthetic, washable bedding material such as 'Vetbed' is ideal.

- Puppies that have not received colostrum may be started on their vaccination course sooner than normal.

Normal development

- Puppies' eyes usually open at between 10–14 days.

- At this time the puppies begin to be more mobile. Any puppy which does not show increasing activity at this time should be checked over for possible abnormalities.

- The puppies can be handled more by different family members now. They can also be introduced to other animals in the household. All dogs which the puppies come into contact with should, of course, be fully vaccinated. This is an important part of the socialisation process and should help to produce a happy, well-adjusted adult dog.

- Weaning is started at about 3 to 4 weeks, when most puppies will begin attempting to lap fluids. A puppy milk substitute should be used at this stage (in puppies that have previously been suckled by the bitch), gradually introducing puppy food made sloppy with water. 4 to 5 small meals a day should be given. Weaning is normally complete by 6 to 8 weeks.

Preventative medicine

- First worming treatment is normally at 2 weeks, and worming is repeated every 2 weeks up until 3 months of age. A veterinary-approved wormer for puppies should be obtained from your veterinary clinic.

- Dew claws on the back feet, if present, are normally removed before 1 week of age by the veterinary surgeon. It is a small operation and causes only minor discomfort. Front dew claws are sometimes removed but these rarely cause problems in most dogs and can usually be safely left alone.

- First vaccination courses are given at the time suggested by your veterinary clinic. This is often at 8 and 12 weeks, but sometimes an earlier vaccine is also given. It is important that a complete vaccination course is received for a full immunity to occur (see Infectious Diseases, Chapter 1).

The new home

- Puppies are normally re-homed after 8 weeks.

- Health insurance policies should be taken out at this time.

- Always ensure that the new owner receives vaccination documents, worming schedule, pedigree (if appropriate) and details of further veterinary appointments to complete the primary vaccination course.

Tail docking

Several dog breeds have traditionally had their tails docked while puppies. Examples include Spaniels, Boxers, Corgis and Bulldogs. In the UK, tail docking is generally no longer carried out by veterinary surgeons except for medical reasons, such as a damaged or paralysed tail. Breeds traditionally accepted as being docked are now seen with their complete tails. The move against tail docking has not however been without controversy, and docked dogs are still encountered – many of these may have been docked by breeders or owners keen to remove the tails

Docking a tail without use of proper or sterile instruments carries the risk of infection, which could be potentially serious, as well as causing considerable pain and distress to the dog. Many previously docked dogs look even better with their tails – they have a more balanced appearance and their owners can enjoy that most fundamental means of dog communication: the tail wag.

CHAPTER 16

Dog Behaviour and Behaviour Problems

Common symptoms of behaviour problems
- Anxiety/fear • Aggression • Disobedience
- Inappropriate urination or defaecation
- Destructive behaviours
- Territorial or defensive behaviours

Every dog is different, has its own 'personality' and reacts to the world in its own unique way. Some dogs are naturally outgoing and inquisitive of places, people and animals whereas others are quieter and more retiring. Whenever dog owners get together, they can talk endlessly about their own pet's unique habits and routines. This is one of the greatest pleasures in owning dogs; it allows us to recognise that they are, indeed, all individuals and that our relationship and bonds with them can be varied and interesting. No two dogs, even of the same breed or from the same litter, are very similar in anything other than overall appearance.

What Makes a Dog's Character?

Undoubtedly, a substantial part of a dogs' character and behaviour is genetically determined. In a general sense, all dogs share certain basic behavioural characteristics which make them respond like dogs. This is despite the huge variation in size, shape and stature that exists in modern domestic dogs. Underneath all that, there is something essentially 'doggy' that can be recognised in any dog, whether it is a Chihuahua or a Great Dane. These basic behaviours are common to all members of the dog family, and can be seen in purest form in wild members of the family such as

wolves. This is important because, surprisingly, many of the behaviour problems that appear in domestic dogs have their roots in these very basic instincts. While most dog owners may not like to think of their pets as being close to wild dogs, in a behavioural sense, this is very true! Wolves, of course, are surrounded by superstition and 'bad press' but, as natural history films show, they display many of the qualities we recognise in our pet dogs: affection, loyality, respect to 'superiors', etc.

As well as the basic behaviours inherited from their wild ancestry, behaviour is also influenced by the breed of dog (or breeds, in the case of crossbreeds). For generations, dogs have been specifically bred for a huge variety of different purposes and appearances. The most obvious example of this is the very strong herding instinct that is seen in Border Collies. Even if these dogs have been born in a city and never seen a sheep in their lives, the desire to herd animals or objects together can be extremely strong and can result in them trying to herd together other dogs which they meet on walks, or indeed any animal that will move in response to them. Terrier breeds, such as the Jack Russell, were originally bred to seek out hunted animals underground. Behaviour characteristics that were bred for include determination, high levels of activity and a degree of fearlessness.

Two Border Collies at work. Even Border Collies born in the city may exhibit the herding instinct.

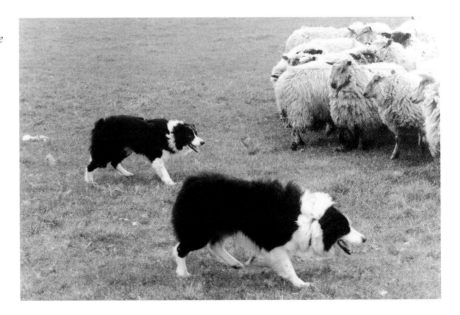

A certain part of a dog's character, then, is also influenced by its breed, but this is by no means everything because if that was the case *every* Border Collie would live to herd animals and *every* Jack Russell Terrier would be fascinated by underground burrows. We know that this is not the case: some Collies are frightened of sheep and some Jack Russells are lazy, placid dogs who could never be persuaded to go down a burrow after another animal.

Other influences on character and behaviour

The inherited aspects mentioned above provide a 'baseline' of basic dog behaviour and responses. But a large part of how individual dogs respond to their environment, to people, and to other dogs and other animals, depends on behaviours which are formed *after* birth. After birth and as the young dog matures, basic behaviour patterns are moulded into the individual patterns that we see in different dogs. Thus to truly understand behaviour we have to take account of these influences: inherited and acquired.

The character of a dog is made up by the interaction of many different aspects of behaviour and experience.

Early behaviour in puppies

Even in young puppies, differences in behaviour can be seen by the observant owner. At around the time of weaning, some puppies will be more confident and outgoing than others – they may run to greet strangers or investigate new places much more readily than some of their litter mates. Other puppies may be much more retiring, staying near their mother or in the nest area, or else they may adopt a position somewhere between these two extremes!

Early behaviour	Adult character	Potential problems
Inquisitive	Confident; outgoing	Assertive; dominant
Retiring	Quiet; loyal	Nervous; frightened

These very early differences in behaviour can provide clues about future personality. Note however that these cannot be considered hard and fast rules, only indications about *possible tendencies* in these dogs. The reason for this is because of the crucial effects on behaviour which occur during the first few months of independent life after weaning. This is the time during which the influence of the owner is all-important in moulding the dog's future character.

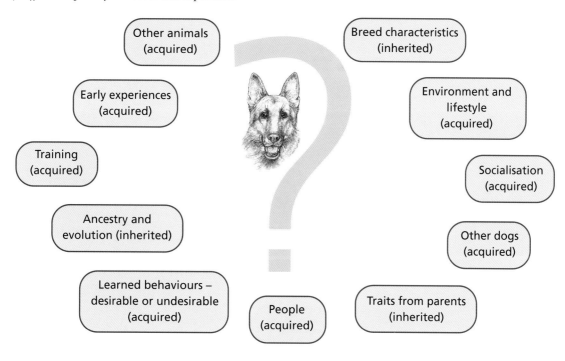

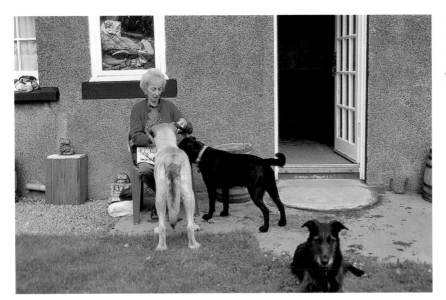

Individual dogs vary in their confidence and behaviour. Some are more outgoing and forward than others in their approach to people.

Checklist for a Well-adjusted Pet Dog

It is possible to draw up a list of basic characteristics which should be present in a well-adjusted pet dog to allow both dog and owner to get the most out of life in a stress-free way.

- The dog should generally be free from extremes of behaviour. It should be neither nervous, anxious or frightened nor assertive, dominant or aggressive.

- The dog should be well socialised with other dogs and people, allowing the owner to predict confidently how the dog will react in situations when unfamiliar people or animals are met. Difficulties with other dogs or other people are a major problem for many pet dog owners and can seriously undermine the enjoyment of owning a dog. Early socialisation (see below) can prevent these problems developing in the first place.

- The dog should be able to be left unattended in its usual environment in the knowledge that it will settle without showing destructive behaviour, excess barking or other associated problems of separation anxiety.

- The dog should not be defensive or protective over food, toys or sleep areas. In other words, it should be possible at any time to remove food from the dog, to take away its toy or to move the dog from an area where it is sleeping without the dog showing any signs of aggression or over-protection.

- The dog should have reasonable basic obedience such that lead walking is possible without excess pulling and such that the dog will sit still to be examined by the owner, veterinary surgeon or groomer. Off the lead, the dog should come within a short time of being called.

- Although most dogs have one person they bond particularly with, there should be no question of a pet dog reacting unpredictably towards any family member, especially children. It is a dangerous situation if children are fearful of a dominant dog and cannot, for example, move the dog in order to get past.

Early Socialisation in Puppies and Young Dogs: a Crucial Period

Not everyone gets a dog when it is a puppy. Many pet dogs are acquired at an older age, particularly those obtained from rescue societies or kennels, and the vast majority of these dogs make excellent pets. If a puppy is obtained, however, the owner has a unique oppor-

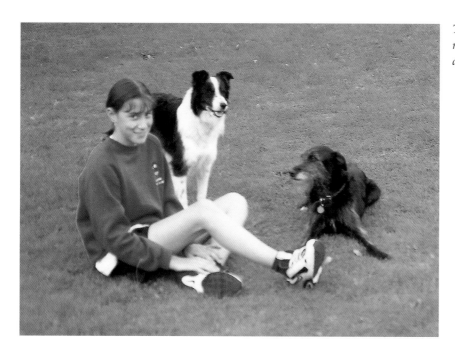

The family dog should be relaxed and dependable with all age groups.

tunity – and responsibility – to ensure that the dog grows up to be as sociable and well-adjusted as it could be.

A few simple guidelines can help lay the foundations for stress-free dog ownership.

1. From as early an age as possible, the puppy should be introduced to different people and situations. Ideally, this should begin even before weaning. From 3 or 4 weeks of age, supervised handling of the puppies by adults and children of both sexes should be encouraged. Only a few minutes at a time is required.

2. After weaning, and in the new home, socialisation should be continued. The puppy can interact with vaccinated dogs and cats and, once fully vaccinated itself, can be introduced to the outdoor world, to cars, public places and transport, friends' or relatives' houses, strange sounds and smells.

3. The puppy's life should not be a constant whirl of new experiences however; rather these things should happen gradually – a new experience every few days – and should be carried out in a calm, unhurried way, giving the puppy time to investigate, explore and learn.

4. From the very beginning, the owner and family members should be in complete control of feeding. Basic obedience can be started, encouraging the puppy to sit and wait quietly before food. Occasionally, the food should be removed from the puppy while it is eating and then given back after a few minutes.

5. Similarly, although the puppy must have a bed area, any member of the family should be able to move the puppy at any time. Toys should occasionally be taken off the puppy while playing in order to reinforce owner dominance.

6. Attention and petting should not always be given when demanded. It is important that puppies are occasionally ignored so that they learn to be comfortable and relaxed by themselves. Regular short periods of being left alone should ensure that behaviour problems caused by separation anxiety (such as chewing, howling or messing in the house) do not occur in adulthood.

7. Socialisation with other dogs is important. Puppy classes, organised at many veterinary practices, are an ideal way of gaining this experience, though they should if possible be supplemented with further interactions in between the formal classes. During

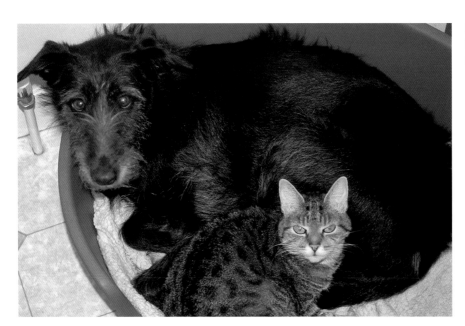

If a dog and cat are kept, it helps if they are well socialised!

these classes, expert advice is on hand regarding normal behaviour and common puppy medical problems.

It is natural that some dogs will be more dominant or submissive than others, and this will be visible during interactions with other puppies and young dogs during puppy classes or play. Yelps and small squabbles are part of the learning process as the puppies gradually acquire the knowledge of how to communicate adequately with each other. Gradually the normal behaviour code should be built up without abnormalities or extremes of aggression or nervousness occurring.

The important thing is to observe and encourage normal behaviours and reactions between dogs. Owners of puppies which appear to be more dominant can if necessary take steps to ensure that this dominance does not become out of hand (see box). Similarly, owners of puppies tending towards nervousness can take special steps to introduce new experiences very gradually and unthreateningly.

Why is owner dominance so important?

Unforced dominance is the key to a happy dog, content with its place in the social hierarchy of the family. The reason is simple: this is the way in which wild dog societies are organised. Every member knows his or her place and is content to stay there. Anxiety or stress only arises when the hierarchy is upset. Domestic dogs, although far removed from their wild counterparts in appearance, have most of the instincts that are present in their predecessors and react to them accordingly.

Dominance does not mean punishment; real aggression is rare in wolf packs. Rather, dominance is gently reinforced by establishing priority over basic require-ments such as food, sleep areas and play. This is why these aspects are particularly important in developing puppies: in a subtle but effective way, they inform the developing puppy of its place in (human) society. A dog which knows its place is usually secure and content.

Within any family situation, a dog must occupy the *lowest* rung on the ladder of importance, i.e. below all human members of the family, adult or child. This is why anyone should be able to displace the dog from food, bed or play – to ensure that a happy stable relationship is maintained. Note that these actions should be carried out gently but firmly. They are not part of a game, but a crucial part of the young dog's education. Well-performed, they lay the foundations for an ideally behaved family pet.

The Newly-acquired Adult Dog

Many dogs are acquired as adult animals. In this case, much of the dog's fundamental behavioural and personality traits will already be formed. This does not mean that they cannot be changed because, above all, dogs are adaptable animals, but special considerations do apply. Specific problems are dealt with later in this chapter.

General considerations when acquiring an adult dog

- If possible, find out about the dog's background and any special problems. Trial periods may be possible, during which time you can assess whether the dog suits you and your family, or whether any unmentioned difficulties are present.

- Be aware that re-homing can be a stressful time for the adult dog. Give the dog time to settle and do not expect too much initially. 1–2 weeks is a reasonable time to allow for settling in.

- It can be very satisfying to give a rehomed dog a 'second chance' and to see the dog's character blossoming as it gradually gains confidence in its new home.

- Obvious problems such as aggression, dominance and extreme nervousness should be tackled early on, and with expert advice. These may affect any decisions about whether you can keep the dog. Remember that as the owner of a dog, you have a responsibility to ensure that the dog is safe and not a threat to other people or dogs.

Commonest Behavioural Problems in Dogs

AGGRESSION

Aggression in dogs is a complex problem and can have a number of causes. It is not simply the case of the dog just being 'bad' or 'wicked'. Aggression is a type of behaviour that is brought about by defined circumstances. The usual types of aggression are detailed below.

Dominance aggression to owner or family

This is a common form of aggression in dogs, often tolerated for a long time by owners who may eventually, and in desperation, request euthanasia of their pet because it has bitten a relative or child. In affected dogs, it is usually provoked by approaching the dog while it is eating, resting or guarding a toy. A dominant aggressive dog may also, for example, refuse to move from an owner's bed or chair.

This type of aggression reflects a failure of early socialisation (see earlier) and emphasises the necessity of ensuring that pet dogs are never allowed to become possessive over objects, places or, indeed, people.

Treatment outline

Expert help may be required but treatment depends on depriving the dog of initiative and control in the key areas of feeding, resting and exercise/play. Punishment is usually futile and could also be dangerous.

- The dog should be barred from sleeping in the bedroom and should instead be provided with a dog bed in another room.

- Periods of separation from the rest of the family should be implemented – the dog should be quietly taken to another room and left there for intervals. When reunited with the family, this should be done without fuss or attention. The dog is studiously ignored.

- Approaches made by the dog for attention, play, walks or food should be ignored by all members of the family. The dog can still have all these things but they must be initiated by the owner or members of the family at times when the dog is *not* seeking attention of any form. As treatment proceeds, requests for attention by the dog can be answered but only after the dog has responded to an obedience command.

- Obedience commands should be made before all feeding. The feeding time may be altered, i.e. the dog is not fed when he is expecting it.

• In male dogs, castration should be considered.

The overall aim is to reinstate the dog in its proper subordinate role in the household. Consistency is paramount. There is no point in one person implementing treatment if other family members are unwittingly undoing the good work; everyone must understand the objectives and work to achieve them if success is to result.

Aggression to other dogs

This, too, can be a complex disorder, often involving elements of territorial, fear and dominance aggression.

Treatment outline

Again, expert help may be required since slightly different approaches are used for different dogs.

• Castration should be carried out in male dogs.

• The owner should impose stronger dominance control over the aggressive dog in order to try to place the dog in a more stable subordinate role. The methods described above for dominance aggression are appropriate.

• Under careful supervision, and using a muzzle and 'Halti' head collar, aggressive dogs can be introduced to non-aggressive ones and distracted from

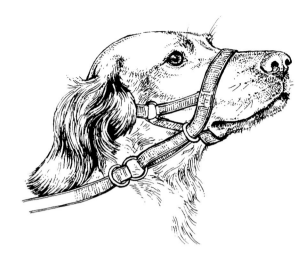

A 'Halti' is a humane way of controlling excitable dogs.

the undesirable behaviours. Useful distracting techniques include loud noises (e.g. whistles) and jets from a water pistol. Positive behaviours are well rewarded.

• This is a carefully staged process which must be repeated often with different dogs and in different situations.

A combination of the above techniques is usually effective in most dogs.

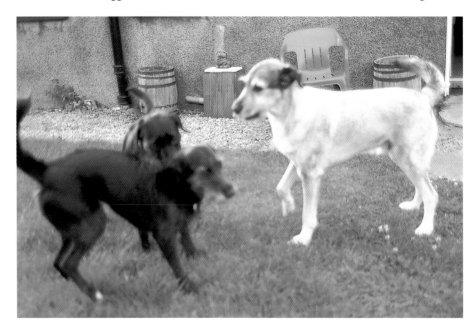

Three dogs at play, showing subtle signs of dominance and submissiveness that reinforce hierarchies.

Other dogs in the same house

Dogs are sometimes aggressive to another dog within the same household. In this situation, the owner should intervene and reinforce the dominant status of the dog which appears to be higher up in the pecking order. The reinforced dog receives generally preferential treatment: it is fed first, has its lead put on first, gets into the car first and is spoken to first, etc. The aim here is to try to create a stable hierarchy and, although it may seem 'unfair' that one dog is going to be preferentially treated, a stable pecking order is necessary for overall harmony! Many squabbles are in fact caused by the less dominant dog challenging the dominant one. The aim is to avoid all such interactions. The owner must 'take sides' in order to try to resolve this situation because if it cannot be sorted, the only alternative is rehoming one of the dogs.

Aggression to strangers or visitors

This is a type of territorial defence – a relic of natural defensive behaviours that are seen within wolf packs. In a real sense, the dog believes he is protecting his 'pack', i.e. the family. Although this does have a somewhat endearing quality to it, and is even erroneously encouraged by some owners, this can be a highly problematical behaviour and causes more trouble than it is worth.

> ❗ There is always the risk that serious injury could arise from this type of behaviour and could, justifiably, lead to euthanasia of the dog. Never take undue risks with a dog that may bite someone – fit a muzzle.

Treatment outline

- There is sometimes an element of dominance aggression in this behaviour, so owner dominance should be increased (see above) and castration considered.

- A muzzle must be used if the dog is in any way liable to bite strangers.

- Treatment consists of gradual introduction of strangers to the house while the dog is controlled using a lead, muzzle and 'Halti' headcollar.

- Initially, strangers should not approach the dog but should enter slowly, quietly and in a 'matter of fact' way, not making direct eye contact with the dog.

- Ideally, they would chat quietly with the dog's owner, while the dog slowly approaches and investigates them. During these interactions, the owner should give the dog obedience commands, telling the dog to sit, lie, etc. Rewards are given for appropriate responses. If safe to do so, the visitor can give commands and reward with treats when the dog obeys.

- This process must be built up slowly and repeated often in order to break down undesirable behaviour responses. Understanding friends are useful! Try to encourage a variety of people to visit, and at different times.

- Removal of the muzzle should be carried out after several sessions, when you are sure biting is not likely. The dog is still controlled using the lead and 'Halti' by the owner.

- With persistence, this behaviour can be improved. Patience – and safety – are the crucial factors.

Fearful aggression

This type of problem may be seen at the veterinary surgery: a normally sociable and placid dog bites because it is frightened or has been accidentally hurt. If fear is the only cause of the aggression, none of the other patterns described above is shown.

Treatment outline

- This problem is treated by gradually building up confidence in an unthreatening way. For example, the dog can be brought to the veterinary surgery (if that is the source of the problem) frequently, made a fuss of and given treats without any examination or restraint being carried out. In this way, the dog is gradually 'desensitised' to the stressful experience. (Most owners are only too glad not to have to return after a stressful experience with their dog at the vet, however to tackle the problem properly, harmless visits are necessary.)

257

- The same principle applies to other situations: build up tolerance by frequent, non-threatening exposure to the frightening situation. Exposure times should be very short initially (even just a few seconds), gradually increasing in length as confidence grows.

Predator aggression

This type of aggression could in some respects be thought to be 'natural'. It is seen, for example, in dogs chasing rabbits or squirrels (or cats). It is not however inevitable that dogs see these animals as prey; many dogs live peacefully alongside other species in the same house.

Undoubtedly, there are some strong breed influences here. Certain breeds – such as the sighthounds like Greyhounds and Lurchers – are strongly 'programmed' to chase and the sight of an animal running will provoke the chase response as instincts take over. Thus a Greyhound could live happily with a pet cat at home, yet still desire to chase one that ran away when outside. Breeds, and individual dogs, vary somewhat.

Variations of this behaviour can include chasing other things which some dogs view as prey: bicycles, cars, joggers, etc. Chasing farm animals such as sheep, poultry etc. can be a particular problem in the countryside and dogs have been shot by farmers while doing this.

Treatment outline

- There are usually few problems with other pets in the house. Dogs usually co-exist happily with cats (and, often, rabbits too) that they are used to. It is more difficult to guarantee that they will not chase unfamiliar animals outside, although if they do share a house with another species they are probably less likely to chase a member of that species outdoors.

- To a certain extent, general obedience training can help but this is not foolproof as many generally obedient dogs will not respond if they start chasing.

- Punishment by fright or surprise can help here, e.g. if a dog chases geese or swans and is attacked by one, this may well prevent future occurrences. Indeed, the dog may become frightened of them. However this cannot be relied upon to happen and

you should never deliberately allow your dog to chase another animal, even if you are hoping that a fright to the dog will be the result. The chased animal could become badly stressed or injured.

- Administration of shocks via electric collars has been tried in persistent chasers. It is controversial but may be very effective if properly applied in a controlled, knowledgeable way.

- Desensitisation using techniques described above for aggression towards other dogs can be successful. This depends on adequate facilities and controlled exposure to the animals concerned, and can only be justified when the animals used for the exercise are not unduly stressed by it.

> ## Summary of approaches for aggression
>
> In treating aggression it is important to identify what type of aggression is occurring and then to apply specific treatments directed at that. A consistent, co-ordinated approach is essential. Everyone involved must understand the objectives and work to achieve them. Predator-type aggression can be difficult to treat.
>
> Expert advice can help in all cases but unmanageable aggression may mean that euthanasia is the only sensible course of action.

DESTRUCTIVE BEHAVIOURS AND SEPARATION ANXIETIES

This group of behaviour problems occurs when dogs are left alone and can include:

- Chewing or destroying carpets, furniture, etc

- Excessive barking or howling

- Urinating or defaecating in the house

- Other behaviours in rarer cases, e.g. self-mutilation

The triggering factor is stress or anxiety caused by the owner leaving the dog. This can be a serious problem for dog owners, restricting their social lives and proving both expensive and frustrating. The problem is prevented in puppies by avoiding over-dependency and by getting the puppy used to being left alone for short periods from a very early age.

Most of the dogs exhibiting this behaviour are highly bonded to their owners – too much so, with the resultant effect that being left alone appears intolerable.

Treatment outline

A progressive schedule of reduction in dependency is important. Do not expect instant results, but perseverance usually pays off.

1. Overall, the dog should be given less of your time. When you are in the house spend less time with the dog and, importantly, when the dog approaches you for attention, do not respond all the time. The dog should be ignored or told to lie in its bed/basket for about 50% of the time when you would otherwise have given attention.

2. Introduce separation while in the home. Leave the dog in another room. Initially, this can be for only a few moments, building up gradually to several minutes, then 10–20 minutes and up to an hour. A low key reward can be given for good, quiet behaviour. Many destructive dogs shut in another room of the house will not destroy things if they can hear you moving around elsewhere in the house, as they will not become unduly anxious. This situation can therefore be manipulated by you to reward good behaviour when the dog has stayed quietly in a room by itself. The useful behavioural result of this exercise is that the effect is extended to relate to the times when you are both out of the room *and* out of the house.

3. Begin a programme of feigned leaving of the house, i.e. put on coat, collect car keys, etc. – but then disorientate the dog by sitting down and reading the paper or having coffee. This desensitises the dog to the subtle trigger signals which it associates with you getting ready to leave. These triggers lead on to the undesirable behaviour. Your exercises here mean that the connection between the triggers and the destructive behaviour is gradually broken down; the dog no longer associates these actions as a cue to start being destructive or noisy. (A similar effect is obtained by suddenly leaving the house for short spells *without* putting on coat, collecting things together, etc. This variation can also be used to good effect.)

4. Build in exits from the house to the training programme. Initially, leave only for a few moments. Literally go out, and come straight back in again. Do this frequently, gradually varying the time you stay away. **It is important that you do not fuss or speak to the dog immediately before you leave or soon after you come back**. Ten minutes or so after your return, the dog can be rewarded quietly.

5. Build up the time you remain away.

6. It is appreciated that a staged approach is not always practically possible. For example, appointments or employment may mean you have to leave the dog for longer than you would like to at that particular phase of its training programme. In practice, this does not seem to affect the outcome. Most dogs will still improve if the rest of the guidelines are followed.

Summary of approaches for separation behaviours

A gradual approach is required with the aim of 'tricking' the dog into being left alone and then rewarding good behaviour, but take care that the periods immediately before leaving and immediately after returning are marked by an indifference to the dog. Do not give undue attention at these times.

Overall, aim to give less attention to the dog in order to encourage it to become slightly more independent.

Note that it is pointless punishing destructive dogs for the damage they have done. They do not associate the behaviour with the punishment.

Drug therapy can be available for difficult cases. This should be used in conjunction with behavioural training, as outlined above, and is often successful.

Many dogs settle better if, for example, a radio or a light is left on. They associate these things with your presence in the house.

NERVOUS AND FEARFUL DOGS

There is a natural spectrum of behaviour in pet dogs, with some individuals being more confident and outgoing than others. These traits can even be recognised in young puppies (see page 251) and are part of the normal range of dog personality types.

Fight or flight

Problems occur when nervousness or fearfulness is so severe that it interferes with daily life and makes unavoidable situations very difficult. Sometimes, nervousness can manifest as aggression (see page 257). In other cases, the dog simply becomes very anxious or even terrified. Symptoms include trembling, panting, scrabbling and struggling to escape (even to the extent of running away from the owner across roads, etc.). In extreme cases, urine and/or faeces may be passed involuntarily. All of these, and aggression, are symptoms of the 'fight or flight' response dependent on a massive release of the hormone adrenaline.

To a large extent, these problems are prevented by a good socialisation process carried out in the young puppy, as described on page 252. When problems in this area arise, several general guidelines should be followed. Expert advice, and sometimes medication, can help in individual cases.

Treatment outline

• *Fear of the veterinary clinic*
First, ensure you are not unwittingly adding to the dog's distress by passing on anxieties of your own! The commonest occurrence of this is in the veterinary surgery when the owner thinks: 'I know he'll be terrified and misbehave. It's going to be embarrassing and difficult. I'll be so glad to get out!'

You own anxieties and subtle nervous behaviours are picked up by the dog. Of course, it is easy to say 'Don't be anxious' but harder to put into practice. Most veterinary staff however are very sympathetic to this problem and will go out of their way to try to help. Veterinary surgery anxiety is best treated by going there more often – not for treatment, but to get the dog thoroughly used to the place (even, if possible, slightly bored by it!). Popping in regularly,

for example to check your dog's weight, coupled with a doggy treat from the reception or nursing staff, can do wonders for this kind of anxiety.

• *Other situations*
In general, the same principles apply to other situations. The aim is to 'decondition' the dog by very gradually exposing it to the fearful situation and breaking down the connection with anxiety-related behaviour. Frequent repetition is necessary. At the beginning only *very short* exposures to the fearful situation are required. Above all, remain calm and detached yourself; this will ultimately give the dog confidence.

POOR TOILET TRAINING

If an adult dog which was previously reliable starts messing in the house, always suspect a medical problem first. This is more likely than a breakdown in toilet training. While the latter can occur in adult dogs – usually in sensitive dogs where some major disturbance in the household or family has occurred – it is, overall, less frequently seen than medical problems in this age group.

Housetraining puppies

A suitable initial house training programme is given below.

• Puppies have poor control over bowel or bladder function until 8–12 weeks of age. Up to this time, excretion is stimulated by the bitch licking the perineal area. House training cannot begin until after this time. Note that it is normal for the bitch to swallow urine and faeces from young puppies.

• Puppies nearly always pass urine and faeces after sleeping, and after eating. In initial training, you must be ready to act at these times (especially early in the morning!).

• Careful observation will allow you to detect subtle signs that the puppy wishes to relieve itself. There may be slight restlessness, a few whines, circling behaviour, etc. You must quickly and calmly lift the puppy outside at these times, or encourage it to walk out.

- It is very likely that the puppy will pass urine and faeces shortly after being taken outside if you have timed your actions correctly. If you give an encouraging command while the puppy is in the act of passing urine or faeces, it will soon learn to associate this with the activity and you should then have a dog which will go to the toilet on command – a very useful thing.

- Always praise copiously when the puppy has gone to the toilet in the correct place.

- Punishment – harsh words or surprise tactics (e.g. water spray or loud noise) – only work if you catch the puppy *in the act* of going to the toilet in the house. It is pointless punishing at any other time and may only confuse the dog.

- Training results in the puppy gradually associating outdoors with passing urine and faeces. There is also an instinctive tendency not to pass urine or faeces in the 'den' area (i.e. the house).

- Training is likely to take several months before it is completely reliable. Usually by about 6 months most dogs are well house trained.

Inadequate housetraining in young dogs

Occasionally, problems arise: the dog never seems to become properly housetrained or is very inconsistent. It is important to rule out medical problems here, especially where urination is concerned, since congenital problems such as ectopic ureter (see page 148) can lead to apparent housetraining problems. The problem may lie elsewhere and no amount of housetraining will help if this is the case.

Assuming medical problems have been ruled out, some additional training can often cure this problem.

Treatment outline

- Avoid all punishment unless the dog is 'caught in the act'. Even then, only harsh words or surprise tactics such as a water spray or a sudden unpleasant noise should be used – no physical punishment.

- Ensure soiled areas are cleaned using an enzyme-based or biological detergent designed to eliminate residual odour from the carpets. These are available from veterinary practices. The reason for their use is because dogs will tend to return to the same spot.

- Make sure your dog's life is organised so that it gets out frequently enough, and that ample praise is given for good behaviour whenever this occurs.

- Restricting the dog, temporarily, to an indoor kennel or cage with a bed and water bowl in it can be an effective training aid. Dogs are very unlikely to soil their own bed area. If the dog tends to soil when you are not in the house, the dog should be placed into its kennel or cage before you leave. On your return, the dog can be taken outside and praised for proper urination or defaecation outdoors. Usually a week or so of this routine will break old associations and form new ones.

- Some dogs may require additional treatment for separation anxiety problems (see earlier).

Urine marking in male dogs

This can be a persistent and difficult problem in a few male dogs. The dog is acting out an instinctive behaviour which involves placing small quantities of urine around its territory boundaries. A new dog in the neighbourhood may provoke this behaviour in a dog which has not previously been guilty of it.

When urine marking occurs within the house, it can be considerably inconvenient. As with other problems of this type, medical problems need to be ruled out. Cystitis, for example, can produce signs rather similar to this.

Treatment outline

- If there is thought to be an element of anxiety or dominance involved (e.g. the dog always indulges in the behaviour when a certain person visits the house) then desensitisation as described under aggression to strangers or visitors (see earlier) can be tried. Muzzles are unnecessary unless the dog is showing aggressive tendencies as well as urine marking.

- Reinforcing the social hierarchy within the home, as for the dominant dog, may also make the dog feel more secure in a subordinate role.

- Punishment in the form of reprimands or surprise tactics (water spray or loud, unpleasant noise) are appropriate if the dog is 'caught in the act'. Physical punishment is not helpful.

- Suitable biological detergents or enzyme-based products should be applied to soiled carpeting or furnishings to eliminate residual odour.

- Hormonal treatment or castration can often be effective.

EATING FAECES (COPROPHAGIA)

This problem causes a lot of distress for owners. It is however a natural phenomenon for bitches to eat their puppies' faeces, and young puppies may also do this out of curiosity. Usually, with toilet training, the problem disappears, especially if the dog is trained to defaecate on command and the faeces are lifted and disposed of.

Treatment outline

- Medical conditions should be ruled out as, occasionally, abnormal appetite can arise due to organ disease or poor digestion.

- Punishment in the form of a verbal reprimand, a squirt with a water pistol or making a sudden noise near the dog can be successful if 'caught in the act'.

- The diet can be bulked with fibre (e.g. raw vegetables) or a high fibre food fed.

- Adding vegetable oil to the diet may help.

- Iron or other dietary supplementation may be used on veterinary advice. The aim is to render the faeces unpalatable rather than treat any presumed deficiency (deficiencies are very unusual if the dog is being fed a good quality food). Once the dog associates the process with an unpleasant taste, the habit usually stops and the supplement can be discontinued.

POOR OBEDIENCE

This topic is a large one and there can be many causes. Consultation with a veterinary surgeon, animal behaviourist or reputable dog trainer who uses humane methods is advisable. It is important to be objective and to understand that your dog may be perceiving your responses in a different way than you think. For example, if your dog has run off chasing rabbits and refused to come when called, and then does eventually come back to you, punishment may not be interpreted by the dog as relating to the initial disobedience.

Persistent disobedience of this type may be able to manipulated and corrected using food rewards. In extreme cases, bowl feeding is reduced in amount by 50%. The remainder of the food is 'earned' by obedient behaviour when out of doors.

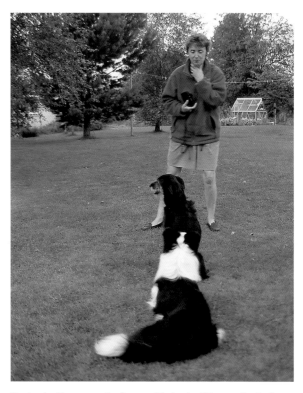

Basic obedience can be fun and helps build a good relationship between dog and owner.

Euthanasia

Introduction

Euthanasia is the painless killing of an animal; in dogs this is usually brought about by means of a lethal overdose of anaesthetic, administered directly into the bloodstream in exactly the same way as routine general anaesthetics are given. The only difference in euthanasia is that a massive dose of a very strong anaesthetic agent is used. The result is that the dog first loses consciousness and then the heart stops, bringing about painless death. The term 'putting to sleep' is often used for painless euthanasia.

For the dog, the process is no more distressing than a simple injection and they are likely to experience the same feelings that we do when receiving a general anaesthetic, usually a sensation of falling backwards or floating, that is not in itself unpleasant.

Euthanasia is one of the most important duties of any veterinary surgeon, since he or she will be called upon to perform this task on an almost daily basis. In most cases it is an act carried out to alleviate suffering, pain or distress in dogs that can no longer be treated effectively. It is thus an act of kindness when quality of life is poor and suffering inevitable. None of this, however, makes the decision to request euthanasia easy for the owner and there is no doubt that 'signing his life away' is the most painful decision one has to make as a pet owner.

As described on the flow chart on page 8, euthanasia becomes necessary when treatment is impossible or ineffective, or when various aspects combine to render quality of life poor. In some ways, decisions regarding euthanasia are easier or more straightforward in cases of severe and unrelenting disease, e.g. terminal cancer. More difficult decisions include older dogs who are thought to have no more enjoyment left in life, and who may have several on-going problems contributing to this, or in healthy dogs which have behavioural problems which the owner is unwilling or unable to manage, e.g. aggression. The hardest decisions of all are situations in which treatment may be available but is impossible due to high cost or impracticibility. For example, a highly specialised operation may be outwith the budget of some owners, an elderly owner may be unable to cope with the demands of a dog with diabetes or other serious disease, or administration and continuity of treatment may be impossible for various other reasons.

Owners of ill older dogs often deliberate for many weeks before requesting euthanasia, and decisions are made harder when old dogs seem to have bad days then good days. In many cases, however, the underlying trend is one of deterioration, and it is here that unbiased veterinary advice can greatly help in making this decision or in reviewing treatment in order to try to maximise the quality of life for a further period.

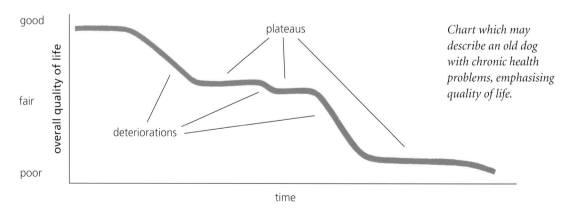

Chart which may describe an old dog with chronic health problems, emphasising quality of life.

good quality of life
• no pain
• bright and interested
• continent

fair quality of life
• pain controllable
• quieter but responsive
• occasional 'accidents'

poor quality of life
• chronic pain
• disinterested
• incontinent

Why can't dogs be allowed to die naturally?

Some dogs, especially old dogs that have perhaps been ill for some time may die naturally at home. Many owners hope that their pet may pass away 'in his sleep'. Unfortunately, this does not happen in the majority of cases and the main worry is that there may be unpleasant fear, suffering or panic before death, which could be distressing for both pet and owner. Euthanasia aims to eliminate this risk by allowing a pain and fear-free death by controlled injection. No one denies the difficulty of making such a decision but, having done it, many owners later view it as the last service they could do for their pet, giving them an easy way out from a life that has become painful or difficult.

When is the Right Time?

There is no simple answer to this question as various factors are involved with each individual dog. Some things which need to be considered and discussed with the veterinary surgeon and family members include:

- The nature of the disease or condition and its likely course and treatability.

- The response of the dog to treatment and, especially, whether pain can be adequately controlled.

- The presence of other distressing symptoms, e.g. breathing difficulty, problems in moving around, incontinence and psychological distress.

- Time for adjustment to the idea of losing the dog: this applies to both adults and children. If possible, without causing the dog further suffering, allowing a day or two to come to terms with the decision can often help people through this difficult time.

At Home or at the Veterinary Surgery?

Most dogs are euthanased ('put to sleep') at the veterinary surgery, where skilled assistance and facilities are to hand to aid the veterinary surgeon to ensure that the process is as peaceful as possible. However, there is no doubt that some owners feel more comfortable having their dog put to sleep at home, in a familiar environment and surrounded by known people and things. In most cases, this should be possible and the veterinary surgeon will make a home visit. This normally entails some additional cost and would need to be arranged for a time at which the veterinary surgeon could safely leave the clinic or hospital premises. Extremely nervous or aggressive dogs may however be difficult to handle at home, and it may be better that they are brought to the surgery at quieter times (such as the end of a clinic) so that additional time can be spent and help provided by nursing staff to reassure and steady the patient while the injection is given.

In certain instances, e.g. if a decision has to be made at night or if treatment is normally received at a busy animal welfare charity hospital, it may be very difficult to arrange a house visit without endangering the lives of other animals being attended to by the veterinary surgeon. In these situations, you may be asked to transport your pet to the clinic in the interests of other animals currently being treated there.

What Happens?

Once the decision to have a pet put to sleep is made, a consent form must usually be signed to confirm that the owner understands and authorises the procedure. Although this can be an upsetting thing to do – many owners feel bad about 'signing her life away' – it is a necessary formality. In this situation, try to remember that the decision is being made in the dog's best interests and that the form is required for ethical and legal reasons.

Usually, the veterinary surgeon will then explain briefly what will happen. In most cases, the dog will be made comfortable sitting or lying on the consulting table or, with larger dogs, perhaps on the floor. Most veterinary surgeons prefer a nurse to hold the dog as it is important that the injection is made correctly into the vein, but owners can be very close too, steadying the head or stroking the dog to provide reassurance. A small quantity of hair is clipped off from a front leg and the area swabbed. The nurse will then 'raise the vein' by applying gentle pressure in the elbow area to allow the veterinary surgeon to make the injection.

When the needle is correctly positioned, the veterinary surgeon will administer the injection. Most owners are surprised at how quickly an anaesthetic takes effect. Usually by the time the injection is being finished, the dog will have lost consciousness; the heart stops soon after. There may be a few deep breaths, even one or two that resemble short gasps. These are breathing reflexes of which the dog is totally unaware. In a few cases, especially in very ill dogs, these irregular breathing reflexes may continue for several minutes after consciousness is lost. They are upsetting only if one is not prepared for them. They happen because, with a sluggish or poor circulation, it takes a little longer for the strong anaesthetic overdose to take full effect. Although consciousness has been lost and the dog is unaware of anything, the breathing (respiratory) system takes longer to shut down. Other common occurrences are small muscular twitches which occur as the body fully relaxes and, occasionally, the passage of urine as the bladder relaxes. The eyes do not close naturally after death.

Should I stay with my dog?

If at all possible, it is preferable to stay with your dog while it is put to sleep. There are two reasons: the first is because it is obviously reassuring for the dog to have someone he knows close by while the injection is being given. The second is because the owner is also reassured by seeing how quick, painless and stress-free euthanasia is. This can be a considerable comfort after the event has taken place.

If however, you cannot bring yourself to stay or if in staying you may become so upset that you would cause anxiety to your dog, then it may be best not to be there, or to arrange for someone else who knows the dog well to take your place. In most instances, owners are glad that they have stayed even although it is naturally upsetting at the time.

If you have to leave your dog with the veterinary staff, you should be reassured that every effort will be made to make the procedure as stress-free as possible for your dog. Remember that veterinary staff have pets themselves: they know what it is like and will do their best to treat your dog like their own.

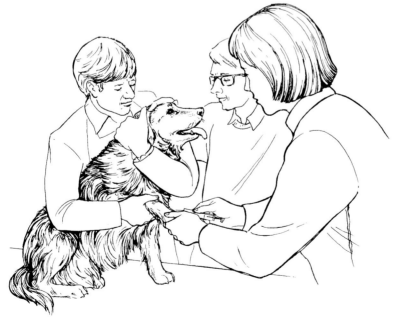

Euthanasia consists of a large overdose of anaesthetic solution injected directly into the bloodstream. The dog literally falls asleep.

The Very Nervous, Distressed or Aggressive Dog

Administering an intravenous (into the bloodstream) injection requires a certain amount of cooperation from the patient, as well as skill on the part of the veterinary surgeon and nurse. Most pet dogs do not find the process frightening or threatening. Sometimes, however, in very nervous, aggressive or distressed dogs, the procedure can be difficult if not impossible to achieve safely. In these situations, most veterinary surgeons will administer a sedative injection first. This small injection, usually given into a muscle or underneath the skin (like a routine vaccination), is simpler to administer and acts like an anaesthetic pre-med. After 20 minutes or so, the dog becomes very sleepy and relaxed and can usually then be safely and easily restrained for the final injection, avoiding stress on the part of the dog, owner and veterinary staff. During this 20 minute period, the owner can sit with the dog in a quiet place, reassuring it while it becomes sleepy. If you feel your dog may be very upset or difficult, you could warn the veterinary clinic in advance so that adequate time can be set aside to allow for sedation before euthanasia.

After Euthanasia has Taken Place

Once death has been confirmed by the veterinary surgeon, most owners wish to spend a few minutes with the body. It is natural to cry at this time and no one should feel awkward or embarassed about this. The veterinary surgeon will have seen this many times before and will be sympathetic. What happens next depends on the preferences of the owner. There are three main options.

Home burial

The body can be taken home for burial in the garden. Although this may be the 'ideal' option, it is often not possible for various reasons. There may not be a suitable garden available, or perhaps the act of burying the body is not possible or practical, e.g. a very elderly dog owner. However, when home burial is possible, it can be a comfort to know that a beloved pet has been laid to rest in a favourite place.

If the body is taken for home burial then it is best to wrap the dog in a large blanket and thick plastic bag (available from the veterinary practice) in case the bladder empties in the car on the way home.

Pet cemetries

Pet cemetries are becoming more popular for owners who feel that burial is the thing they would like for their dog. It is important to visit the cemetry beforehand so that you can see the surroundings, and have costs and procedures fully explained. It may be necessary for you to take your dog's body to the cemetry yourself prior to burial.

Cremation

Cremation is the option followed by most dog owners. Veterinary practices usually use local pet crematoriums who operate to high standards and provide a professional and caring service. The cremation staff collect pets' bodies from the veterinary practice and transport them to the crematorium where they are cremated. Prior to collection by the crematorium, bodies will be placed in impermeable clinical bags and kept in cold storage. This is necessary for hygiene and health and safety purposes at the veterinary practice.

Cremation can be carried out on a grouped or individual basis, depending on the owner's preference, and the ashes may be returned to the owner or scattered by the crematorium staff along with the ashes of other pets. It is usually possible for owners to transport their dog's body to the crematorium themselves if they wish, but bear in mind this may be some distance away and that receiving arrangements should be made with the crematorium beforehand.

The ashes from private cremations can be returned to the owner, who may scatter them or bury them in a suitable place. Private cremations are always more expensive than group cremations and ashes are usually returned to the owner in a small box or casket.

Many pet crematoriums welcome visits by animal owners. Often, this serves to reassure owners that

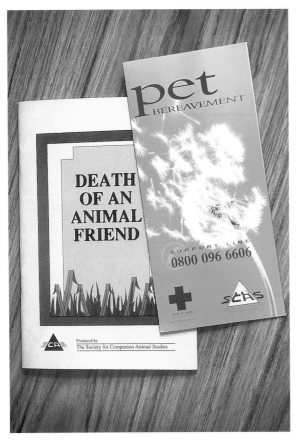

Finding a way of coping with pet loss is necessary after the death of a valued companion.

the crematorium is operating in a professional and respectful way.

Grief after Pet Loss

Loss of any companion animal is a painful and emotional experience. Dogs are long-lived species and loss of a canine companion after living with him or her for many years is a traumatic experience of grief. Such grief after pet death varies somewhat between owners. The severity and duration of symptoms of grief depends on the personality of the dog owner, the strength of the bond that existed between individual and dog, and other factors such as presence or absence of family, carers or close friends. Elderly dog owners without a support network of family or friends are at risk of the most serious effects of grief, as are other

isolated individuals. In these cases, loss of a pet dog can have a major effect on the pattern of that person's life. Without a dog, for example, an old person may have no reason to leave the house, to encounter other people or to follow any sort of regular daily routine. In a few instances, their own health can suffer adversely and they may even perceive that they have no real reason to live any more.

In most cases, however, initial symptoms of acute grief (including feelings of numbness, disbelief, shock and crying) gradually give way to acceptance of the situation and, eventually, an ability to think of the deceased dog without severe emotional upset. There is however no specific time span for this process; what is 'right' for one person may not be so for another and many people have extended periods of grieving and feelings of loss after the death of their dog. Some owners feel ashamed that they should be so upset and are perhaps even surprised at the intensity or duration of their own emotions, but any veterinary surgeon will testify to the range and complexity of the grieving process after pet loss.

Feelings of guilt and anger are also encountered reasonably frequently and often include thoughts such as:

- 'I should have realised she was sick earlier and taken her to the vet sooner.'

- 'I should have sought a second opinion. Perhaps my vet made a wrong diagnosis.'

- 'I let him go on too long before agreeing to euthanasia. His last few weeks were unpleasant.'

- 'I didn't follow the vet's advice exactly – that was what caused her to die. If she hadn't missed that tablet or if she had gone for that operation she might be alive.'

It is important to recognise these thoughts as being part of the grieving process. In many cases, reassurance can be sought from the veterinary surgeon that a correct decision was made at the right time, given individual circumstances. Additional information regarding the nature of the illness, the objectives of diagnostic tests and the prognosis of the condition can often help provide reassurance that a reasonable course of action was followed.

Many owners feel they are somehow to blame for their pet's illness and deterioration and that it was something that they did (or did not) do. Of course, there are cases of genuine neglect and deliberate cruelty with respect to pet animals, but these are very much in the minority. In most cases, one must accept that decisions in medicine are rarely black and white and that recognition of symptoms is difficult enough for veterinary surgeons, let alone owners, so that failure to spot a serious illness is not a failing of pet ownership, merely a fact of the nature of disease. Similarly, decisions about when, and how, to treat individual diseases are not always black or white. A large range of different factors come into play and what may be the correct decision for one owner may not be the correct one for another. Discussing the matter fully with family, friends and veterinary surgeon usually helps to alleviate anxieties that the wrong thing was done.

Response of children

Many owners worry how much or little to tell their children and are anxious about the effect the death of the family dog will have upon them. For many children, this may be their first experience of death and loss and thus is highly significant and important. In general, the best response is to be as open and honest as possible, explaining the nature of the disease and decision in a simple way. Many veterinary surgeons and nurses will be willing to try to help with this and children could be involved in the euthanasia consulta-tion if they wished. In this way expression of their grief is allowed and acknowledged. Children could also be encouraged to come to terms with their grief through actions and ceremony, e.g. writing a story/ poem, painting a picture or using past photographs to tell the story of the dog's life. Burying the dog at home provides an opportunity and focus for this process. Alternatively, burying or scattering ashes, burying the dog's lead and bowl or planting flowers or a tree in a favourite place can be used in the same way to give direction and focus to childrens' grief.

Engaging with the process in whatever way seems appropriate will, for many children, be healthier than avoiding the issue entirely.

Severe grief after pet loss in adults

In situations where the grieving process is especially severe or prolonged, additional help and support should be sought. Grief counselling of this type is becoming an accepted part of modern veterinary practice as the complexities of the human-companion animal bond are investigated. As mentioned above, such additional help may intially simply take the form of extra reassurance from veterinary staff that correct decisions were made, but where this general form of support is insufficient, contact numbers of individuals and organisations who exist to help with the situation of severe grief should be obtained from the veterinary practice. Trained counsellors can then provide support, space and time to allow the grieving owner to finally come to terms with his or her loss.

First Aid

Effective first aid can save a dog's life. The 'ABC' of saving a life, discussed on page 274, is applicable to any animal or, indeed, human. First aid can also prevent other conditions from worsening before professional veterinary advice can be sought. The commonest situation of this type is the dog that injures itself while out on a walk or the non-life threatening condition which occurs at a time when it would be impossible or inconvenient to call out the veterinary surgeon. Chapter 18 provides an outline of basic first aid/medical techniques in different common situations likely to be encountered by the dog owner.

Homoeopathy

Homoeopathy is an ancient form of medicine that utilises very dilute concentrations of drugs and substances to cure illnesses or control symptoms. Homoeopathic medicines in low potency are available 'over the counter' in many pharmacies and health shops, and can be a useful addition to the dog owner's first aid kit. Homoeopathy is available for people on the National Health Service and there are hospitals specialising in homoeopathy in major cities, e.g. Glasgow and London. When homoeopathy could be used by the dog owner in a first aid situation, this is mentioned under the relevant condition.

CHAPTER 18

Practical First Aid and Homoeopathy

for Emergencies and Common Health Problems

How Does Homoeopathy Work?

One of the controversies surrounding homoeopathy is that the precise mode of action of the remedies is not known, although there are several ideas. However, the exact mode of action of some conventional drugs also remains a mystery, so this alone is not grounds for dismissing homoeopathy as a potentially useful form of treatment. There seems little doubt that the technique does work in animals and people, when applied correctly, but the skilled use of homoeopathy requires years of training and a thorough knowledge of disease and medicine in the widest sense. In giving homoeopathic remedies, you are unlikely to do any harm to your pet unless you do not also seek professional advice. In other words, homoeopathy should be seen as a **complementary** rather than **alternative** medicine. Never delay seeking veterinary advice because you have given a homoeopathic product, even if it appears to be working well. You could be risking your dog's health.

In simple terms it is possible that the remedies work by 'showing' the body something which causes a disease in such a way that the body is activated to fight the disease or condition more effectively. There are clear parallels with vaccination here, but in homoeopathy substances are diluted to a much higher extent than conventional vaccines. Thus, to take a simple example, the homoeopathic treatment for arsenic poisoning would be the administration of a highly diluted and activated solution of arsenic. This may seem odd at first – treating a disease using something that would ordinarily *cause* the disease – but the important aspect is the massive dilution process and the chemical or electrical changes that are thought to occur as this takes place. When the remedy is given, the body is then 'shown' arsenic in such a way that it is able to respond better to the toxicity it is suffering from. This same basic principle applies to other diseases and symptoms. An effective prevention and treatment for travel sickness, for example, is Petroleum in homoeopathic preparation, indicating that many dogs experience unpleasant symptoms from the smell of petrol, which they are presumably much more aware of due to a far more acute sense of smell.

Controversy surrounds the subject, yet homoeopathy seems to work much more frequently than would be expected by mere chance. A very effective homoeopathic remedy used a lot in human and animal first aid is Arnica. This remedy is mentioned frequently below and if only one remedy was to be purchased and kept for first aid situations, Arnica would be the best choice. This remedy, when taken for severe muscular bruising, stiffness and bleeding or after dental or any other form of surgery or trauma, seems to be highly effective at relieving symptoms in most cases.

Important word of caution

Homoeopathy is not a substitute for professional veterinary advice and care. Although this form of medicine can be used in the treatment of difficult and chronic conditions, this is best left to veterinary surgeons specialising in the technique otherwise important symptoms that required conventional medical treatments (e.g. intravenous fluid therapy), as well as homoeopathy, may be missed. Unfortunately, dogs' lives have been lost by owners attempting to treat serious conditions homoeopathically, perhaps with the aid of a book or via the internet, when quite different forms of treatment were actually called for. Similarly, you should ensure that any person offering to treat your dog with homoeopathic medicines is a qualified vet as well as a homoeopath. If you have used homoeopathic medicines on your dog as part of simple first aid, let your veterinary surgeon know. They will not interfere with conventional treatments given – this is one of the advantages of homoeopathy in the first aid situation.

Administering homoeopathic medicines and potencies

Homoeopathic medicines are sensitive products and should not be handled as perspiration from human skin may affect them. The easiest way to administer them is to tip a tablet onto a clean dry spoon. Another spoon is then used to crush the tablet into a fine powder, and then the powder is placed on the gums or in the mouth, where it quickly dissolves. Alternatively, a mortar and pestle can be used to powder the tablet.

Certain homoeopathic products are available in solution (e.g. Arnica) and as creams, but the most common form is as tablets. The medicine is quickly absorbed into the system from powdered tablets applied in the mouth.

Homoeopathic medicines come in various potencies. However, over-the-counter products are generally only available in low potency form; higher potencies are for specialist use. The common potencies used in animal first aid, and available from pharmacies, health stores etc., are known as 6C and 30C potencies. Either of these are suitable for first aid use; 30C is of higher potency than 6C. The frequency of dosing may vary depending on the nature of the problem. Generally, more serious conditions require more frequent dosing, sometimes as often as every 10 minutes. Guidelines on frequency of dosing are given under the relevant conditions.

A list of suitable remedies for a basic homoeopathic first aid kit is given below. With just a few common remedies, most of the frequently encountered first aid situations can be treated in a simple, safe way whilst awaiting professional veterinary assessment and care. Arnica and Aconite are mentioned most frequently as these are two remedies particularly appropriate for simple first aid use.

Suggested remedies for basic homoeopathic first aid kit

Most useful	Also useful
Arnica	Carbo veg
Aconite	Ignatia
Apis mel	Pulsatilla
Nux vomica	Petroleum
Arsen alb	

Several other remedies are mentioned in the text.

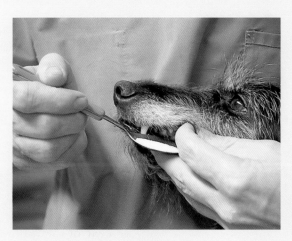

Giving a homoeopathic remedy by placing the powdered tablet into the lip fold. Most dogs readily accept this method.

273

Common First Aid and Emergency Situations

How to handle an emergency

The best advice is to 'Think slow, but act fast'. In other words, try not to panic, make sure your actions are well thought out and then put them into action as quickly as possible.

Above all:

- Never put yourself in a position of danger. Always seek help. Remember that shocked and injured dogs may bite, so be prepared to use a muzzle or place a secure tie around the dog's nose while you are trying to help. This will do the dog no harm and could enable you to provide more effective first aid.

- Take great care near traffic, water or ice. These are potentially highly dangerous situations and people have been killed attempting to rescue dogs. If in doubt, phone for help and observe the situation until a safe attempt at rescue can be made. Never venture onto ice or into deep or moving water.

The 'ABC' Guide to Saving a Collapsed Dog's Life

The 'ABC' routine refers to the sequence that is gone through when you encounter an injured or collapsed dog. By working through the sequence, you attend to the most serious, and life-threatening, conditions first. It ensures you do not concentrate on the wrong thing initially.

A = AIRWAY

The airway is the route for air entering the lungs. Without a supply of oxygen the dog will quickly die, so it is important to ensure there are no obstructions here. This is the first priority when you see a collapsed dog.

Common obstructions to the airway

- Swallowed stones

- Swallowed toys

- Swallowed bones

- Swelling after a sting in the throat

- Vomit in a collapsed dog

Action to take when there is an airway obstruction

1. Examine the nostril, mouth and throat areas.

   - *Warning* Make sure you do not get bitten as semi-conscious dogs will not be aware what they are doing.

2. Hold or prop the mouth open to visualise the throat area. An assistant can help here, e.g. by using loops of a dog lead around the upper and lower jaws to hold open the mouth, or else use any convenient object to wedge between the teeth in order to avoid being bitten.

3. Pull the tongue well forward.

4. Remove any objects seen. Balls are best removed by pushing forwards and upwards from the underside of the throat area.

5. Seek veterinary help immediately.

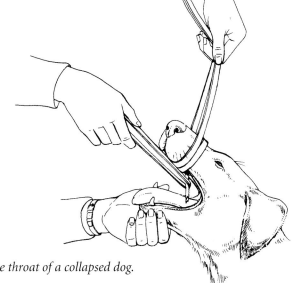

> ### Homoeopathic First Aid
>
> Homoeopathy is not appropriate in airway obstructions. The priority is to remove the physical obstruction. Once the obstruction is relieved, treatment for shock could be started while transporting the dog to the veterinary clinic:
>
> *Aconite*, one tablet crushed onto the gums every 10–15 minutes

Removing an object lodged in the throat of a collapsed dog.

B = BREATHING

Is the dog breathing?

- Look carefully at the chest to detect movements.

- Place your hand or a small piece of cotton at the nostrils to detect air flow.

Action to take when there is no breathing

1. Extend the dog's neck and pull the tongue well forward.

2. Close the dog's mouth, cup your hands around the nose and blow forcefully into the nostrils (around 15–20 times per minute).

3. Check for a heart beat by placing the flat of your hand against the chest.

4. If there is none, fold a jersey, towel or other object and place it underneath the dog, between the chest and the floor or ground. Compress the chest wall just behind the elbow (around once every 1–2 seconds).

5. Keep checking for breathing and a heart beat.

6. Seek veterinary help immediately.

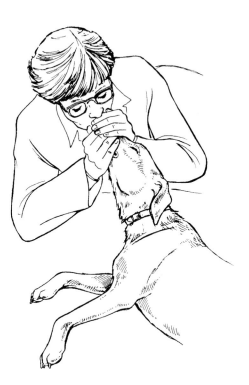

Mouth-to-nose resuscitation of a collapsed dog.

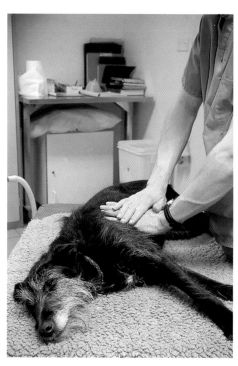

This photograph shows how to compress the chest in a collapsed dog. This technique is combined with mouth-to-nose resuscitation.

Homoeopathic First Aid

Assisting respiration and heart beat using the methods described above takes priority. If extra help is available, or while transporting the dog to a veterinary clinic, treatment for shock and collapse can be given:

Aconite, one tablet crushed onto gums every 10 minutes

Carbo veg, one tablet crushed onto gums every 10 minutes

C = CIRCULATION

Circulation refers to the dog's blood volume. Is there any bleeding?

- Arterial bleeding occurs in waves in time with the heart beat. The blood is bright red and tends to spurt.

- Venous bleeding (commoner) occurs as a continuous slow flow. The blood is slightly darker.

- When there is severe internal or external bleeding, the gums will be pale, even white.

Action to take when there is bleeding

1. Apply firm pressure to the bleeding area for 5–10 minutes using any clean item available, e.g. paper towel, handkerchief, etc. In emergencies, anything can be used as infection is less of a worry than blood loss. Infection can be treated later using antibiotics, but severe blood loss could prove fatal. Make sure the direct pressure you apply is firm enough, is applied over the bleeding point and is continuously maintained.

2. If possible, apply a bandage to the area (easiest on limbs). If blood seeps through the bandage, apply more and firmer layers, do not take off previous layers. Ideal bandages consist of absorbent materials (e.g. cotton wool) and fabric/stretch bandages to hold this firmly in place, but anything can be improvised in emergency situations, e.g. torn sheets, socks etc.

3. Severe bleeding on the lower limbs can be stemmed by applying a firm tourniquet above the bleeding point. Fabric, rope or bandage can be used. The material is wound on just firmly enough to slow/stop the bleeding below. The wound is then covered as above.

4. Keep the patient warm and quiet.

5. Seek veterinary advice immediately.

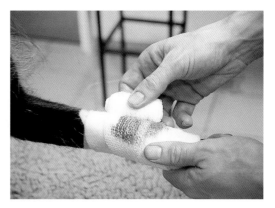

Bandaging is wrapped firmly around a bleeding wound. Improvised bandages may be needed if a first aid kit is not to hand.

Homoeopathic First Aid

Once bleeding has been dealt with, and while transporting the dog to a veterinary clinic, homoeopathic treatment for blood loss and shock can be started:

Arnica, one tablet crushed onto gums every 10 minutes

Aconite, one tablet crushed onto gums every 10 minutes

BITES AND OTHER WOUNDS

These can vary enormously in severity: from mild surfaces grazes to deep penetrating wounds. Often, it is the small, deep puncture wounds which are the most serious, and painful. These may not look as dramatic as gaping, open gashes, but often the potential for serious damage such as abscesses and cellulitis is greater with puncture-type wounds. Especially worrying are bite wounds of this type in the chest area inflicted by large dogs on smaller ones. These can be life-threatening injuries if they cause lung collapse or bruising of the heart muscle.

FIRST AID First aid is appropriate in dogs which seem well other than having the skin wound.

Check that the breathing seems normal, that the dog is bright and responsive, able to move around and willing to eat and drink. In these instances professional veterinary treatment is not immediately necessary. The wounds can be carefully clipped of hair and bathed using copious amounts of tepid saline or water. A routine veterinary appointment can be made and homoeopathic treatment started in the meantime. Open wounds should be covered or bandaged if bleeding is severe.

If there are signs of severe pain, breathing irregularity, shock or distress, urgent help should be sought.

HOMOEOPATHIC FIRST AID Two common remedies are very useful in this situation. Aconite and Arnica are invaluable for shock and bruising. Both can be given every hour until veterinary advice is sought. Ideally give both together for the first 2 hours then switch to Arnica alone.

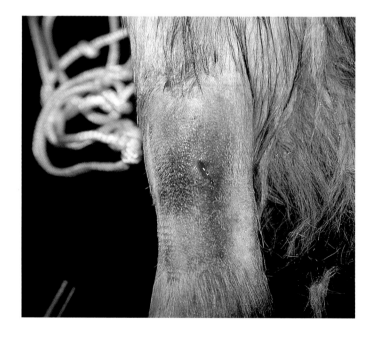

A small puncture wound in a stray dog. Underneath, the damage was much worse: the tibia (shin bone) was broken.

BURNS AND SCALDS

The commonest causes of this injury are accidents involving spilt hot water and dogs which have encountered fires at home. Often, the extent of skin damage in this type of injury is much worse than it initially appears. All dogs which have been burned should receive urgent veterinary assessment as they can quickly enter shock and may also be suffering severe pain.

FIRST AID If possible the scalded or burned area should be showered in cool/cold water and/or ice packs applied. Ice packs (e.g. frozen peas) can be held over the area while the dog is transported to the veterinary clinic.

HOMOEOPATHIC FIRST AID Treatment for shock is indicated: Aconite, one tablet every 15 minutes. Apis mel, as for stings, can also be useful for this injury.

CHOKING/OBJECT STUCK IN THROAT

Signs of this life-threatening problem are gagging, retching, salivating, difficulty breathing and incessant pawing at the mouth.

FIRST AID See under 'Airway' in the ABC guide to saving a life, above. Unless you can safely restrain the dog to allow wide opening of the mouth and retrieval of the stuck object, it is best to proceed immediately to a veterinary clinic. If you are attempting removal – and this should be tried if at all possible in serious emergencies – the dog's mouth can be wedged firmly open (e.g. using a piece of wood) or held open by an assistant using a looped dog lead or chain around the upper and lower jaws to allow clear examination of the mouth and throat. Firm restraint will be necessary to help the distressed dog.

If the dog collapses and appears comatose, swift removal of the object followed by resuscitation as described above may well be successful.

Sharp objects such as fish hooks are best removed under anaesthetic by the veterinary surgeon. They are unlikely to cause rapid death by suffocation in the same way as a ball or other large object lodged in the throat.

EYE INJURIES

Eye injuries should always be urgently assessed by a veterinary surgeon due to the catastrophic consequences of blindness. Blunt injuries are usually more dangerous than sharp penetrating ones, as more general damage is done to the eye. Squash faced breeds, especially Pekinese, are susceptible to prolapse of the eyeball, and these breeds should never be lifted by the scruff of the neck as the tension on the skin tends to open the eye orifice and displace the eyeball forwards, risking prolapse.

FIRST AID Only limited first aid should be attempted. The eye can be covered with moistened cotton wool or a swab while the dog is taken to a veterinary clinic. Ensure that the dog does not inflict more damage to the eye during transportation.

In cases of prolapse of the eyeball, it may be possible to replace the eye immediately after the incident, before swelling makes this difficult or impossible. An assistant can gently hold the eyelids apart while the dog owner pushes the eye back into the socket using a moistened pad or swab. If the dog struggles, abandon the attempt and go straight to the veterinary clinic.

HOMOEOPATHIC FIRST AID Many remedies work well for the eye but their choice should be left to the specialist veterinary surgeon. Effective first aid treatment can be started using Aconite and Arnica every 10–15 minutes before veterinary attention is sought.

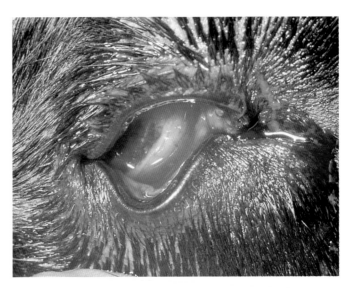

Eye injuries should always be treated as emergencies owing to the great sensitivity of this organ.

FEAR AND ANXIETY

This problem is covered in Chapter 16, Behaviour Problems, for more general causes of fear and anxiety. In otherwise normal dogs, excessive fear can be brought on by sudden frightening events. The commonest one is the letting off of fireworks, and some dogs suffer weeks of distress around November in the run up to Guy Fawkes night or at other times of the year when fireworks are used, such as New Year. For the extreme case, sedatives can be obtained from the veterinary surgeon, assuming there are no clashes with other medication the dog is receiving.

First aid Reassurance, avoiding taking the dog outside, playing music or having the television on and the presence of another animal that is not bothered by the fireworks can all help. Some owners have placed cotton wool plugs in their dogs' ears. There is obviously a slight risk these could be inserted too deeply, requiring veterinary attention for removal, so this is best avoided.

Homoeopathic first aid Fear and anxiety can be a complex response. It may be possible to find a remedy that works well for an individual dog's problems, but this is a specialist task, though undoubtedly worth it in many cases. More general remedies include: Aconite (for thunder/loud bangs); Pulsatilla (for shy, timid dogs); Gelsemium (fear of the car); Ignatia (fear of being alone, also bereavement); Silicea (fear of veterinary premises). Dosing should, ideally, be started before the frightening stimulus and repeated at 1–2 hour intervals.

Many more remedies can be tried for fears and anxieties as this type of homoeopathic prescribing works on 'mentals' (i.e. psychological states), which vary greatly between individuals. Expert help from a practising veterinary homoeopath can often be worthwhile.

FITS/CONVULSIONS

Fits and convulsions are discussed fully in Chapter 10. These symptoms can be caused by nervous system disease (e.g. epilepsy and brain tumours, see pages 180, 184), poisonings (e.g. slug baits containing metaldehyde), infectious diseases (e.g. distemper, page 21) and metabolic problems (e.g.eclampsia in lactating bitches, page 242). The veterinary surgeon will try to establish a cause for the fits but the first aid action remains the same.

First aid Ensure that the fitting dog cannot damage itself: remove dangerous objects and obstructions from the vicinity. The room should be darkened and kept quiet. Typical fits caused by epilepsy last around 5 minutes (see page 180), but other causes may lead to continuous fitting, for which emergency treatment must be sought. When transporting the fitting dog, hold the patient firmly but gently, perhaps wrapped in a blanket. Ensure that there is a good supply of air.

In very pregnant or recently whelped bitches, eclampsia should always be considered as a cause of fits/convulsions.

Homoeopathic first aid A variety of homoeopathic medicines may be tried with epilepsy, particularly if the patient is proving difficult to stabilise with conventional drugs, but prescribing these is a specialised procedure. If eclampsia is the cause, Calc phos, one tablet powdered onto the gums every 10 minutes, can be used while transporting the dog to the veterinary surgery for a life-saving injection of calcium.

HYPERTHERMIA/HEATSTROKE

The commonest cause of this potentially fatal condition is a dog being shut inside a car. Temperature and humidity can increase rapidly inside in a car, even when the weather outside is not particularly hot. Windows and/or sun roofs should always be left open or, better still, remove the dog from the car except for short periods.

Other causes of hyperthermia are:

- Muzzled dogs which are unable to pant.

- Dog having fits or convulsions: the muscular energy involved in this causes hyperthermia. Many bitches suffering from eclampsia have very high temperatures.

- Over-exercised or excited dogs, especially in hot weather.

- Overweight dogs and brachycephalic breeds such as Boxers, Bulldogs, Pugs, etc. These breeds have anatomically compressed upper respiratory systems which prevent efficient heat loss in stressed states or warm environments.

- Infections may result in very high temperatures.

First aid Immediate cooling is necessary using cool water sprays, soaks or wet towels. Air fans are also helpful. When applying water, concentrate on the feet, face and chest areas. Offer water or oral hydration replacement fluids to drink, ideally with ice cubes added.

NOSEBLEED

This occurs occasionally in dogs, most often as a result of trauma while running/playing or after violent sneezing.

First aid Keep the dog quiet and elevate the nose slightly. Cold packs over the nose can help.

Homoeopathic first aid Arnica is a useful remedy here; Carbo veg can be used if the bleed is associated with severe sneezing. Both should be given every 5–10 minutes until bleeding stops.

POISONING

Dogs may eat or drink a wide variety of poisons. They may lick dangerous substances off their paws or coat, eat dead animals which have been poisoned (and thus poison themselves) or actually ingest dangerous substances directly, e.g. slug baits. Dogs may also eat human medicines left within their reach.

Various symptoms can be produced, depending on the poison. Severe vomiting, diarrhoea, salivating, weakness, collapse and fits/convulsions are amongst the commoner ones. Caustic substances may cause ulceration of the mouth, nose and throat areas. Rat poisons may interfere with blood clotting and cause internal or external bleeding which can prove fatal.

FIRST AID If you have witnessed a dog taking in poison, or suspect that this has recently happened, the dog should be made to vomit. A concentrated solution of salt or baking soda should be given by mouth; this will often provoke vomiting and will limit further absorption of the poison into the dog's system.

However do not waste valuable time if you cannot manage to administer the emetic. Veterinary help should be sought immediately. If at all possible, take a sample of the poison (wear gloves) or the chemical container with you so that the veterinary surgeon knows what they are dealing with and what antidote, if any is available, to give.

Any contamination of the coat or feet should be copiously shampooed and rinsed off and the dog must be prevented from licking the affected areas. If acid, alkali or caustic burns to the mouth have occurred, it may be possible to repeatedly swab out the mouth using water-soaked cotton wool wads if the dog's temperament will allow.

HOMOEOPATHIC FIRST AID Advanced homoeopathy can utilise potentised preparations of toxins to help the body recover from a poisoning episode. This depends on knowing what the original toxin was, and is not applicable to the first aid situation. In most cases, general supportive therapy using conventional medicine and antidotes (when available) is the most appropriate course of action for poisonings.

ROAD TRAFFIC ACCIDENT AND FRACTURES/ DISLOCATIONS

Dogs involved in road traffic accidents can be assumed to be in shock. After checking through the 'ABC' routine, follow the guidelines for shock below.

FIRST AID If fractures are present, it is safer to move the dog on a board or blanket stretcher. Signs of fractures include inability to stand or walk, abnormally shaped legs or joints and open wounds on the legs. Bone dislocations produce similar signs.

In most cases, it is best not to try to apply a splint to a suspected broken leg or dislocated joint. Instead, try to encourage the dog to adopt the most comfortable position and take care that the injured area is not moved or stressed when lifting the dog. Sometimes, dogs may prefer to lie on the fractured leg since the ground underneath acts as a splint and prevents painful movement of the fractured bone ends below the skin.

- *Warning* It is safest to apply a makeshift muzzle when attempting to move or examine any dog that has been involved in a road traffic accident as the dog may bite if inadvertantly hurt while being helped. Any suitable material (e.g. tie, shoe laces) can be tied securely around the dog's nose if a proper muzzle is not available. In most cases, this will not interfere with breathing and will allow more effective first aid to be carried out.

HOMOEOPATHIC FIRST AID Arnica is particularly indicated when there are fractures, bruising, tissue damage or bleeding. It can be given along with Aconite, repeating every 10 minutes until veterinary attention is sought.

Serious fracture of the humerus following a road traffic accident.

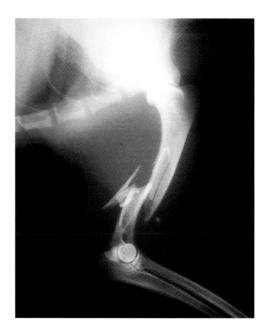

SHOCK

Shock is the medical term for life-threatening changes which can occur in the bodies of injured or very ill animals. The main problem in shock is failure of organ and tissue function due to lack of oxygen. Shocked animals are usually collapsed, cold and poorly responsive to stimulation. The gums may be pale or bluish and breathing may be rapid and irregular or very slow. Shock can arise from many different types of injury and disease; it can be gradual or sudden in onset. A common cause of shock is internal or external blood loss (haemorrhage) or profound dehydration arising from protracted vomiting and diarrhoea, especially in small patients.

FIRST AID Shocked patients should be taken to a veterinary clinic as soon as possible. The 'ABC' routine above should be followed and any obvious bleeding stopped. The dog should be warmed up, e.g. covered with blankets, use of warm water bottles, use of bubble wrap insulation, etc. Attempts should be made to keep the dog conscious, such as talking to it, reassuring it, and so on. If possible without distressing the dog, the patient should be positioned with the head slightly lower than the rest of the body.

Have someone warn the veterinary practice that you are on your way with a collapsed dog.

HOMOEOPATHIC FIRST AID Aconite is useful in shock; in dogs which appear comatose Carbo veg can be used. Powder should be applied to the gums every 10 minutes. If bleeding is present, Arnica can be given in addition to the other two remedies.

SNAKEBITES

Although most snakes will take cover when humans or dogs approach, inquisitive dogs may provoke a snakebite, usually receiving this on the nose, muzzle or feet areas. In the UK, adder bites can occur and in other countries and climates, a wide variety of poisonous snakes may be encountered.

Swelling often occurs at the site of the bite and this can be very severe and rapid in onset. As toxins are absorbed into the dog's body, other symptoms may then occur. This obviously depends on the species of snake that has bitten, and also the quantity of venom received, but symptoms such as vomiting, disorientation, fits, dilated pupils and shock/collapse are all possible.

FIRST AID First make sure that you are not at risk yourself. A threatened snake will strike out at anything which approaches. Call your dog from a distance or distract its attention by means of shouting, throwing objects, etc.

Only general first aid measures can usually be applied whilst veterinary advice is sought as quickly as possible. The main priorities are to keep an open airway and encourage breathing. Treatment and resuscitation for shock may be required at the veterinary clinic if large doses of toxin have been received.

If antitoxins are available, these may be administered if it is known which species of snake caused the bite. It is not usual for UK vets to keep doses of adder antitoxin unless bites occur frequently in the local area.

HOMOEOPATHIC FIRST AID Arnica and Aconite are appropriate and useful remedies. Aconite should be given first, one tablet every 5–10 minutes, whilst transporting the dog to a veterinary surgeon. After 3–4 doses of Aconite switch to Arnica, 1 tablet every 20 minutes until professional attention is received.

If snakes are frequently encountered, Cedron and Echinacea may be added to the first aid kit and used if a bite occurs.

SPRAINS/STRAINS

Sprains or strains can occur in athletic dogs exercising vigorously or in other animals when they perform an incoordinated movement or after a minor fall. Various structures can be affected: muscles, tendons or ligaments – the supporting 'soft tissue' structures which surround and connect the bones and joints of the skeleton.

Sprains and strains usually produce a fairly mild lameness although occasionally the limp or pain can be more severe, especially at first. It is often difficult to be sure that more serious injury (e.g. fracture/dislocation or ligament rupture) has not occurred, so veterinary examination is advisable to rule these out especially if the problem does not seem to be clearing up quickly. X-rays may be needed.

FIRST AID Strict rest and restricted lead exercise are very important. The dog should be confined to one room and exercised on the lead for toilet purposes only. Usually this needs to be kept up for 7–10 days to give the injured muscles, tendons or ligaments time to recover fully. Beware of allowing the dog to do too much too soon, especially if painkillers have been prescribed – this could result in a return of the problem, perhaps worse than before. Applying cold packs (e.g. bags of frozen peas) to affected areas for 20 minutes 4 times daily can often help a great deal in the first few days; alternating hot and cold treatments can also be beneficial. After a suitable period, a gradual return to more normal exercise is allowed.

HOMOEOPATHIC FIRST AID Homoeopathy has a good reputation for these types of injury and by far the most useful remedy is Arnica. One tablet given 4 times daily for 3–5 days will help most cases considerably. Other remedies, such as Rhus tox, are also possible but in general Arnica should be reached for first in every case.

STINGS AND ACUTE ALLERGIC SKIN REACTIONS

Bee, wasp or nettle stings are relatively frequent in summer and early autumn. Sometimes the dog is seen being stung by an insect, at other times a sting is inferred from soft swellings around the face, muzzle or paws or, in short-coated dogs, on the body. Nettle rash (urticaria) is also seen in dogs and is an acute allergic-type reaction that can occur when contact is made with nettles or various other plants. The dog's skin comes out in blotches of raised swollen skin.

In most instances, stings are not life-threatening and simple first aid may be the only treatment that is needed. The swellings disappear over a day or two. The exception is any sting or suspected sting in the throat area caused by the dog attempting to swallow an insect. This can lead to swelling of the throat which could be sufficient to cause suffocation, and is obviously an emergency.

FIRST AID Bathing affected areas in cold water or applying ice packs helps reduce the swelling. Wasp stings, being alkaline, should be bathed with a dilute acid such as vinegar or lemon juice; bee stings are acidic and should be bathed with bicarbonate of soda. Look carefully for the bee sting which remains in the dog and remove it with tweezers if possible. Wasp stings are retracted after the sting has been made.

HOMOEOPATHIC FIRST AID Apis mel tablets can be given; one tablet is crushed onto the gums 4 times daily for 2 days. The stung area can also be bathed in Hyper-cal solution or Arnica lotion.

For nettle rash or a general skin reaction, Urtica is given: 1 tablet 4 times daily for 2 days.

SURGERY

Surgery is a controlled form of trauma which, though often necessary to control or cure disease, also causes some tissue damage. Skilled surgeons cause the minimum of tissue damage in order to achieve the objectives of the operation, but certain operations inevitably lead to postoperative discomfort. Particularly significant procedures are:

- Abdominal surgery, especially when wide retraction of the abdominal muscles are required, e.g. in overweight dogs

- Orthopaedic surgery

- Ear surgery, which is notoriously painful

- Oral and maxillofacial surgery, including dentistry

Dogs receiving major surgery should be treated with potent painkillers prescribed or injected by the veterinary surgeon. Even so, some post-operative discomfort may remain and become apparent at home.

FIRST AID Dogs recovering at home should be kept warm and quiet. Appetising food and clean water should be available (though intake may be reduced for a day or two). They should be taken out to empty bladder and bowels frequently, assisted and supported as necessary. Four times a day is required. Ensure they have plenty of soft bedding and allow them to rest quietly, away from noise and inquisitive children.

- **Warning** Do not be tempted to administer additional painkillers using human medicines, e.g. aspirin, ibuprofen. These may clash with drugs your dog has already been given in the veterinary hospital, causing serious side-effects. Homoeopathic medicines are safe to use in these situations, but in seriously ill dogs or dogs recovering after major operations, it is sensible to clear their use with your veterinary surgeon first.

HOMOEOPATHIC FIRST AID Arnica is the tried and trusted remedy for post-operative pain, bruising and muscle spasm. There is a good case for using it before and after any surgical operation, including dental extractions. It can be given every 1–3 hours during the first day, reducing to 4 times a day for the following 2–3 days.

Staphysagria can be used alongside Arnica. Its main indication is for surgery of the reproductive or urogenital tract. It is a good remedy to use, with Arnica, in female dogs recovering from overiohysterectomy (spay)operations.

TRAVEL SICKNESS

Dogs unused to car travel may experience unpleasant symptoms of nausea, salivation and anxiety. Sometimes, these symptoms can be lessened by careful acclimatisation of the dog to car travel, starting with extremely short (several minute) journeys and plentiful reassurance. Otherwise, anti-sickness tablets can be obtained from the veterinary surgeon. A frequent side-effect is mild sedation, making this treatment unsuitable for show or performance dogs.

HOMOEOPATHIC FIRST AID Petroleum is the remedy of choice here; Borax can also be tried. If fear of the car is present, Gelsemium should be given. Start treatment one hour before travel begins and repeat at hourly intervals during travel.

VOMITING AND DIARRHOEA

Dogs vomit quite readily and this is a common symptom encountered in veterinary practice.

Vomiting is discussed fully in Chapter 6. It can be a symptom of both mild, self-limiting conditions and of more serious underlying disorders. First aid is only appropriate in milder conditions in which:

- The dog is bright, alert and active

- The dog seems keen to eat and drink

- There is no apparent pain; some dogs become a little anxious just before vomiting, probably due to nausea.

Many cases of simple gastritis (mild inflammation of the stomach) present as a bright, alert dog with vomiting and diarrhoea. This may follow a sudden change of food type or over-eating of rich foods, e.g. at Christmas time, and is a common symptom in many dogs.

FIRST AID Water only should be given for 12 hours, followed by bland food and then a gradual weaning back to normal diet over 3–5 days. Suitable bland food includes cooked chicken and rice, cooked fish and rice or scrambled egg (made with water, not milk) and rice. Do not offer milk to drink. This treatment will be successful in most cases although it may take a day or two for symptoms to completely disappear.

HOMOEOPATHIC FIRST AID Nux vomica is useful if the vomiting and diarrhoea is caused by overeating or rich food. Arsen alb is another useful remedy. Treat every 2 hours until symptom relief.

Index